Dysarthria and
Apraxia of Speech

Dysarthria and Apraxia of Speech

Perspectives on Management

edited by

Christopher A. Moore, Ph.D.
Department of Communication
Division of Communication Disorders
University of Pittsburgh
Pittsburgh

Kathryn M. Yorkston, Ph.D.
Department of Rehabilitation Medicine
University of Washington
Seattle

and

David R. Beukelman, Ph.D.
Department of Special Education and Communication Disorders
University of Nebraska-Lincoln
Lincoln

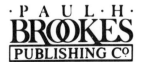

·P·A·U·L·H·
BROOKES
PUBLISHING CO.   Baltimore · London · Toronto · Sydney

Paul H. Brookes Publishing Co.
P.O. Box 10624
Baltimore, Maryland 21285-0624

Typeset by The Composing Room of Michigan, Inc., Grand Rapids, Michigan.
Manufactured in the United States of America by
The Maple Press Co., York, Pennsylvania.

Library of Congress Cataloging-in-Publication Data
Dysarthria and apraxia of speech : perspectives on management /
  edited by Christopher A. Moore, Kathryn M. Yorkston, David R.
  Beukelman.
      p.   cm.
  Outgrowth of the Clinical Dysarthria Conference held in San
Antonio, Tex. in 1990.
  Includes bibliographical references and index.
  ISBN 1-55766-069-7
  1. Articulation disorders — Congresses.   2. Apraxia —
Congresses.   I. Moore, Christopher A., 1956–   .   II. Yorkston,
Kathryn M., 1948–   .   III. Beukelman, David R., 1943–   .
IV. Clinical Dysarthria Conference (1990 : San Antonio, Tex.)
  [DNLM: 1. Apraxia — congresses.   2. Dysarthria —
congresses.   WL 340 D9973   1990]
RC424.7.D94   1991
616.85′52 — dc20
DNLM/DLC
for Library of Congress   90-15163
                                                              CIP

Contents

Contributors

The Editors

Christopher A. Moore, Ph.D., Department of Communication, Division of Communication Disorders, 303 Salk Hall, University of Pittsburgh, Pittsburgh, PA 15261

Christopher A. Moore is Assistant Professor of Communication Disorders at the University of Pittsburgh and a speech scientist whose primary research interests are normal and disordered speech motor control. He received his doctorate from Purdue University in 1985. He has published papers on parkinsonian speech and psychoacoustic performance of patients with neuropathology. His current research involves imaging of the vocal tract using nuclear magnetic resonance and the physiologic development of speech coordination.

Kathryn M. Yorkston, Ph.D., Department of Rehabilitation Medicine RJ-30, University of Washington, Seattle, WA 98195

Kathryn M. Yorkston is Head of the Division of Speech Pathology and Professor in the Departments of Rehabilitation Medicine and Adjunct Professor of Speech and Hearing Sciences at the University of Washington. Her publications have focused on clinical research in acquired neurologic communication disorders in adults. She has written and edited texts that include *Clinical Management of Dysarthric Speakers*, *Recent Advances in Clinical Dysarthria*, and *Communication Disorders Following Traumatic Brain Injury: Management of Cognitive, Language, and Motor Impairments*.

David R. Beukelman, Ph.D., 202F Barkley Memorial Center, University of Nebraska-Lincoln, Lincoln, NE 68583-0738

David R. Beukelman is Barkley Professor of Communication Disorders and Co-Director of the Barkley Augmentative Communication Center, Department of Special Education and Communication Disorders at the University of Nebraska-Lincoln. He is Director of Research and Education of the Communication Disorders Division of the Meyer Children's Rehabilitation Center. Dr. Beukelman received his doctorate from the University of Wisconsin-Madison. From 1975 to 1985 he was Director of Speech Pathology Services and the Augmentative Communication Center at the University of Washington Hospital in Seattle. Dr. Beukelman's primary research and clinical interests have been in the areas of dysarthria and augmentative communication.

The Chapter Authors

Scott Adams, Ph.D., Speech and Swallowing Laboratory, The Toronto Hospital, 399 Bathurst Street, Toronto, Ontario M5P 2S8, Canada

Scott Adams is Speech Scientist at the Speech and Swallowing Laboratory of the Toronto Hospital. His research interests are acoustic and physiologic characteristics of motor speech disorders, with a primary emphasis on Parkinson's disease. He also maintains an interest in coordination, rate, and timing as they affect models of speech production.

Linda A. Alp, M.A., Alta Bates-Herrick Hospital, Berkeley, CA 94553

Linda A. Alp is a speech-language pathologist at Alta Bates-Herrick Hospital in Berkeley, California. Previously she was a research speech-language pathologist in the Dysarthria Laboratory of the Veterans Administration Medical Center, Long Beach, California. Ms. Alp's research interests include computerized and instrumental analysis of normal and disordered speech. She received her M.A. from the University of California-Santa Barbara.

Suzanne Apeldoorn, M.H.Sc., Department of Communication Disorders, West Park Hospital, Toronto, Ontario M5P 2S8, Canada

Suzanne Apeldoorn is a clinical speech-language pathologist in the Neurologic Rehabilitation Unit at West Park Hospital. Her duties also include work with continuing care units and coordinating bedside feeding and the swallowing assessment program. She received her M.H.Sc. from the University of Toronto.

Julie M. Barkmeier, M.A., Wendell Johnson Speech and Hearing Center, University of Iowa, Iowa City, IA 52242

Julie M. Barkmeier is a speech pathologist in the Department of Otolaryngology Speech Physiology Laboratory at the University of Iowa Hospitals and Clinics. Her primary responsibilities involve research and speech physiology analysis of voice disordered individuals. She is a consultant speech pathologist for the University of Iowa Cochlear Implant Program and is a doctoral candidate in the University of Iowa Speech and Hearing Program.

John E. Bernthal, Ph.D., Barkley Memorial Center, University of Nebraska-Lincoln, Lincoln, NE 68583-0738

John E. Bernthal is Professor and Chair of the Department of Special Education and Communication Disorders, and Director of the Barkley Augmentative Communication Center at the University of Nebraska-Lincoln. Dr. Bernthal holds a Ph.D. from the University of Wisconsin-Madison. His primary research and clinical interests have involved phonologic delay and disorders in children.

Allen E. Boysen, Ph.D., Audiology and Speech Pathology Services, Department of Veterans Affairs, Washington, DC 20420

Allen E. Boysen is Director of Audiology and Speech Pathology Services of the Department of Veterans Affairs, Washington, D. C. He received his Ph.D. from the University of Oklahoma Health Sciences Center. His interests include the development of model dysarthria programs that link perceptual and instrumental measurements of speech.

Michael P. Cannito, Ph.D., Department of Speech Communication, CMA 7.204, University of Texas at Austin, Austin, TX 78712-1089

Michael P. Cannito is Assistant Professor of Communication Sciences and Disorders in the Department of Speech Communication at the University of Texas at Austin. He teaches courses in the disorders of speech and language and is coordinator of the speech production laboratory of the College of Communication. He received his doctorate from the University of Texas at Dallas, specializing in disorders of neuromotor function and neurolinguistics.

Patricia Dowden, M.S., Children's Hospital of Eastern Ontario, 401 Smyth Road, Ottawa, Ontario K1H 8L2, Canada

Patricia Dowden is a doctoral candidate in the Department of Speech and Hearing Sciences at the University of Washington. She is also Coordinator of the Clinic for Augmentative Communication at the Children's Hospital of Eastern Ontario and Ottawa Children's Treatment Centre. Her research interests include augmentative communication and the speech of individuals with severe dysarthria.

Michele J. Eliason, Ph.D., School of Nursing, University of Iowa, Iowa City, IA 52242

Michele J. Eliason is Assistant Professor at the University of Iowa School of Nursing. She is a neuropsychologist with research interests in learning disability and social interaction in children.

Karen Forrest, Ph.D., Department of Communicative Disorders and Waisman Center, 565 Waisman Center, University of Wisconsin-Madison, Madison, WI 53705

Karen Forrest is Assistant Scientist at the Department of Communicative Disorders, University of Wisconsin-Madison. Her research centers on sensorimotor influences on speech production of neurologically normal and disordered adults. Additional research interests include the acoustic characteristics of speech development in normal and phonologically disordered children.

Bruce R. Gerratt, Ph.D., Audiology and Speech Pathology Service (126), Veterans Administration Medical Center, Wilshire and Sawtelle Boulevards, Los Angeles, CA 90073

Bruce R. Gerratt is Assistant Chief of the Audiology and Speech Pathology Service of the Veterans Administration Medical Center, and Associate Professor in Residence of the School of Medicine, University of California-Los Angeles. His research interests include normal and disordered physiologic properties of laryngeal function and the relation of these properties to acoustic and perceptual measures of the sounds produced.

Vicki L. Hammen, Ph.D., Department of Rehabilitation Medicine, University of Washington, Seattle, WA 98195

Vicki L. Hammen is Research Speech-Language Pathologist in the Department of Rehabilitation Medicine at the University of Washington. Her research interests are in the area of motor speech disorders, with particular emphasis on acoustic and physiologic analysis.

Wayne R. Hanson, Ph.D., Audiology and Speech Pathology Service, Veterans Administration Medical Center, Sepulveda, CA 90073

Wayne R. Hanson is Chief of the Audiology and Speech Pathology Service at the Veterans Administration Medical Center, Sepulveda, California. He received his Ph.D. from the University of Oklahoma Health Sciences Center. A Fellow of the American Speech-Language-Hearing Association, Dr. Hanson has numerous publications in the area of neurogenic communication disorders.

E. Charles Healey, Ph.D., Barkley Memorial Center, University of Nebraska-Lincoln, Lincoln, NE 68583-0738

E. Charles Healey is Associate Professor of Speech-Language Pathology in the Department of Special Education and Communication Disorders at the University of Nebraska-Lincoln. The author of numerous papers and articles in the field of voice and fluency disorders, Dr. Healey serves as editorial consultant for the *Journal of Speech and Hearing Research* and was the State of Nebraska recipient of the 1985 Clinical Achievement Award for the Advancement of Clinical Practice. He is a Fellow of the American Speech-Language-Hearing Association.

Donnell F. Johns, Ph.D., Division of Plastic Surgery, Southwestern Medical School, University of Texas at Dallas, 5323 Harry Hines Boulevard, Dallas, TX 75235-9031

Donnell F. Johns received his doctorate in Speech Pathology from Florida State University and was a post-doctoral Fellow at the Mayo Graduate School of Medicine. He is a Fellow of the American Speech-Language-Hearing Association and is currently Professor of Surgery and Director of Clinical Research in the Division of Plastic Surgery, University of Texas Southwestern Medical School at Dallas. He is also a Clinical Professor of Otorhinolaryngology and Director of the Center for Craniofacial Reconstruction at the Children's Medical Center of Dallas.

Linda S. Jordan, Ph.D., Department of Neurology, University of Iowa Hospitals and Clinics, Iowa City, IA 52242

Linda S. Jordan provides speech-language assessments and remediation for patients with communication problems associated with neurogenic disease or trauma. Her research interests include descriptions of dysarthrias and treatment strategies for aphasia and apraxia.

Raymond D. Kent, Ph.D., Department of Communicative Disorders and Waisman Center, University of Wisconsin-Madison, Madison, WI 53705

Raymond D. Kent is Professor of Communicative Disorders at the University of Wisconsin-Madison. Dr. Kent's research concerns are intelligibility and quality in speech disorders, especially in the dysarthrias associated with amyotrophic lateral sclerosis, Parkinson's disease, stroke, cerebellar disease, and cerebral palsy. His publications include approximately 100 research articles, two co-authored books, and two edited books.

Karen K. Kenyon, M.S., 2116 West Faidley Avenue, P. O. Box 9804, Grand Island, NE 68802-9804

Karen K. Kenyon is a speech-language pathologist in private practice in Grand Island, Nebraska. She works primarily with persons with CVA and with traumatic brain injury patients, but she also works with individuals with vocal fold pathologies and neurogenic speech and language disorders.

George V. Kondraske, Ph.D., Human Performance Institute, Box 19180, University of Texas at Arlington, Arlington, TX 76019-0180

George V. Kondraske is Professor of Electrical and Biomedical Engineering at the University of Texas at Arlington (UTA), is an Adjunct Professor of Neurology at the University of Texas Southwestern Medical Center at Dallas, and serves as Director of the Human Performance Institute at UTA. His research is directed toward measurement, modeling, and understanding of human performance.

Julie M. Liss, Ph.D., Department of Communication Disorders, 115 Shevlin Hall, University of Minnesota, Minneapolis, MN 55455

Julie M. Liss has research interests in motor speech disorders, speech production characteristics of geriatric individuals and individuals with cleft palate, and in the anatomical characteristics of the speech articulators.

Christy L. Ludlow, Ph.D., Speech and Voice Unit, National Institute on Deafness and Other Communication Disorders, National Institutes of Health, 9000 Rockville Pike, Building 10, Room 5D-38, Bethesda, MD 20892

Christy L. Ludlow is Chief of the Speech and Voice Unit of the National Institute on Deafness and Other Communication Disorders at the National Institutes of Health. Her work involves research in the pathophysiology and treatment of speech and voice disorders and in laryngeal modeling. She has also been investigating the effects of botulinum toxin in treating several types of speech and voice disorders, including spasmodic dysphonia, stuttering, and orolingual-mandibular dystonia.

Erich S. Luschei, Ph.D., Department of Speech Pathology and Audiology, Laboratory of Speech and Language Neuroscience, University of Iowa, Iowa City, IA 52242

Erich S. Luschei is Professor of Speech Pathology and Audiology at the University of Iowa. He is a neurophysiologist who studies the neuromuscular and sensory processes that control the larynx, tongue, and mandible. He uses experimental approaches in his work, which ranges from the study of tongue strength in normal and disordered speakers to basic neurophysiologic studies of laryngeal control in anesthetized animals.

Malcolm R. McNeil, Ph.D., Department of Communicative Disorders and Waisman Center, University of Wisconsin-Madison, Madison, WI 53705

Malcolm R. McNeil is Professor of Communicative Disorders at the University of Wisconsin-Madison. He works in the general area of neurogenic speech and language disorders, and his research in aphasia has included auditory information processing and comprehension, and assessment and differential diagnosis of aphasia. His recent work in aphasia, apraxia, and dysarthria focuses on the phonologic versus phonetic description and explanation of these disorders.

E. Jeffrey Metter, M.D., The Baltimore Longitudinal Study of Aging, Gerontology Research Center, National Institute on Aging, 4940 Eastern Ave., Baltimore, MD 21224

E. Jeffrey Metter is the Medical Officer for the Baltimore Longitudinal Study of Aging, which is an internationally recognized study of human aging. It is part of the intramural research program of the National Institute on Aging. Formerly he was Associate Professor of Neurology of the School of Medicine, University of California-Los Angeles, and a staff neurologist at the Veterans Administration Medical Center, Sepulveda, California.

Donald A. Robin, Ph.D., Department of Speech Pathology and Audiology, Laboratory of Speech and Language Neuroscience, University of Iowa, Iowa City, IA 52242

Donald A. Robin is Associate Professor of Speech Pathology and Audiology at the University of Iowa. He teaches, conducts research, and treats patients in the area of neurogenic communication disorders. His research interests include the measurement of strength and fatigue of oral structures, auditory psychophysics, and attention.

John C. Rosenbek, Ph.D., Audiology and Speech Pathology (126), William S. Middleton Memorial Veterans Hospital, 2500 Overlook Terrace, Madison, WI 53705

John C. Rosenbek is Chief of Audiology and Speech Pathology at the William S. Middleton Memorial Veterans Hospital, and Adjunct Professor in the Department of Neurology and in the Department of Communication Disorders at the University of Wisconsin-Madison. Dr. Rosenbek's particular research interests are oral motor disorders, including dysphagia, dyspraxia, and dysarthria.

Geralyn M. Schulz, M.A., Speech and Voice Unit, National Institute on Deafness and Other Communication Disorders, National Institutes of Health, 9000 Rockville Pike, Building 10, Room 5D-38, Bethesda, MD 20892

Geralyn M. Schulz is a research speech pathologist at the Speech and Voice Unit of the National Institute on Deafness and other Communication Disorders at the National Institutes of Health. Her work involves research in the pathophysiology and treatment of speech and voice disorders. Recently this has focused on patients with orolingual-mandibular dystonia.

Robert L. Schum, Ph.D., Department of Speech Pathology and Audiology, University of Iowa, Iowa City, IA 52242

Robert L. Schum is a clinical psychologist and Adjunct Associate Professor in the Department of Speech Pathology and Audiology at the University of Iowa. His primary area of interest is the psychological implications of communicative disorders.

Lori B. Somodi, Department of Speech Pathology and Audiology, Laboratory of Speech and Language Neuroscience, University of Iowa, Iowa City, IA 52242

Lori B. Somodi is a student in speech and hearing sciences. She is a research assistant in the Laboratory of Speech and Language Neuroscience at the University of Iowa. Her research involves motor control of the tongue in normal and disordered speakers.

Helen Southwood, Ph.D., Department of Speech and Language Pathology and Audiology, University of Wyoming, Laramie, WY 82071

Helen Southwood is Assistant Professor in the Department of Speech and Language Pathology and Audiology at the University of Wyoming. Her research interests are in the area of neurogenic communicative disorders, focusing on acoustic and perceptual characteristics of dysarthria.

Paula A. Square-Storer, Ph.D., Graduate Department of Speech Pathology, Faculty of Medicine, University of Toronto, 88 College Street, Toronto, Ontario M5G 1L4, Canada

Paula A. Square-Storer is Chairperson of the Graduate Department of Speech Pathology of the Faculty of Medicine, University of Toronto. She has taught in the area of communication disorders of neurologic origin in that program for the past decade. Her research has focused on apraxia of speech, and she is editor of the text *Acquired Apraxia of Speech in Aphasic Adults.*

Sheela L. Stuart, M.A., Barkley Memorial Center, University of Nebraska-Lincoln, Lincoln, NE 68583-0738

Sheela L. Stuart is a doctoral candidate in Communication Disorders at the University of Nebraska-Lincoln. From 1982 to 1986 she was Department Head of Speech Pathology Services and the Augmentative Communication Center of Crippled Children's Hospital and School in Sioux Falls, South Dakota. From 1986 to 1988 she was Supervisor for Speech Pathology Services of Sioux Valley Hospital in Sioux Falls, South Dakota.

James A. Till, Ph.D., Veterans Administration Medical Center, 5901 East Seventh Street, Long Beach, CA 90822

James A. Till is Director of the Dysarthria Laboratory of the Veterans Administration Medical Center, Long Beach, CA. He is Associate Clinical Professor of the Division of Otolaryngology-Head and Neck Surgery, University of California-Irvine. Dr. Till has published articles in the *Journal of Speech and Hearing Research*, *Journal of Speech and Hearing Disorders*, and in other journals. His current work concentrates on computer-assisted evaluation of speech disorders and analyses of diagnostic profiles.

Gary Weismer, Ph.D., Department of Communicative Disorders and Waisman Center, University of Wisconsin-Madison, Madison, WI 53705

Gary Weismer is Professor of Communicative Disorders at the University of Wisconsin-Madison. His research interests include speech production characteristics of persons with motor speech disorders and construction of an acoustic tool for the understanding of speech intelligibility deficits.

Robert T. Wertz, Ph.D., Audiology and Speech Pathology Service (126), Veterans Administration Medical Center, Martinez, CA 94553

Robert T. Wertz is Chief of the Audiology and Speech Pathology Service of the Veterans Administration Medical Center, Martinez, CA. He is also Adjunct Professor of the Department of Neurology of the School of Medicine, University of California-Davis. His research interests involve the management of neurogenic communication disorders, including appraisal, diagnosis, prognosis, and treatment efficacy.

Marilyn Seif Workinger, Ph.D., Marshfield Clinic, 1000 North Oak Avenue, Marshfield, WI 54449

Marilyn Seif Workinger is Manager of the Section of Speech-Language Pathology at the Marshfield Clinic, Marshfield, Wisconsin. She received her Ph.D. from the University of Wisconsin-Madison. Children and adults who have neurologic disorders of speech are her primary clinical, research, and teaching focus.

Preface

Dysarthria and Apraxia of Speech: Perspectives on Management was written to provide speech-language pathologists, researchers in neuromotor speech disorders, and graduate students with recent clinical and research developments in the field of neuromotor speech disorders. The content appeals to a wide range of readers by highlighting new perspectives on clinical and research activities involving neuromotor speech disorders, investigations of speech intelligibility, characteristics of specific neuromotor speech disorders, and physiologic and acoustic descriptions of dysarthria and apraxia of speech.

The impetus for this effort comes from the Clinical Dysarthria Conference. Since it was first held in 1982, this biennial conference has encouraged the integration of clinical experience and research in the fields of dysarthria and other neuromotor speech disorders. The key to this integration is dissemination of information beyond the 50 to 100 conference participants. The first Clinical Dysarthria Conference was followed by a book, *Clinical Dysarthria*, edited by Bill Berry and published in 1983. The fourth Clinical Dysarthria Conference was also followed by a book, *Recent Advances in Clinical Dysarthria*, edited by Kathryn Yorkston and David Beukelman. In 1990, the conference was broadened to include apraxia of speech and was held in San Antonio, Texas. *Dysarthria and Apraxia of Speech: Perspectives on Management* contains many of the presentations that were well received by participants at that conference. A review of the Contents reveals the diversity of the participants in this conference, and a biographical sketch for each author is included in this work. This diversity is not only characteristic of the field of motor speech disorders, but is also one of its greatest strengths. Each chapter was accepted following two peer review procedures. First, the program committee of the Clinical Dysarthria Conference reviewed all presentation proposals. Only those proposals accepted by the committee were presented at the conference. Second, the three editors of this book reviewed all manuscripts submitted for publication and only those accepted by all three editors were included in this volume.

Dysarthria and Apraxia of Speech: Perspectives on Management contains five sections. The first, Perspectives, comprises three chapters that offer new and thoughtful views on the field. Most significantly, each perspective is demonstrated by the author(s) in their later chapters in this volume. In Chapter 1, Erich Luschei presents the perspective that objective nonspeech measurement should be included in clinical assessments of persons with neuromotor speech disorders. In Chapter 2, Gary Weismer and Julie Liss argue that neuromotor speech disorders are better understood by studying data from individual subjects rather than by reducing data within diagnostic categories and obscuring individual variability. In

Chapter 3, Christy Ludlow questions the extensive use of standardized measures and outlines research strategies effective in the neuromotor speech disorders.

The second section, Intelligibility, contains four chapters relating to clinical measurement. Vicki Hammen, Kathryn Yorkston, and Patricia Dowden introduce a new measurement tool, the Index of Contextual Intelligibility, in Chapter 4, and report the impact of semantic context on different dysarthric speakers, which varies with the severity of the dysarthria and, to a lesser extent, with the size of the semantic category. Chapter 5 continues the analysis by examining the perceptual features that distinguish intelligible from unintelligible speech productions. They report that severely dysarthric speakers do not exhibit similar changes when most intelligible and least intelligible word production are contrasted. In Chapter 6, Julie Barkmeier, Linda Jordan, Donald Robin, and Robert Schum study the influence of speaker appearance on intelligibility ratings by inexperienced and experienced judges. They conclude that inexperienced listeners may be influenced by components other than how much information can be understood when rating speech intelligibility. In Chapter 7, Bruce Gerratt, James Till, John Rosenbek, Robert Wertz, and Allen Boysen report on the use, clinical value, and attitudes toward various computerized and noncomputerized assessment procedures for the evaluation of dysarthric speakers in Department of Veterans Affairs Medical Centers.

Section III, Specific Disorders, contains four chapters. In Chapter 8, Sheela Stuart, David Beukelman, Karen Kenyon, E. Charles Healey, and John Bernthal present a case study of a teenage female with severe dysarthria due to Reye's syndrome and the effect of speaking rate reduction on her speech performance. In Chapter 9, Marilyn Seif Workinger and Raymond Kent review the parameters that differentiate the dysarthrias in children with spastic and athetoid cerebral palsy, and they conclude that experienced listeners are able to make perceptual distinctions between the two groups. In Chapter 10, E. Jeffrey Metter and Wayne Hanson describe the hypokinetic, spastic, and ataxic characteristics of dysarthric speakers with progressive supranuclear palsy. The variability among speakers is documented. Donald Robin and Michele Eliason describe, in Chapter 11, the speech production and prosodic characteristics of children with neurofibromatosis. They report that these children have a constellation of cognitive deficits and speech patterns, which are characterized by spatial difficulties, neuromotor speech production problems, and an impairment in the ability to convey accurately prosodic intent in both linguistic and emotive contexts.

The fourth section, Physiology, contains five chapters. Chapter 12 by Karen Forrest, Scott Adams, Malcolm McNeil, and Helen Southwood highlights differences in motor control among three different groups of speakers with neurogenic communication disorders. In Chapter 13, Donald Robin, Lori Somodi, and Erich Luschei describe a new device to measure nonspeech tongue strength and endurance. They report preliminary data from normally speaking adults, normally speaking children, and children with developmental apraxia. James Till and Linda Alp, in Chapter 14, describe procedures for conducting aerodynamic and temporal measures during the monologue speech of normal and dysarthric speakers. Although the dysarthric speakers had disparate neurologic etiologies, they presented similar speech signs and symptoms regarding mean air flow values, respiratory volumes, pauses, and breath group patterns. In Chapter 15, Michael Cannito, George Kondraske, and Donnell Johns discuss five quantitative measures of oral-facial function. Their results show that speakers with spasmodic dysphonia differed from matched normal controls on clinical ratings of oral-facial motor dysfunction but not on somatosensory examination. In Chapter 16, Geralyn Schulz and Christy Ludlow studied the effects of botulinum toxin injections on hypotonic muscles of persons with orolingual-mandibular dystonia. They report that the effects of botulinum toxin on speech production and intelligibility of these patients can be objectively assessed. Two of the acoustic and two of the perceptual measures reflected changes in the patients following botulinum toxin treatment.

Section V, Apraxia of Speech, reflects the new area of conference concern. In Chapter 17, Gary Weismer and Julie Liss describe a method by which acoustic representations of disordered speech may be qualitatively examined and described. They report that persons with apraxia of speech demonstrate exaggerated articulatory gestures and misdirected formant trajectories for some vocalic events. In Chapter 18, Paula Square-Storer and Suzanne Apeldoorn report on the articulatory and prosodic characteristics of apraxic speech using perceptual and acoustic measures. In Chapter 19, John Rosenbek and Malcolm McNeil suggest that the field of motor speech disorders consider setting aside the assumptions about dysarthria and apraxia until more data are collected from normal and abnormal groups. An effort could then be made to develop one or more "strong" neuromotor syndromes in both dysarthria and apraxia of speech. Such a syndrome would be defined as one in which neuromuscular abnormalities are identified in predictable distribution across functional components and are related to a pattern of perceptual speech abnormalities with sufficient frequency to suggest a causal relationship.

Because this volume is an outgrowth of the Clinical Dysarthria Conference, we wish to acknowledge the efforts of the many individuals who were responsible for planning and organizing the 1990 Conference. The program committee included Anne H. B. Putnam-Rochet, Christy Ludlow, Gary Weismer, and Christopher Moore, Chair. They deserve credit for developing an excellent program that reflected the wide interests and contributions of individuals involved with neuromotor speech disorders. No conference can be successful without the considerable efforts of a local arrangements committee. Our thanks must go to Deane Vogel, Michael Cannito, and Anthony Salvatore who managed to make our stay in San Antonio a very enjoyable one.

Dysarthria and
Apraxia of Speech

SECTION I

PERSPECTIVES

IN THIS SECTION, three leaders in speech motor control research respond to an invitation to identify and address some essential questions facing scientists and clinicians. They form these questions: Can speech be studied and understood in the context of nonspeech behaviors? Can such observations be standardized? Can researchers and clinicians employ diagnostic categorization usefully, or does the "ubiquitous variability" of speech defy the reduction of grouped observations to general principles and patient populations? What scientific methods are essential to answering these most basic questions? Luschei (Chapter 1) responds with a call for a large, carefully standardized data base of nonspeech behaviors. Weismer and Liss (Chapter 2) take a different view and suggest that the essential characteristics of speech motor control are best described with isolated speech productions by individuals. Ludlow (Chapter 3) provides a framework for clinical research by outlining specific procedures and methods to be adopted in evaluating treatment of dysarthria and apraxia. Most importantly, these authors have each taken the bold step of applying these ideas empirically and have demonstrated the utility of each approach in this volume (Chapters 13, 16, and 17).

Chapter 1

Development of Objective Standards of Nonspeech Oral Strength and Performance
An Advocate's Views

Erich S. Luschei

THE READER OF this chapter should be warned in advance that the author (henceforth "I") is not an expert in the area of objective measurement of oral strength and performance, and that, except for a chapter in this volume, co-authored with Donald Robin and Lori Somodi, I have no publications on the subject. I have become very interested in the topic, however, and strongly feel that our ability to help people with speech disorders can be greatly facilitated by developing standards based upon instrumentation and procedures that are available and applicable to clinics as well as research laboratories. Objective measurements and norms based on large numbers of observations would help in refining diagnostic categories, monitoring progression of a disorder, and assessing the effect of intervention therapy, as well as ultimately helping in understanding the basic process of speech production.

Let me note first of all that the need for objective measurements of articulator strength and coordination has been recognized by many previous investigators in speech-language pathology. Palmer and Osborn (1940) attempted to measure tongue strength by measuring the pressure the tongue could exert on a hard rubber ball placed in the mouths of various types of speakers. While their results unfortunately were flawed technically in several ways, the basic approach has the potential for being quite useful. More recently, Dworkin (1980), Dworkin and Aronson (1986), Dworkin, Aronson, and Mulder (1980), Dworkin and Culatta (1985), and Posen (1972) published results of studies of tongue strength, measured as isometric force, in both adult and child normal and disordered speakers. Barlow and Abbs (1983) also developed an instrumentation system for measuring strength and performance of the tongue, lips, and mandible. Barlow and Netsell (1989) have shown how a sophisticated instrumentation system of this type can be used in a clinical setting to understand further the problems of dysarthric speakers.

To be perfectly honest, my knowledge of these studies came "after the fact." My own personal interest in methods to develop normative standards for oral strength gradually arose from technical questions posed by several colleagues, and from my own fascination with instrumentation systems for measuring physiological variables. Working with Donald Robin and Lori Somodi, I helped develop a prototype of a portable and inexpensive device to measure objectively tongue strength and endurance (see Robin, Somodi, & Luschei, chap. 13, this volume). My experience with this project is not, however, the motivation for this chapter. Rather, it is the experience encountered with the review of our project for the Clinical Dysarthria Conference that stimulated my thinking. Although Donald Robin, Lori Somodi, and I were granted the opportunity to present our findings at the conference, the comments of the reviewer who evaluated our submission for the conference came as quite a shock. To quote, "My opinion about this proposal is that it is motivated by a real clinical concern for objectivity and accessibility. . . , but that it begs the question of the relevance of the measures to speech disorders." The reviewer continued, "They [the authors] should be aware that participants at the conference . . . will demand more of a rationale for this technique than the typical blind acceptance that non-speech tasks are a reasonable part of a diagnostic battery." The reviewer then suggested examination of criticisms raised in a recent review of maximum performance tasks written by Kent, Kent, and Rosenbek (1987).

After careful study of the Kent et al. (1987) paper, and after hearing many remarks from scientists and clinicians at the conference who are involved in the study and/or treatment of dysarthria, I have begun to appreciate the honest candor of the reviewer's remarks, and the experience from which they arose. There are at least three basic reasons why, I think, many people in the field are reticent to embrace a proposal for the development of standards of oral strength and performance.

1. Studies on this subject have not, so far, produced methods or standards that are perceived as generally useful clinically.

2. Advocates of objective measurements and standards have perhaps "oversold" the concept and created an impression that the goal is to replace the clinician's experience and skill with machines and numbers.
3. For many people, it is not obvious how measures of oral strength, resistance to fatigue (endurance), and maximal performance (speed) in nonspeech tasks are related to the requirements of speech articulation.

I cannot, in the space allotted, address these reasons in any depth, but I would like to comment on them. My reasons are simple: I *am* optimistic about the potential worth of objective measurements of simple nonspeech motor tasks, including those that require maximum performance, to clinicians who have to understand and treat dysarthria. Here are some things to think about.

OBJECTIVE MEASUREMENT IS A BASIC APPROACH OF SCIENCE

Many, if not most, of the things we know in science and the health professions that help people and allow us to understand very complex processes have derived, in the beginning, from the application of objective measurements made in the currency of commonly accepted "units." Such measurements typically have been compiled, often by contributions from scientists all over the world, until a large data base is available. At this stage, a data base of this type has a certain empirical value, but it does not really explain the process in question. However, it does allow a person to take an individual sample of the process (e.g., a patient) and make a good guess whether it is "significantly" different from other samples with respect to this particular data base. We can often use this information to make good "clinical" decisions even if we don't know everything there is to know about the process. Consider an example. Suppose someone claims that a piece of shiny yellow metal is pure gold. How does one know this person is telling the truth, without being an expert chemist? A very useful test would be to weigh the metal and measure its volume to calculate its density. We know the density of pure gold because we have a book compiled by chemists who had very elaborate ways of determining what pure gold is. If the piece of metal has the same density as gold, then it *might* be gold. However, if its density is 3 standard deviations from the mean density of gold, then a very good guess would be that the metal is not gold. A good clinical decision would be to decline the offer to purchase the piece of metal.

When we can recognize really deviant samples, we can study those specimens with the question "Why?," and our knowledge of the subject may advance. Progress in science has often followed a very whimsical path, but many success stories have started with objective measures of simple aspects of the phenomenon in question. I am quite confident that careful measurements of simple oral behaviors may one day make significant contributions to our understanding of motor speech control. Because it hasn't happened yet is no reason for being pessimistic.

Let me present another familiar example, partly because it reinforces my point about the potential usefulness of standardized measurements, and partly because it also illustrates the point that measurements and normal standards are an *aid* to the clinical process, not a *substitute* for it. Consider the problem of a patient who can't seem to understand what is said. Could it be the patient doesn't hear? If we want an answer to that question, we can obtain a very good estimate of the person's ability to hear because of the invention of the audiometer, which tests the limits of a person's ability to detect very simple, physically specified, stimuli. Should a clinician order a hearing test just because we have that wonderful ability? He or she could, I suppose, but let common sense prevail. Is there reason to believe the person understands the clinician's language? Is there a possibility that the person had a stroke? Can the person hear a clap of the hands? When other reasonable explanations for a problem can be eliminated, and the clinician is still unsure of the cause of the problem, then measurement and standards become very useful. However, qualitative tests of speech and nonspeech oral behaviors that clinicians have used for years continue to be important and useful even if objective methods and standards exist.

MEASUREMENT OF ORAL MAXIMAL PERFORMANCE: AN IMPERFECT BEGINNING

Scientists interested in speech and its disorders have been making simple measures of motor performance for many years. This body of work has recently been reviewed and evaluated by Kent et al. (1987). I would recommend the paper to anyone who has not already studied it. Quite a few measures are considered, but there is a subset of measures that has been studied by a number of investigators: maximum phonation duration; pitch range; maximum expiratory pressure; maximum sound pressure level (a shout); strength of the tongue, lips, and jaw; and maximum syllable repetition rate. I won't try to review this review, but I would like to comment on some of its general conclusions.

Both intra-subject and inter-subject variability is large. To quote Kent et al. (1987):

The issue of variability should not be underestimated. For some measures at some ages (e.g., maximum phonation duration for young children), the range of normal values is nearly an order of magnitude. It is abundantly clear from the literature on measures of maximum performance that instructions to the subject can strongly affect the data. (p. 382)

Intra-subject variability should not be large. If it is, and the source of the variability cannot be found and eliminated, then it seems unlikely that much use can be made of the measurements. I am in complete agreement with the comment on instructions. They should be given in a highly standardized way, and should be detailed in the published results. Motivation and experience with the task also affect maximum performance. It would be helpful, perhaps, to have investigators with an interest in maximum performance agree on a standard procedure. Other investigators in various disciplines have met to develop common procedures. Let me suggest an example of how one might proceed in a measure of maximum performance. Ask the subject, clearly and simply, to perform the task as "long as possible," or as "hard as you can." Make two measurements, recording both, but interpreting the highest as the maximum. Do not give feedback between these responses, or comment on performance. Then ask the subject to perform the task once more and "try as hard as you can to go longer (harder, faster)." One could call the third performance the "motivated" performance and report the typical percentage change in the measurement.

Now let me confess that we have not used this motivated third trial in our preliminary study (Robin, Somodi, & Luschei, chap. 13, this volume). It is a post hoc thought, and it is just a guess whether it is useful. The point is that human variables such as motivation will always be there, but we can try to neutralize them by standardization, or specifically manipulate them to assess their influence. Experiments could be done to determine which standardized instructions produced the least variability or had the best controls for motivation. Refining procedures in science sometimes takes a long time and requires help from many people.

Inter-subject variability may simply be part of the data. There is no doubt that we can weigh people accurately, but the range of weights that might be encountered among a group of middle-age males in the state of Iowa is impressive. Such variability greatly weakens the ability to detect "abnormality" if factors cannot be identified that account for much of the variability. It seems to me that these circumstances should lead us to search for variables that can be combined to form a mathematical model that is able to account for much of the intersubject variability. For example, one could ask people about their daily food intake and activity pattern as well as weigh them. A 300-pound 6-foot Iowan male would not be unusual in most circumstances, but if it was known that such Iowan males ate 3,000 calories a day and read magazines for exercise, one would have a very different clinical impression when it was noted that a particular 300-pound male ran laps and ate diet entrees.

Kent et al. (1987) suggest that maximum performance measures might not be relevant to speech because "speaking under ordinary circumstances does not tax the performance capabilities of the speech system" (p. 382). These authors subsequently modify this suggestion, however, by noting the need for timing of articulation, which can be affected by speed of movement. They note that "the temporal sequencing of speech may be performed at rates that allow for a small margin of error — a margin that is occasionally exceeded by many talkers" (p. 382). Let me consider the first comment, that strength and power exceed that required for ordinary speech. This view arises because, I think, we usually measure strength of articulatory muscles in a highly artificial way (i.e., under static isometric conditions). The tongue of normal people, either adults or children (and interestingly they do not differ much in this regard) can produce an isometric anterior push of 15–20 N (Dworkin et al., 1980; Dworkin & Culatta, 1985; Posen, 1972). We never push with the tongue in this manner during speech, so how can this measurement be relevant? Normal speech movements require, particularly of the tongue, very high rates of muscle fiber shortening. The tongue is a muscular hydrostat. Contracting muscle fibers cause compartments within the tongue to constrict in one dimension, and the fluid that is displaced has to move to other regions of the tongue where muscle fibers are relaxed. This is a "clever" way of making muscle fibers, whose only active response is to contract, move things in one of several different directions without using bones. We don't often think of it, but it is an old trick, "invented" to move tentacles and elephant trunks as well as tongues. Because of this feature, however, the tongue muscle has to operate against a large viscous load. The situation is like opening a door with a dashpot, a device that keeps the door from banging shut when it is released. Although it does not take much force to open the door slowly or hold it open, it requires a very large force to move the door rapidly. Thus, there is reason to believe that a significant fraction of the strength we measure in the tongue during a static isometric behavior may be used during normal speech to get the tongue to its proper positions in a timely manner. This conjecture has been given strong support by the observations of Dworkin et al. (1980). They found very strong negative correlations between maximum isometric tongue force and the severity of articulation defects and maximum rates of /pʌ/, /tʌ/, and /kʌ/ in patients with amyotrophic lateral sclerosis.

Jaw muscles are another matter. The power of these muscles so far exceeds the requirements for speech that I doubt that they ever impose limitations on speech movements. I personally regard having a person

would be useful. One measure that has been used to assess coordination of the articulators is maximum repetition rate or diadochokinetic rate. Kent et al. (1987) provide an enlightened discussion of this measure. They conclude, basically, that it is not a very useful measure. The appeal is that it is simple to measure: you need a stopwatch, the ability to count, and an "ear" that can detect failure of production accuracy or substitutions. These perceptual judgments, however, introduce a source of variability that one hopes to avoid in the development of objective standards. For this purpose, one really needs spectral analysis of sounds to see if they are, in fact, being properly produced. This analysis also allows attention to the variability of both timing and amplitude of the sounds, as illustrated by the study reported by Tatsumi, Sasanuma, Hirose, and Kiritani (1979). I personally, however, would not advocate a measure of coordination that emphasized abnormally high rates of production. Maximum rates of coordinated, practiced movements are not limited by the nervous system. They are limited by the time it takes to alternatively shorten and lengthen muscle fibers. This process is greatly limited by the internal workings of muscles. To achieve high syllable repetition rates, even for adequate production, subjects must drive their muscles with "everything they've got," and most subjects probably change their mode of production to a state that has little to do with speech. Amplitudes of movements of slow and massive articulators, such as the jaw, may decrease dramatically. I don't know whether all people do what I do when I produce /pʌ/ at high rates, but I never stop voicing; my /pʌ/s are produced by a steady stream of air through a static larynx. This stream continues during the brief period of lip seal to recharge the intraoral pressure to produce the plosive. Thus, only the labial system is actually moving rapidly. In this case, coordination is greatly simplified, rather than "stressed," by the rapidity of the task. The pattern of articulator coordination is completely different from normal production of /pʌ/.

If I were to try to develop a "pure" standard test for motor speech coordination, I would look at the variability of sequencing of articulators, and variability of their amplitude characteristics during repetitions of a simple syllable like /pʌ/, /tʌ/, or /kʌ/, or, if an adult, the trisyllable /pʌtʌkʌ/. I would have the speaker time repetitions to a metronome set at a rate of 2 per second, or what is found to be a preferred repetition rate among most normal speakers. One could use elaborate instrumentation, but to keep things simple, I would measure intraoral pressure with a good transducer system (high-frequency response >100 Hz) and a microphone placed at a standard position in front of the lips. Such a high-frequency pressure transducer would allow detection of the onset of voicing from the intraoral pressure record, which may occur in some individuals before lips part for the plosive. An extraoral microphone alone may fail to detect such an event. From the timing and amplitude relationships of intraoral pressure and acoustic signals and their token-to-token variability, I would predict that one could learn a great deal about the inherent ability of a person to coordinate his or her articulator muscles. I would expect considerable inter-subject variability in the pattern of coordination. More informative, I think, would be variability of the pattern within an individual. Remember that the essence of highly developed athletic skill, which we attribute to excellent motor coordination, is the ability to perform a complex sequence of movements in exactly the same way each time. Consider the tennis serve, the basketball free throw, or the delivery of a bowling ball. An individual's pattern may be unique but nonetheless very reproducible from one attempt to the next if he or she has normal motor coordination.

CONCLUSIONS OF THE REVIEW BY KENT ET AL.

The major conclusion of Kent et al. (1987) is "that the data base is generally inadequate for confident clinical applications" (p. 384). They go on to call for a "second generation of speech production measures." Although I am not sure if their plan calls for measures of speech-like responses, with less emphasis on simple behaviors and strength, I think an important point is that they do not call for abandonment of this effort, but for its refinement. I am in agreement with Kent et al. (1987), but I also think we must not leave the impression that the "first generation" was a failure. It has been a good start, and the investigators deserve a good deal of credit. It is worth noting that there are only 20 studies published on maximum phonatory duration, probably the most studied maximum performance measure. By comparison, there were over 100 papers published in 1989 on the pineal gland! Compared to most areas of scientific investigation relevant to human health and happiness, oral strength and nonspeech performance have hardly been touched.

FUTURE EFFORTS

Two words come to mind in thinking about the future of the effort to develop good performance standards in the area of speech motor control. One is technology, and the other is cooperation. Modern instrumentation makes it possible to measure variables with an ease and reliability that our teachers never dreamed of. Applications of technology to motor speech control are well illustrated by the tongue strength instrumentation system developed by Dworkin et al. (1980), and the multipurpose oral performance instrumentation system developed by Barlow and Netsell (1989). These are well suited to the study of dysarthric speakers, and I suspect they and their refinements will become standard in research and teaching. They are not, however, "field instruments," and widespread application of information gained by normalization of performance standards will be enhanced by development of an inexpensive, easy to use, portable instrument specifically designed for speech pathologists, or anyone who wants to objectively measure certain motor capacities in humans. These two basic approaches to instrumentation (sophisticated, expensive, and fixed location versus simple, inexpensive, and portable) are not inherently in competition. They may, in fact, complement each other in important ways.

Whatever course we take in the development of normative standards, it will be useful to cooperate with one another. For one thing, any one investigator generally will have access to limited populations (i.e., children, elderly, patients with swallowing problems). Another area of cooperation could be in developing procedures for giving instructions and controlling the variables related to practice and motivation. It is too early to call for a convention to develop an "ANSI Spec" for speech-language pathologists, but I firmly believe that day will come.

REFERENCES

Barlow, S.M., & Abbs, J.H. (1983). Force transducers for the evaluation of labial, lingual, and mandibular motor impairments. *Journal of Speech and Hearing Research, 26,* 616–621.

Barlow, S.M., & Netsell, R. (1989). Clinical neurophysiology for individuals with dysarthria. In K.M. Yorkston & D.R. Beukelman (Eds.), *Recent advances in clinical dysarthria* (pp. 53–82). Boston: College-Hill Press.

Blair, C., & Smith, A. (1986). EMG recording in human lip muscles: Can single muscles be isolated? *Journal of Speech and Hearing Research, 29,* 256–266.

Dworkin, J.P. (1980). Tongue strength measurement in patients with amyotrophic lateral sclerosis: Qualitative vs quantitative procedures. *Archives of Physical Medicine and Rehabilitation, 61,* 422–424.

Dworkin, J.P., & Aronson, A.E. (1986). Tongue strength and alternate motion rates in normal and dysarthric patients. *Journal of Communication Disorders, 19,* 115–132.

Dworkin, J.P., Aronson, A.E., & Mulder, D.W. (1980). Tongue force in normals and in dysarthric patients with amyotrophic lateral sclerosis. *Journal of Speech and Hearing Research, 23,* 828–837.

Dworkin, J.P., & Culatta, R.A. (1985). Oral structural and neuromuscular characteristics in children with normal and disordered articulation. *Journal of Speech and Hearing Disorders, 50,* 150–156.

Kent, R.D., Kent, J.F., & Rosenbek, J.C. (1987). Maximum performance tests of speech production. *Journal of Speech and Hearing Disorders, 52,* 367–387.

Palmer, M.F., & Osborn, C.D. (1940). A study of tongue pressures of speech defective and normal speaking individuals. *Journal of Speech Disorders, 5,* 133–140.

Posen, A.L. (1972). The influence of maximum perioral and tongue force on the incisor teeth. *Angle Orthodontist, 42,* 285–309.
Tatsumi, I.F., Sasanuma, S., Hirose, H., & Kiritani, S. (1979). Acoustic properties of ataxic and parkinsonian speech in syllable repetition tasks. *Annual Bulletin of the Royal Institute of Logopedics and Phoniatrics* (Tokyo), *13,* 99–104.

Dysarthria and Apraxia of Speech:
Perspectives on Management
edited by Christopher A. Moore, Ph.D., Kathryn M. Yorkston, Ph.D.,
and David R. Beukelman, Ph.D.
copyright © 1991   Paul H. Brookes Publishing Co., Inc.
Baltimore · London · Toronto · Sydney

Chapter 2 _____

Reductionism
Is a Dead-End
in Speech Research
Perspectives on a New Direction

Gary Weismer and Julie M. Liss

A TOPIC THAT has received substantial attention in various scientific fields in the 1980s is that of levels of analysis (see Bunge, 1977). In a global sense, this refers to the fact that any process or system can be formally or functionally partitioned into different levels. This chapter discusses this issue, both in general terms and in terms directly applicable to speech production. Our discussion of levels of analysis will lead into consideration of reductionistic trends in scientific research, and the implications for development of a model of speech production. We conclude the chapter by arguing that the levels of analysis problem has direct relevance to measurement issues that concern speech researchers, but may be less relevant in the development of a *control* model of normal and disordered speech production. This last point is illustrated by a preliminary model of speech production that is conceptually different from the typical sequence models that promote reductionistic thinking.

As a simple example of the levels of analysis issue, consider possible approaches to the study of the effects of air pressure in balloons. One could examine certain *macroscopic* characteristics of the pressure (viewer perceptions of the "stretch" of the balloon with different pressures, or general compliance functions relating pressure increments to volume with changes in balloon thickness) or certain *microscopic* effects (local porosity

_____

This work was supported by NIH Grant NS 18797.

functions with air pressure changes, or air particle speeds dependent on reflection characteristics of balloon material). The point is that different levels of analysis may be chosen to examine the effects of pressures on balloons, and that each level ultimately would provide evidence that balloons tend to get bigger as they are inflated.

In biological processes, and particularly in the area of motor control, the levels of analysis issue is very relevant and has a varied history. When the early advances in animal neurophysiology were made by people such as Sherrington (1900), it seemed reasonable that the experiments in which more or less direct measures of motor physiology were made (recording from motor cells in the cortex, or in subcortical motor nuclei, or even EMG) would provide a complete understanding of how people controlled movements. These early experiments, and the rapid advances that were made over the next 50–70 years, precipitated a "cult of technique," meaning that motor neurophysiologists tended to take a condescending view of scientists engaged in behavioral research on motor control (see Gardner, 1985). To paraphrase the general attitude as we understand it, the motor neurophysiologist might evaluate the results of an experiment in which tapping consistency is shown to be different for digits of the left and right hands by saying, "So what, you've shown a difference in tapping consistency between the hands, but you don't know why — you have no idea of what the mechanism is. What's worse, you'll never know about the mechanism if you insist on using those silly telegraph keys in your experiments. All behavioral phenomena are eventually traceable to nervous system states, so why even bother with the behavioral observations?" You will recognize the person making this statement as a *reductionist*, or, to use Bunge's (1980) terminology, a *physicalist*, a person who practices an extreme form of the reductionist program. As Gardner (1985) pointed out, this view held the scientific community spellbound until people started looking past the technological issues, and asking how well the reductionist observations were doing at *explaining* behavior, and the answer was, miserably. Many microscopic facts had been accumulated, and incredible technological advances had been made, but the sum of all of these reductionist observations still could not make good sense of macroscopic levels of movement behavior.

In an attempt to clarify further this issue of reductionism in movement research, consider a basketball analogy concerning the motor control required for free throw shooting. Could you, under any circumstance, envision a fruitful line of inquiry in the absence of a basketball, or of the goal? Would you submit a grant application that claimed that the best — the most basic — way to study the skill of free throws is to have a basketball player stand in the middle of your laboratory and simulate free throws while the electromyographic and kinematic activity of the effectors was monitored? Or, monitor the same variables in the presence of the goal and ball, but regard the *behavior* (i.e., shooting the ball, the success) as trivial and uninteresting, and perhaps a scientific pseudoproblem[1]?

Now consider that we have our own little reductionist-realist issue in the area of speech production research in general, and motor speech disorders in particular. The traditional sequential model of speech production, as proposed by Netsell (1973) and extended by Abbs (1988), has served as a basis for conceptualization of levels of analysis in speech production (Figure 1). Inherent in this model is the notion that levels closer to the CNS (e.g., nerve impulses, and muscular events) are a more basic reflection of the mechanisms underlying speech production. The notion of "more basic" has been considered by some investigators to mean that observations at levels closer to the CNS are preferable to observations made downstream from the CNS. How many times have you heard this: "Well, these are only perceptual observations, they don't really tell you much about the speech production deficit." Or, "Of course, acoustic observations are useful to a point, but they don't tell you much about the underlying movements, because the relationships between acoustics and movements are ambiguous." This message has been conveyed many times and has taken many forms. For example, Sussman, Marquardt, Mac-Neilage, and Hutchinson (1988) make a statement that observations at the motor level of the speech production process are preferable simply because they are "basic." They do not tell you what they are basic to, but we can assume basic means "closer" to the nervous system when compared to other levels of analysis (such as acoustic or perceptual). Sharkey and Folkins (1985) motivate their study of articulatory behavior in children by noting that whereas this issue has been studied acoustically, the actual movements should really be studied. They do not say why this is the case. Apparently, it is obvious to them that movements are more basic, and presumably, for a theory of speech production, more valuable. Hunker

---

[1]The term scientific pseudoproblem is borrowed from William Barrett's book, "The Illusion of Technique," published in 1979, and deserves attention within the context of this chapter. Barrett outlines the development, in the early 1900s, of a philosophical technique called "mathematical logic." The technique, which was developed and published by the reknowned philosophers Bertrand Russell and Alfred North Whitehead, was designed to provide a mechanism — a straightforward decision procedure — to answer *all* philosophical questions. Stated otherwise, Russell and Whitehead believed that their technique *reduced* all philosophy to mathematics. If a problem could not be addressed by the technique, it was a *pseudoproblem* — that is, not worthy of serious inquiry. This technique, which was supposed to revolutionize philosophy, was abandoned — indeed, renounced — by its creators within 30-some years because it failed to solve the fundamental problems of philosophy. Neurophysiology waited 30 or so more years before it, too, abandoned the strict reductionist orientation and admitted the field of "cognitive neurosciences" to the legitimate theater of scientific inquiry. Much of the explanation for the abandonment of reductionism in philosophy and neurophysiology is that people began to realize that some questions (perhaps most) of genuine importance would not be answerable within a reductionist framework.

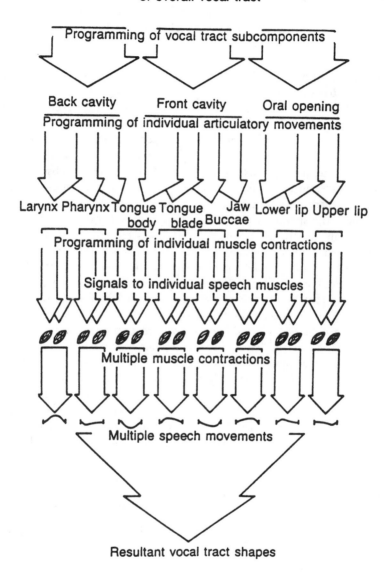

Temporal spatial specification
of overall vocal tract

Programming of vocal tract subcomponents

Back cavity   Front cavity   Oral opening
Programming of individual articulatory movements

Larynx Pharynx Tongue Tongue   Jaw Lower lip Upper lip
              body   blade Buccae
Programming of individual muscle contractions

Signals to individual speech muscles

Multiple muscle contractions

Multiple speech movements

Resultant vocal tract shapes

Figure 1. A typical sequence model of speech production. (From Abbs, J.H. [1988]. Neurophysiologic processes of speech movement control. In N.J. Lass, L.V. Mc Reynolds, J.L. Northern, & D.E. Yoder (Eds.), *Handbook of speech-language pathology and audiology* (p. 158). Toronto: B.C. Decker; reprinted by permission.

and Abbs (1984) follow this line of thought when they offer the following syllogism to guide the study of dysarthria:

1. Dysarthria is a movement disorder.
2. The ultimate understanding of movement disorders for assessment and treatment must be based on analyses of aberrations in movement and muscle contraction.
3. The assessment and treatment of dysarthria ultimately can be understood only at the movement and muscle contraction level of analysis. (p. 70)

Although this line of logic is obviously flawed because of the arbitrary nature of the major premise, a number of people in our field seem to think that a motor level of analysis, meaning a level that looks at movement and muscle activity, is automatically preferable to other levels of analysis, such as aerodynamic, acoustic, and perceptual. To further emphasize the prevalence of this attitude, here is a quote from a recently published chapter on speech physiology:

> The phenomenon of motor equivalence flexibility, coupled with the vocal tract modeling data of Stevens and House, also suggest the difficulty of attempting to discern articulatory movement patterns via analyses of the acoustic signal. Fundamentally, there is no unique relation between parameters of the speech acoustic signal and movements of the vocal tract. This lack of relationship is not to suggest that the acoustic signal is a useless global index of speech output, but rather that such analyses are limited for making inferences to underlying speech movement or neural control processes. (Abbs, 1988, p. 160)

In other words, these authors assume that the movement level of analysis is more basic, more "informative," than the acoustic level. Incidentally, the quote misrepresents the "nonuniqueness" problem: The nonuniqueness problem has always been stated in terms of *vocal tract area functions*, not movements.

We submit that this orientation to understanding speech production in normal and disordered speakers is not supported by research to date, is flawed on grounds of logic and common sense, and can only do harm to our advancement as a science if we continue to believe it. In an effort to clarify our position that acoustic and perceptual observations are as likely to produce valuable information as EMG/movement observations, we will present relevant philosophical considerations and selected evidence from acoustic, aerodynamic, and perceptual investigations.

Our philosophical position on levels of analysis derives from scientists such as Bunge (1977, 1980), Vogt, Stadler, and Kruse (1988), and

Yates (1982). We propose that the levels of a system or process cannot be ranked in terms of importance, because a level cannot be fully predicted from the preceding level. Reductionism — wherein the research program is aimed at ranking levels of analysis — implies that all observations at one level of analysis can be reduced to, or predicted from, observations at a different level. For example, the reductionist orientation in speech production would claim that any acoustic observations can, with the proper amount of research, be predicted completely by appropriate observations at the EMG/movement level, thus trivializing observations at the acoustic level. The few attempts that have been made to relate articulatory *positions* to acoustics have not met with great success (cf. Perkell & Nelson, 1985), and the future does not appear to be particularly promising in this regard, given that acoustic output is a product of sets of movements that are transformed into a tube shape. Now, the relationship between the movements and the tube shape are decidedly complex, nonlinear, and thus analytically intractable (at least at this point), and herein lies the rub. The form of the vocal tract shape (the area function) is not reducible to movements, but is an emergent function of those movements. Emergent means that the resulting area function is a new product of the sets of movements and boundary constraints that occur in the vocal tract. The area function is not "possessed" (in Bunge's 1977 terms) by the movements (e.g., brain cells do not possess memories, but memories are an emergent function of the action of collections of brain cells), but is a new form that derives from complex interaction among the movements. This is why, in the view of researchers such as Bunge, levels of a process are not ranked in importance, because the levels have their own identity, and they are not reducible to other levels (see Kelso & Schoner, 1988). In this sense, movement, aerodynamic, acoustic, and perceptual levels of analysis of the communication process should share equal billing in attempts to construct theories of normal and disordered speech production. Gardner (1985), echoing the sentiments of Mehler, Morton, and Jusczyk (1984), has a wonderful anti-reductionist statement: "One cannot have an adequate theory about anything the brain does unless one also has an adequate theory about that activity itself" (p. 286).

In the theory of normal and disordered speech production, we have two related issues that bear on the reductionist-realist problem. First, some ardent reductionists have built their careers studying single articulators — for example, the lower lip (or lower lip plus jaw), or a plane of movement at the approximate location of the tongue dorsum. An implicit assumption in these studies — especially when sweeping theoretical claims are based on single articulator observations — is that motor control of the *system* can be modeled from the behavior of a single articulator. Sometimes the logic in these studies attempts to be even more encompassing, evidenced by a recent claim that observations of reduced lower lip elevation in /vavavavava/ sequences produced by speakers with Parkinson's disease provides an explanation of the perception of hypokinetic dysarthria (Caliguiri, 1989). Some years ago, Gay (1973) showed that the lips and tongue respond differently to changes in speaking rate, and Adams (1990), in his dissertation, replicated and extended Gay's findings by showing that in five speakers, the tongue tip and lower lip have qualitatively different responses to speaking rate manipulations. (Indeed, he shows that opening and closing gestures of these articulators respond differently to rate manipulations.) When the system is broken into its components and these are assessed in an orthogonal way, it cannot be assumed that the behavior of an individual component models the behavior of other components. Second, it cannot be assumed that the sum of individual components somehow yields an overall system performance. The operative word here is *system:* The system is not possessed by any of its components but emerges from them. Netsell (1983) has written that it is likely that the speech mechanism is greater than the sum of its parts in the context of expressing concern about such tasks as, "Wag your tongue back and forth," then, "Pucker your lips." Fant (1982) has stated the "well established metaphor of studying speech motor control by EMG techniques as 'driving a nail into a computer with the hopes of finding out how it is organized' " (p. 273).

To summarize, we have argued that under the traditional model of speech production and its associated levels of analysis (see Figure 1), any given level is no less important than any other for understanding the speech production process. This position is somewhat at odds with that of investigators who believe that analyses performed at levels closer to the CNS are preferable to those farther away. In closing, we would like to take our argument one step further and illuminate a path for continued development of the ideas presented in this chapter.

Although we have borrowed liberally from philosophical perspectives offered by Bunge (1977, 1980), Vogt et al. (1988), and Yates (1982), levels of analysis for the speech production process, and the interactions between these levels, are likely to be infinitely more complex than the analysis problems approached by these philosophers in other biological processes, such as heartbeat and respiration (Yates, 1982). Some investigators (Kelso, Saltzman, & Tuller, 1986) have tried to adapt these schemes, which are based on simpler biological processes, in a fairly direct way to speech production. However, we feel it is important to question and evaluate the concepts of "levels" and "emergence" as they apply specifically to speech production.

In our view, the issues of levels and emergence in speech production reflect a model of speech production that shows what can be measured, but not necessarily *how* the process actually occurs. For example, the traditional model (Figure 1) suggests that the acoustic waveform results from the sequence of nerve impulses, or muscular events/structural movements. Our position is that the acoustic waveform is an *emergent* of articulatory movements, because measurement of the movements cannot predict the acoustic waveform. What cannot be gained from either sequence, however, is the *process* by which the acoustic waveform is produced. More specifically, the levels of analysis that permit measurement are not necessarily isomorphic with, or predictive of, the levels at which you conceptualize *control* of a process. Because something can be measured (e.g., electromyographic activity of individual muscles) does not mean that the measured phenomenon is represented in the control scheme for the behavior (see Riccio & Stoffregen, 1988, for similar thoughts on the control of stance). Instead, the levels at which control is conceptualized should be based on the behavioral goals of the mechanism (Kelso & Schoner, 1988; Riccio & Stoffregen, 1988). To expand on the general position offered in this chapter, we believe that the concept of emergence is basically relevant to the relations between various levels or grains of measurement in a system *and need not play a prominent role in the specification of control strategies for that mechanism.*

A PRELIMINARY (REDUCTION-FREE) MODEL OF SPEECH PRODUCTION

If we were to develop a *control model* of speech production, we would begin by reversing and revising the traditional sequence models described above. Figure 2 shows a first sketch of such a model. Several logistical aspects of this model should be mentioned before content is discussed. First, this is not a sequence model in the traditional sense. Whereas there is a global sequence of events, (i.e., acoustic/perceptual goals give way to a pool of processes ["domain of muscular collectives"] that eventually result in a series of vocal tract shapes), the core of this preliminary model is interactive and heterarchical (see Kelso & Tuller, 1981). Second, in this sketch, there is no treatment of either the units or structure of sequencing, such as that discussed by Shattuck-Hufnagel (1983), but the model could eventually accommodate such components. Third, the selection of components was not guided by measurement considerations (i.e., levels of analysis), but rather by the prospective components of control.

According to contemporary theorists such as Bunge (1980) and Riccio and Stoffregen (1988), control strategies of action systems are organized according to the goals of those systems. Investigators of general motor control are beginning to structure experimental efforts around such thinking (van Sonderen, Gielen, & Denier van der Gon, 1989). In the case

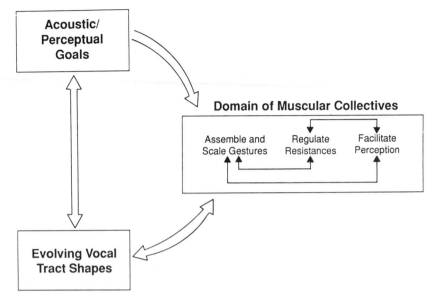

Figure 2. Sketch of a heterarchical model for speech motor control.

of speech, clearly the goal is to generate an acoustic waveform matched to the needs of the listener. Thus, the driving point of the model in Figure 2 is the acoustic/perceptual goals and products. In service of these goals, a domain of muscular collectives, encompassing several related processes, produces the output of the vocal tract. Three of these processes are identified in Figure 2. The process of assembling and scaling gestures recalls work by Bell-Berti (1980), Fowler (1985), Kent 1987), and Perkell (1986). The regulation of resistances has been described both empirically and theoretically by Warren (1986). Facilitation of perception, which has not been addressed comprehensively in any model or theory of speech production, involves the interface between the acoustic signal and aspects of the signal that are perceptually most salient.

Note that this preliminary model presented in Figure 2 gives the acoustic/perceptual levels a certain priority, because together, they comprise the target representation. Perceptual analyses of speech production generally have not been held in high esteem by speech investigators because these analyses are said to lack objectivity and do not require great technical sophistication. As may be gathered from the *facilitate perception* category in the domain of muscular collectives (Figure 2), we regard certain perceptual processes as critical for speech motor control. For example, consider the issue of lexical decisions in speech perception. Listeners use certain strategies to optimize the correctness of those decisions. One strategy is *focused search*, in which listeners do not attend to the entire incoming signal, but rather search for *islands of reliability*, or high yield portions of the signal such as stressed words, word onsets, and regions of abrupt spectral change. Cutler (1976) and Cutler and Foss (1977) have shown that listeners use aspects of timing and fundamental frequency profiles to predict the location of an upcoming stressed word, a strategy that could make the listener's processing task highly efficient (attention cycling). Pisoni and Luce (1986) have presented speech perception research demonstrating that lexical access is organized by word onsets. When these perceptual results are linked with acoustic and aerodynamic data indicating, for example, priority for word-initial articulatory precision and more prominent acoustic and aerodynamic events in word-initial obstruents than in production of word-medial or word-final stops (Kohler, 1984; Stathopolous & Weismer, 1985), there appears to be an adequate basis for incorporation of perception issues in a model of motor speech control.

We believe that certain long-standing issues in speech production are handled more effectively by this conceptualization (Figure 2), than by the traditional sequence model (Figure 1). For example, the role of afference in our models is not reactive, but directly serves the perceptual goals. That is to say, the afferent information in our model is "smart" in the sense that it is driven by the adjustment of the system to meet the laws of adequate message transmission. Moreover, our model explains typical repetition-to-repetition movement variation as a natural consequence of subordinating the domain of muscular collectives to the laws of acoustics. Whereas this may seem to be simply a restatement of motor equivalence in speech production (Abbs & Gracco, 1984; Edwards, 1985), we view it not as a mechanism of control, but as a phenomenon of collective behavior. Investigators who consider motor equivalence as a mechanism of control do so because of what they believe is the goal of control (i.e., articulatory positions or trajectories). In our view, motor equivalence is no more than a description of the phenomena of muscular activities, or movements, subordinated to acoustic/perceptual goals identified in Figure 2. In fact, we argue that the repetition-to-repetition variability observed at the muscular activity or structural movement level is inconsequential because the only relevant variability (i.e., relevant for the control model) occurs at the level of acoustic/perceptual goals.

CONCLUSIONS

Other scientific disciplines have come to the realization that reductionist research programs will not provide an understanding of complex phenomena, and this is especially so in the behavioral sciences. Researchers in our field have believed that physiological techniques would reveal a reduced set of phenomena that would explain all levels of speech production. The lesson from our literature, as well as from the more general scientific community, suggests that we should move away from this perspective. By a preliminary model, we attempt to show how a nonreductionistic approach to speech science might reveal important insights about speech production.

REFERENCES

Abbs, J.H. (1988). Neurophysiologic processes of speech movement control. In N.J. Lass, L.V. McReynolds, J.L. Northern, & D.E. Yoder (Eds.), *Handbook of speech-language pathology and audiology* (pp. 154–170). Toronto: B.C. Decker.

Abbs, J.H., & Gracco, V.L. (1984). Control of complex motor gestures: Orofacial muscle responses to load perturbations of the lip during speech. *Journal of Neurophysiology, 51,* 705–723.

Adams, S.G. (1990). *Rate and clarity of speech: An x-ray microbeam study.* Unpublished doctoral dissertation, University of Wisconsin – Madison.

Barrett, W. (1979). *The illusion of technique.* Garden City, NY: Anchor Press.

Bell-Berti, F. (1980). Velopharyngeal function: A spatial-temporal model. In N.J. Lass (Ed.), *Speech and language: Advances in basic research and practice* (pp. 291–316). New York: Academic Press.

Bunge, M. (1977). Levels and reduction. *American Journal of Physiology: Regulatory, Integrative and Comparative Physiology, 233,* R75–R82.

Bunge, M. (1980). *The mind-body problem: A psychobiological approach.* Oxford: Pergamon Press.

Caliguiri, M.P. (1989). The influence of speaking rate on articulatory hypokinesia in Parkinsonian dysarthria. *Brain and Language, 36,* 493–502.

Cutler, A. (1976). Phoneme-monitoring reaction time as a function of preceding intonation contour. *Perception & Psychophysics, 20,* 55–60.

Cutler, A., & Foss, D.J. (1977). On the role of sentence stress in sentence processing. *Language and Speech, 20,* 1–10.

Edwards, J. (1985). Contextual effects on lingual-mandibular coordination. *Journal of the Acoustical Society of America, 78,* 1944–1948.

Fant, G. (1982). Some remarks from the viewpoint of speech research. In S. Grillner, B. Lindblom, J. Lubker, & A. Persson (Eds.), *Speech motor control* (pp. 273–277). Oxford: Pergamon Press.

Fowler, C.A. (1985). Current perspectives on language and speech production: A critical review. In R.G. Daniloff (Ed.), *Speech science* (pp. 193–278). San Diego: College-Hill Press.

Gardner, H. (1985). *The mind's new science: A history of the cognitive revolution.* New York: Basic Books, Inc.

Gay, T. (1973). Effect of speaking rate on labial consonant production. *Phonetica, 27,* 44–56.

Gracco, V.L. (1988). Timing factors in the coordination of speech movements. *Journal of Neurosciences, 8,* 4628–4639.

Hunker, C.J., & Abbs, J.H. (1984). Physiological analyses of Parkinsonian tremors in the orofacial system. In M.R. McNeil, J.C. Rosenbek, & A.E. Aronson (Eds.), *The dysarthrias: Physiology, acoustics, perception, and management.* San Diego: College-Hill Press.

Kelso, J.A.S., Saltzmann, E.L., & Tuller, B. (1986). The dynamic perspective on speech production. *Journal of Phonetics, 14*, 29–59.

Kelso, J.A.S., & Schoner, G. (1988). Self-organization of coordinative movement patterns. *Human Movement Science, 7*, 27–46.

Kelso, J.A.S., & Tuller, B. (1981). Toward a theory of apractic syndromes. *Brain and Language, 12*, 224–245.

Kent, R.D. (1987). The iceberg hypothesis: The temporal assembly of speech movements. In J.S. Perkell & D.H. Klatt (Eds.), *Invariance and variability in speech processes* (pp. 234–242). Hillsdale: NJ: Lawrence Erlbaum Associates.

Kohler, K.J. (1984). Phonetic explanation in phonology: The feature fortis/lenis. *Phonetica, 41*, 150–174.

Mehler, J., Morton, J., & Jusczyk, P. (1984). On reducing language to biology. *Cognitive Neuropsychology, 1*, 83–116.

Netsell, R. (1973). Speech physiology. In F.D. Minifie, T.J. Hixon, & F. Williams (Eds.), *Normal aspects of speech, hearing, and language* (pp. 1–19). Englewood Cliffs, NJ: Prentice-Hall.

Netsell, R. (1983). Speech motor control: Theoretical issues with clinical impact. In W. Berry (Ed.), *Clinical dysarthria*. San Diego: College-Hill Press.

Perkell, J.S. (1986). Coarticulation strategies: Preliminary indications of a detailed analysis of lower lip protrusion movements. *Speech Communication, 5*, 47–68.

Perkell, J.S., & Nelson, W.L. (1985). Variability in production of /i/ and /ɑ/. *Journal of the Acoustical Society of America, 77*, 1889–1895.

Pisoni, D.B., & Luce, P.A. (1986). Speech perception: Research, theory and the principal issues. In E.C. Schwab & H.C. Nusbaum (Eds.), *Pattern recognition by humans and machines: Speech perception* (pp. 1–50). New York: Academic Press.

Riccio, G.E., & Stoffregen, T.A. (1988). Affordances as constraints on the control of stance. *Human Movement Science, 7*, 265–300.

Sharkey, S.G., & Folkins, J.W. (1985). Variability of lip and jaw movements in children and adults: Implications for the development of speech motor control. *Journal of Speech and Hearing Research, 28*, 8–15.

Shattuck-Huffnagel, S. (1983). Sublexical units and suprasegmental structure in speech production planning. In P.F. MacNeilage (Ed.), *The production of speech* (pp. 109–136). New York: Springer-Verlag.

Sherrington, C.S. (1900). The muscular sense. In E.A. Schafer (Ed.), *Textbook of physiology, Vol. 2* (pp. 783–883). London: Pentland.

Stathopolous, E.T., & Weismer, G. (1985). Stress, word gradient, and oral airflow in children and adults. *Journal of Phonetics, 13*, 343–355.

Sussman, H.M., Marquardt, T.P., MacNeilage, P.F., & Hutchinson, J.A. (1988). Anticipatory coarticulation in aphasia: Some methodological considerations. *Brain and Language, 35*, 369–379.

van Sonderen, J.F., Gielen, C.C.A.M., & Denier van der Gon, J.J. (1989). Motor programmes for goal-directed movements are continuously adjusted according to changes in target location. *Experimental Brain Research, 78*, 139–146.

Vogt, S., Stadler, M., & Kruse, P. (1988). Self-organization aspects in the temporal formation of movement gestalts. *Human Movement Science, 7*, 365–406.

Warren (1986). Compensatory speech behaviors in individuals with cleft palate: A regulation/control problem? *Cleft Palate Journal, 23*, 251–260.

Yates, F.E. (1982). Outline of a physical theory of physiological systems. *Canadian Journal of Physiology and Pharmacology, 60,* 217–248.

Dysarthria and Apraxia of Speech:
Perspectives on Management
edited by Christopher A. Moore, Ph.D., Kathryn M. Yorkston, Ph.D.,
and David R. Beukelman, Ph.D.
copyright © 1991   Paul H. Brookes Publishing Co., Inc.
Baltimore · London · Toronto · Sydney

Chapter 3

Measures and Designs for Research in Dysarthria
Pitfalls and Opportunities

Christy L. Ludlow

IN THE 80s great advances have been made in developing speech measurement techniques. Measures of airflow, air pressure, muscle activity, isometric force, articulator movement, and acoustic properties are now possible in many clinical and research settings. In some research centers, x-ray microbeam and magnetometry systems provide simultaneous measures of movements at several points within the vocal tract. With magnetometry systems for personal computers, complete transduction systems may soon become widely available.

The value of developing batteries of measures with standards for obtaining these measures is recognized (see Luschei, chap. 1, this volume). Normative data needs to be acquired for each measure, similar to testing hearing threshold in audiology, to support comparisons of patients to normal standards. As a result, measures could be used in a variety of settings to determine degree of impairment and to evaluate treatment effects. This approach has been compared to use of an audiogram in hearing.

PITFALLS

Understanding Patient Problems

Availability of standardized measures has not necessarily benefitted patient care. The most common hearing disability, presbycusis, is also the least well understood, though it is usually described using standardized audiologic test batteries. Testing speech intelligibility and completing an audiogram do not necessarily predict hearing aid use. Hearing scientists now know that much signal processing is done at the end organ stage and that the auditory system performs complex signal processing at several levels. It is understandable, then, that pure tone tests may not predict how well persons with aging auditory systems might perceive, process, and recognize complex acoustic signals, such as speech. Hearing is a dynamic and interactive process involving simultaneous forward and backward processing at many levels of the CNS. Standardized tools of audiology such as the audiogram were developed with much simpler concepts of auditory physiology that concentrated on detection of simple, pure tones. Continued use of the audiogram as a standard may limit and obscure addressing such complex clinical problems as difficulties that aging adults have with detecting, perceiving, and processing complex speech signals.

Similarly in speech pathology, the development of a battery of standardized measurement tools for assessing speech production may not contribute to our understanding of patients' speech disorders. In fact, such measurement might even limit our understanding of their problems.

To further demonstrate this point, I would like to draw on some of my personal experience. I first attempted to measure speech production in dysarthria when I was asked to participate in a study comparing Sinemet with bromocriptine in a multidisciplinary study of Parkinson's disease. A review of the literature suggested the aspects of speech production that might be affected (Canter, 1963, 1965a, 1965b; Darley, Aronson, & Brown, 1969; Logemann, Fisher, Boshes, & Blonsky, 1978). To make the measures as objective and reliable as possible, I developed speech tasks from which to measure particular aspects of speech production (maximum phonation time, intensity and frequency control, rate of syllable repetition and sentence production, timing changes for stress contrasts, intonation contours, and speech initiation latency). Objective acoustic measures were developed to measure each aspect of speech production from patient tapes. By the time I had analyzed the speech and made measures in one condition for 3 patients, the rest of the research team had completed the analysis and published their results. We continued with the analysis, however, and published several papers demonstrating how these acoustic measures could be standardized (Ludlow, Bassich, & Connor, 1985), how they related to perceptual ratings of patients' speech (Ludlow & Bassich, 1984), how the measures differentiated the hypokinetic dysarthria in Parkinson's disease from Shy Drager syndrome or multiple systems atrophy (Ludlow & Bassich, 1983), and how the measures could discriminate between patients with and without central nervous system deficits (Bassich, Ludlow, & Polinsky, 1984). We also gathered and published a great deal of normative data on control speakers of different ages (Ludlow et al., 1985).

Nevertheless, after a great deal of work and development of valid, objective, reliable, and standardized methods of assessing speech in patients with Parkinson's disease, we did not have any greater understanding of the speech production disorder in Parkinson's disease or how to treat it. We had demonstrated that laryngeal control is probably the most affected part of the vocal tract, but Logemann et al. (1978) had already demonstrated that using a simple clinical rating scale. We had not furthered our understanding of *how* laryngeal control in Parkinson's disease is impaired. We had found that patients with Parkinson's disease were particularly impaired in producing glottal stops in the middle of voicing for repetition of the vowel /i/. Other researchers had documented voicing offset errors, such as differentiating /is/ from /iz/ (Weismer, 1984). Using fiber-optic viewing, Hanson, Gerratt, and Ward (1984) reported vocal fold bowing in patients with Parkinson's disease, which suggest a lack of muscle tension. Our results and those of Weismer (1984) suggest that the vocal folds move more slowly than normal for adduction in glottal stops and voice offset.

To better understand the physiologic bases for dysarthric patients' speech disorders, we need to focus on the pathophysiology of their motor control. Simply describing how these patients differ from normal speakers, rather than examining their underlying motor control disorders, will not improve patient care. With this in mind, thoughtful selection of meaningful measures is of paramount importance to the study of dysarthria.

Selection of Measures

For a measure to be useful in studying a speech disorder, its validity for specifically quantifying one particular attribute of speech motor control is paramount. Again, let me illustrate this with some personal experience. My co-workers and I went to great pains to measure jitter and shimmer in Parkinson's disease and multiple systems atrophy, and we found that jitter was not affected in Parkinson's disease, but was affected in multiple systems atrophy (Ludlow, Coulter, & Gentges, 1983). But what did that tell us? Jitter and shimmer can be increased by different aspects of vocal behavior. They can be increased in unilateral vocal fold paralysis with glottic incompetence; in vocal fold asymmetry because of nodules, polyps, or carcinoma (Ludlow, Bassich, Connor, Coulter, & Lee, 1987); and by excessive tension in vocal folds that produces overadduction, as in spasmodic dysphonia (Ludlow, Naunton, & Bassich, 1984). These measures are not specific to a particular attribute of glottic function during phonation since they can reflect hyperadduction, hypoadduction, and asymmetric adduction. Furthermore, these are not valid measures of glottic abnormalities because they do not reliably discriminate between individuals with normal and pathologic larynges (Ludlow et al., 1987). Such measures should not be used in assessment since they are neither specific nor valid.

If we are successful in developing standardized measures with standard administration, assessment of speech motor control could become highly prescribed. In the wrong hands, this could result in a "cookbook" approach to speech function assessment. Speech pathologists might function as technicians, administering a battery of tests in a highly routine manner, rather than as clinicians. Although a reasonable balance is likely between the current state and that situation, we must encourage professional judgment and emphasize the need for problem solving during patient assessment rather than merely administering a prescribed battery of tests.

OPPORTUNITIES

Conceptual Models of Dysarthria

The field of dysarthria needs to develop theoretical concepts regarding the disorders in our patients. One approach by Marsden (1985) proposed a hierarchical serial model of motor control with stages of planning, programming, and execution. These stages are based on normal motor behavior, however, and may assume that disorders are confined to one particular stage of processing (e.g., programming). This approach may be useful in cases such as discrimination of dyspraxia (programming) from dysarthria (execution), although this dichotomy may now be in question. In any case, we should not assume that difficulties in dysarthric patients are confined to certain levels in a serial processing model. Rather, the dysarthrias may be varieties of pathophysiology resulting in execution disorders.

Another framework uses functional components (Netsell, 1986), which determine the parts of the vocal tract most affected. This approach may be useful in some focal disorders such as spasmodic dysphonia, but the implicit assumption is that speech execution is the linear sum of its component parts. An example would be if a clinician wanted to understand posture problems in patients with Parkinson's disease and tested isometric force during sustained leg extensions. This measure probably would not be instructive since posture depends upon control and integration of both sensory and motor components. Rather, to understand these problems, integrative aspects of postural control need to be addressed, not integrity of the individual components. In dysarthria, testing muscle strength or respiratory capacity may be useful only for assuring that individual components are intact. Studying these components while varying parameters of movement control may be more useful. For example, in patients with Parkinson's disease, comparing articulatory movements of whispered and spoken productions of the same syllables can determine if vocal fold movements are difficult for these patients to integrate with supraglottic patterning. Only patients' abilities to control distinct components of the speech motor control system should be examined independently. These abilities might include the modulation of brain stem reflexes during volitional movement and their ability to adjust movement patterns in response to various demands.

Research Goals in Dysarthria

Selection of measures should be based on research goals in dysarthria. Two reasonable goals are:

1. To increase our understanding of patients' disorders and problems
2. To improve treatments for these patients

If our goal is to better understand patients' speech disorders, then the purpose of measuring speech production is either: 1) to analyze the disorder, or 2) to relate the disorder to the disease process, the neuropathology. Standardized measurement techniques may not add new information to knowledge of a disorder, and standardized measurements that are available are not necessarily measures that best serve our research goals.

If our goal is to determine the relation between the neurologic disorder and dysarthria, care must be taken to select measures of speech motor control specific to the disorder. For example, to relate positron emission tomography measures of caudate metabolism to dysarthria in Parkinson's disease, measures that reflect an important attribute of that type of dysarthria should be used. Glottal resistance may reflect breathy hypophonia, an important feature in Parkinson's disease, while nasal accelerometry, a measure of velopharyngeal competence, would not. Furthermore, if our goal is to improve treatment for dysarthria, we need specific measures that best reflect the patients' communication impairments.

Analyzing Motor Control Disorders

To analyze a speech motor control disorder, three questions should guide selection of a measure:

1. Do we know what this is a measure of?
2. What new information will this measure reveal about the disorder?
3. Why do we want to know about this aspect of the disorder?

Relating Motor Control Disorders and Neuropathology

To relate a patient's motor control disorder to a neurologic abnormality, measures that represent the patient's speech motor control abnormality must be selected. Three questions should be asked when selecting these measures:

1. Does this measure quantify an attribute important to this disorder?
2. Do these measures represent all aspects of the patient's speech impairment?
3. Is the patient impaired, relative to normal, on this measure?

Assessing Treatment Benefits

Different selection criteria should be followed when selecting measures for assessing the benefit of new treatment approaches:

1. Does this measure reflect the speech communication impairment?
2. Does this measure tell us how the treatment works?
3. Does this measure patient or listener perceptions about the disorder?

Designs To Meet Research Goals in Dysarthria

Just as the measures must be selected to meet research goals, so the research must be designed also to meet those goals. In dysarthria, as in other areas of speech pathology research, considerable debate has focused on whether to use single subject or group experiments. Since each design is best suited for a different purpose, research goals should guide selection of appropriate designs. The design most frequently used in dysarthria research compares a patient group with a normal control group, similar in age and sex, to determine distinctive attributes of the patient group. If differences are found, it is concluded that the measurements are important in describing that patient group's motor control disorder. It may be, however, that any neurologically impaired patient group would differ from normal on those measurement attributes. Therefore, a better design would be to compare a group of patients with other motor control disorders to the original group to determine if the original group only differs from normal on those measurements. Using the research goal as the guiding rationale, the following are recommendations for research designs in studying the motor speech disorders of dysarthric patients.

Designs for Identifying
the Attributes of Motor Speech Disorders

1. Comparisons of the targeted patient group with several other patient groups to determine if a measurement attribute is specific to the targeted group
2. Comparisons within patients during different clinical states to determine if the measurement attribute varies with the disease state and is therefore a component of the disorder

3. Comparisons within patients at stages in disease progression to determine if those measurement attributes change with the disease process
4. Comparisons between patients with and without the same neuropathology to determine if that measurement attribute is affected by any neurologic disease or is affected only by a particular pathology

These comparisons are useful for determining if a particular measurement attribute characterizes a particular type of dysarthria. Such approaches to identifying distinctive attributes are more valid than the frequently used approach that compares a patient group with a normal control group. Correlations between the extent of neuropathology and measurement attributes may not be specific to an experiment group but characteristic of any patient group and, therefore, may not identify specific attributes of a disorder.

Determining the Pathophysiology of Motor Control Disorders

Understanding the pathophysiology of motor speech disorders is necessary to develop new treatments. Hypertonia at rest, spasmodic co-contractions, action-induced muscle hypertonia, exaggerated stretch reflexes, reduced long-latency reflexes, disinhibition of afferent reflexes, increased central conduction times, and cortical hypometabolism are all indications of types of pathophysiology that can contribute to movement disorders. These symptoms require distinct treatments to control abnormalities, such as medication to enhance or block various neurotransmitters, or botulinum toxin injections to peripherally reduce dystonia in selected muscle groups.

The purpose here is to determine which abnormalities contribute to the movement disorder, not what is specific to the disorder.

1. When disorders are task specific, individual patient comparisons of motor control during affected and nonaffected tasks will be useful.
2. When disorders are focal to one or several components of the motor speech system, an examination of afferent and efferent reflexes, muscle activation, and voluntary control of affected and unaffected components in individual patients may help distinguish the physiological abnormalities that contribute to the problems of affected components.
3. Group comparisons of patient groups with known types of pathology with normal controls can be used to determine the aspects of motor control affected by pathology of the cortical, subcortical, and peripheral motor systems. Relevant are the integrity of afferent and efferent responses, evoked sensory and motor potential latencies and amplitudes, and cortical and subcortical metabolism.
4. When treatment is effective in reversing a motor control abnormality, within-patient physiologic studies before and after treatment can de-

termine which physiologic abnormalities change with improvement in speech.

Developing New Treatment Approaches

Single subject designs are useful in preliminary studies to develop new treatments. Study of the effects of a treatment in a single subject requires multiple measures during treatment and nontreatment phases. A single pre–post test in a single subject is not adequate to study if the treatment has been effective, since additional changes occurred between the two trials. Therefore, either an ABAB design with reiterative crossover or withdrawal, multiple baselines, or long-term follow-up with treatment withdrawal are necessary *at minimum* to study a new treatment in individuals.

Single-subject studies are useful for evaluating the effects of treatment in individuals, but they do not support conclusions regarding a group. Therefore, the next stage in developing a new treatment must be to apply it to a group using various designs during different stages in treatment development (Table 1). An open trial, including only an experimental group with pre–post measures to determine treatment parameters such as frequency, duration, and side effects, is useful only in choosing treatment guidelines for subsequent studies. This method does not support any conclusions about treatment benefits. Treatment effects can be studied with controlled designs using repeated baseline measures, a nontreated control group, or reiterative phases of treatment and treatment withdrawal. Without random assignment to treated and nontreated groups, however, no generalization can be made of the effects of treatment to patients other than those studied.

Evaluating New Procedures or Treatments

Clinical trials to evaluate efficacy of surgical procedures or therapy without administration of placebo include random assignment between experimental and control groups (Table 1). In such designs, blind analysis of results is recommended to avoid measurement bias. In dysarthria, since most measures can be performed off-line, noninformed blind analysis can be easily incorporated.

Medication or injection trials are most amenable to single blind trials where the patient does not know if the placebo or medication has been administered. In double blind trials, neither the patient or the experimenter knows which has been administered. There is great advantage in the placebo phase since most patients show some spontaneous improvement associated with high expectations of a new treatment. In double blind crossover studies, each patient undergoes the placebo and the treatment,

Table 1. Characteristics of treatment evaluation research designs

Design and purpose	Pre–Post and Follow-up	Nontreatment controls	Random group assignment	Noninformed (blind) evaluation	Noninformed patients	Noninformed experiments
Open trial	X			yes		
Controlled studies	X	X	yes	yes		
Surgical or nonplacebo trial	X	X	X	yes		
Single blind	X	X	X	yes	X	
Double blind	X	X	X	X	X	X

X = included feature, yes = recommended feature.

randomly assigning the placebo or treatment first. This is a control for order effects and the high expectations of a new treatment. The literature on dysarthria contains few, if any, controlled single or double blind trials. These trials are used to evaluate new surgical and medication treatments in life-threatening diseases where treatment withdrawal can alter life expectancy, so there is little justification for not using such trials for evaluating dysarthria therapies.

In conclusion, many opportunities exist for increasing our knowledge and understanding of motor speech disorders and for developing and evaluating new treatments. Our efforts need to meet these research goals rather than to emphasize measurement standardization, which in itself will not increase understanding or assist in developing new treatment approaches. Unless measurements are selected carefully to meet our particular research, assessment, and treatment needs, they will not serve us or our patients well.

REFERENCES

Bassich, C.J., Ludlow, C.L., & Polinsky, R.J. (1984). Speech symptoms associated with early signs of Shy-Drager Syndrome. *Journal of Neurology, Neurosurgery and Psychiatry, 47,* 995–1001.

Canter, G.J. (1963). Speech characteristics of patients with Parkinson's disease: I. Intensity, pitch, and duration. *Journal of Speech and Hearing Disorders, 28,* 221–229.

Canter, G.J. (1965a). Speech characteristics of patients with Parkinson's disease: II. Physiological support for speech. *Journal of Speech and Hearing Disorders, 30,* 44–49.

Canter, G.J. (1965b). Speech characteristics of patients with Parkinson's disease: III. Articulation, diadocho-kinesis and overall speech adequacy. *Journal of Speech and Hearing Disorders, 30,* 217–224.

Darley, F.L., Aronson, A., & Brown, J.R. (1969). Differential diagnostic patterns of dysarthrias. *Journal of Speech and Hearing Research, 12,* 246–269.

Hanson, D., Gerratt, B.R., & Ward, P.H. (1984). Cinegraphic observations of laryngeal function in Parkinson's disease. *Laryngoscope, 94,* 348–353.

Logemann, J., Fisher, H., Boshes, B., & Blonsky, E. (1978). Frequency and co-occurrence of vocal tract dysfunctions in speech of a large sample of Parkinson's patients. *Journal of Speech and Hearing Disorders, 48,* 47-57.

Ludlow, C.L., & Bassich, C.J. (1983). The results of acoustic and perceptual assessment of two types of dysarthria. In W.R. Berry (Ed.), *Clinical dysarthria* (pp. 121–154). San Diego: College-Hill Press.

Ludlow, C. L., & Bassich, C.J. (1984). Relationships between perceptual ratings and acoustic measures of hypokinetic speech. In M. McNeil, J. Rosenbek, A. Aronson (Eds.), *The dysarthrias: Physiology, acoustic, perception, management* (pp. 163–196). San Diego: College-Hill Press.

Ludlow, C.L., Bassich, G.J., & Connor, N.P. (1985). An objective system for assessment and analysis of dysarthric speech. In J. Darby (Ed.), *Speech and language evaluation in neurology: Adult disorders* (pp. 393–425). New York: Grune & Stratton.

Ludlow, C.L., Bassich, C.J., Connor, N.P., Coulter, D.C., & Lee, Y.J. (1987). In T. Baer, C. Sasaki, & K. Harris (Eds.), *Laryngeal function in phonation and respiration* (pp. 492–508). Boston: Little, Brown.

Ludlow, C.L., Coulter, D.C., & Gentges, F. (1983). The differential sensitivity of frequency perturbation to laryngeal neoplasms and neuropathologies. In D.M. Bless & J.H. Abbs (Eds.), *Vocal fold physiology: Contemporary research and clinical issues* (pp. 381–392). San Diego: College-Hill Press.

Ludlow, C.L., Naunton, R.F., & Bassich, C.J. (1984). Procedures for the selection of spastic dysphonia patients for recurrent laryngeal nerve section. *Otolaryngology-Head and Neck Surgery, 92*, 24–31.

Marsden, C.D. (1985). Defects of movement in Parkinson's disease. In P.J. Delwaide & A. Agnoli, (Eds.), *Clinical neurophysiology in parkinsonism* (pp. 107–115). Amsterdam: Elseview Science Publishers.

Netsell, R. (1986). *A neurobiologic view of speech production and the dysarthrias* (pp. 2–3). San Diego: College-Hill Press.

Weismer, G. (1984). Articulatory characteristics of parkinsonian dysarthria: Segmental and phrase-level timing, spirantization, and glottal-supraglottal coordination. In M. McNeil, J. Rosenbek, & A. Aronson (Eds.), *The dysarthrias: Physiology, acoustic, perception, management* (pp. 101–130). San Diego: College-Hill Press.

Dysarthria and Apraxia of Speech:
Perspectives on Management
edited by Christopher A. Moore, Ph.D., Kathryn M. Yorkston, Ph.D.,
and David R. Beukelman, Ph.D.
Paul H. Brookes Publishing Co., Inc.
Baltimore · London · Toronto · Sydney

SECTION II

INTELLIGIBILITY

THIS SECTION CONSIDERS limits, capabilities, and practices in the description and measurement of speaker intelligibility. Factors such as semantic context, listener experience, and the speaker's physical appearance have long been recognized as important contributors to intelligibility. Similarly, severely dysarthric speech is recognized as difficult to assess, since most instruments are designed to test a range of capabilities without probing small, but significant, differences among speakers who exhibit severe impairment. These factors are now addressed in standardized assessment. Additional factors in assessment are application and perceived value of established methods. Perceptions of clinical value, effectiveness, availability, and use of current assessment procedures are compared in a comprehensive survey of clinical practice in Department of Veterans Affairs Medical Centers. Together, the chapters in this section comprise a clear definition of the state of the art in assessment of motor speech disorders.

Chapter 4

Index of
Contextual Intelligibility
Impact of Semantic
Context in Dysarthria

Vicki L. Hammen,
Kathryn M. Yorkston, and Patricia Dowden

MANY FACTORS INFLUENCE the intelligibility of dysarthric speakers. Some factors do not relate to motor activity of speaking, but relate to such external factors as the semantic context provided by natural communicative situations. Berry and Sanders (1983) suggest that the predictability of the situation may allow listeners to fill in portions of a message that are not understood. The impact of semantic context on speech intelligibility is particularly important for severely dysarthric individuals, who may use augmentative communication approaches in some situations, but whose natural speech may also be an important component of communication (Yorkston, Beukelman, & Bell, 1988). Documenting intelligibility of the natural speech of severely dysarthric speakers is a difficult task. Traditional sentence and word intelligibility tasks, such as the Computerized Assessment of Intelligibility of Dysarthric Speech (Yorkston, Beukelman, & Traynor, 1984), require randomly selected target words to be transcribed orthographically by naive judges. For the severely dysarthric population, these tasks may underestimate seriously the functional

This work was supported in part by Grant #H133B80081 from the National Institute of Disability and Rehabilitation Research, Department of Education, Washington, D.C. The authors wish to thank Kathleen Smith, Tracy Porter, Julie Ferre, Beth Fournier, Lynn Farrier, Inge Anema, and Melissa Honsinger and the staff of the Departments of Speech Pathology at the University of Washington Medical Center and Harborview Medical Center for their assistance.

level of speech performance, because scores on these types of tasks are frequently near zero. The communicative environments in which severely dysarthric individuals use speech consist of semantically predictable, conversational settings. Therefore, in an effort to mimic some of the features of these communicative environments, the Index of Contextual Intelligibility (ICI) task was developed.

This chapter poses the question: What is the effect of semantic context on speech intelligibility for dysarthric individuals? More specifically, does the effect vary as a function of the severity of dysarthria? Finally, does the effect vary as a function of the size of the semantic category used to provide the context?

INDEX OF CONTEXTUAL INTELLIGIBILITY: METHODS

Data Base Development

The first step in development of the Index of Contextual Intelligibility (ICI) data base was identification of 60 common semantic categories. These categories were given to 4 respondents who provided 15 words for each category. Respondents were staff members or research technicians in the Department of Rehabilitation Medicine at the University of Washington. The pool of words they generated was sorted and the frequency of occurrence was determined for each word within a category. A final set of 12 words for each of 60 categories was obtained by selecting items most frequently listed by the respondents. Words provided by 3 or 4 respondents were always included in the final word list. If additional words were needed to complete a set of 12, they were selected randomly from words provided by at least two respondents. When completed, the data base contained 720 words (60 categories × 12 words per category).

Examples of semantic categories and words appear in Table 1. The majority of the data base consisted of single words, and if a two-word item was used, it represented a single concept, such as Mother's Day.

Table 1. Examples of context phrases and words from the ICI

Context phrases	Words
Something men wear	Coat, shorts, socks, sweater, undershirt, vest, hat, jacket, pants, shirt, shoes, tie
Kind of ice cream	Banana, cherry, coffee, mint, mocha, neopolitan, pecan, raspberry, chocolate, peach, strawberry, vanilla
Holiday	Father's Day, Independence Day, New Year's Day, Christmas, Easter, Halloween, Labor Day, Memorial Day, Mother's Day, Thanksgiving, Valentine's Day, Veterans Day
Type of bird	Crow, parakeet, bluejay, cardinal, owl, sparrow, eagle, hawk, parrot, robin, seagull, heron
Color	Black, blue, brown, grey, green, orange, pink, purple, red, tan, white, yellow

Sample Generation

Figure 1 illustrates the process by which the samples for administering the Index of Contextual Intelligibility task were generated. The list of 60 categories and 12 words for each category was entered into a spreadsheet/data base program (Microsoft Corporation, 1988). A program was developed to select randomly 1 of the 12 items for each category and randomly order the 60 categories. Because the task was developed as a clinical tool, the same listener may judge multiple ICI tasks completed by different dysarthric speakers. Therefore, only 50 of the 60 possible categories were used for each sample in an attempt to minimize judge expecta-

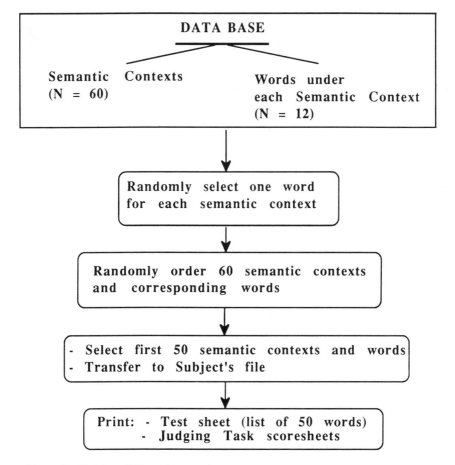

Figure 1. Flowchart of ICI sample generation process.

tion. The 50 semantic categories and the selected word for each category were transferred to a separate subject file for storage. Finally, the list of words for subjects to read and the score sheets used by the judges were provided by the program.

Subjects

Subjects were in- and outpatients served by the speech pathology services of the Departments of Rehabilitation Medicine at the University of Washington and Harborview Medical Centers, Seattle, WA. Many of these individuals were being evaluated in the Augmentative Communication Clinic. These speakers exhibited a level of dysarthria that severely reduced intelligibility and limited their functional communication. Table 2 presents demographic information for the 21 speakers who participated in this study, 10 females and 11 males, ranging in age from 20 to 73 years. The

Table 2. Demographic characteristics and word intelligibility scores for subjects

Subject	Age/gender	Diagnosis	Word intelligibility No context (%)	Speech scale
1	36/F	Cerebral palsy	0	1
2	46/F	Cerebral palsy	0	1
3	30/M	Cerebral palsy	1	3
4	20/M	Traumatic brain injury	1	2
5	24/M	Traumatic brain injury	2	2
6	40/F	Cerebral palsy	4	2
7	29/M	Cerebral palsy	3	2
8	73/F	Myasthenia gravis	3	1
9	42/F	Cerebral palsy	7	2
10	33/M	Cerebral palsy	9	3
11	46/F	Cerebral palsy	15	3
12	38/M	Cerebral palsy	15	2
13	22/F	Cerebral palsy	17	3
14	34/M	Cerebral palsy	25	2
15	23/F	Traumatic brain injury	25	3
16	55/M	Amyotrophic lateral sclerosis	35	3
17	38/M	Cerebral palsy	43	2
18	42/M	Amyotrophic lateral sclerosis	53	2
19	21/M	Cerebral palsy	60	3
20	62/F	Cerebral vascular accident	66	2
21	20/F	Traumatic brain injury	83	3

Speech function was scaled as 1 if speech was used only as a signal, as 2 if speech was functional at times, and as 3 if the subject depended entirely on natural speech.

majority had cerebral palsy as their primary medical diagnosis ($n = 13$). Remaining diagnoses were traumatic brain injury ($n = 4$), amyotrophic lateral sclerosis ($n = 2$), cerebral vascular accident ($n = 1$), and myasthenia gravis ($n = 1$). Speakers were rated on a simple scale of speech function that reflected their speech in natural settings. Three (14.3%) used speech only as a signal to call attention, 10 (47.6%) spoke functionally at times, and 8 (38.1%) depended entirely on natural speech to communicate.

Recording Conditions

Speech samples were recorded in a quiet room as the speakers read the list of 50 words generated by the Index of Contextual Intelligibility program. If a speaker was unable to read the words, the task was completed imitatively.

Judges and Judging Task

The three judges who participated in this project were familiar with dysarthric speech, but were unfamiliar with the speakers who were recorded for this study. The judges were either staff members in the Speech Pathology Department or graduate students from the Department of Speech and Hearing Sciences at the University of Washington. Two judging tasks were completed: 1) No Context and 2) Context. For the No Context task, judges were provided with a score sheet containing item numbers only. They were instructed to listen to each auditory stimulus item twice and then write a response, if possible. Because many of the auditory stimulus items were unintelligible, judges were allowed to guess only if the production suggested a word. This procedure was used to minimize random guessing. Following the No Context task, each judge completed the Context task. Judges read each context cue, which was one of the 50 categories selected for each speaker, then listened to the production twice prior to writing a response. When responding with context, judges were specifically instructed to guess not on the basis of the context phrase alone, but to guess only if speech plus context provided a response.

Experimental Controls

Several factors affecting the interpretation of results were examined: impact of guessing, multiple exposures to the Index of Contextual Intelligibility items, and inter-judge reliability.

To estimate the impact of guessing, five judges who had not scored an Index of Contextual Intelligibility were given lists of 50 context phrases that had been generated for five speakers in this study. These respondents were asked to supply responses based only on the context phrase. The mean accuracy for this Context Only guessing task was 5.6%. Therefore, if the score of the Context task exceeded that percentage, the judges were responding to a combination of the context cue and the individual's speech.

Ideally, the Index of Contextual Intelligibility should be scored by judges assigned to one speaker for the No Context task and to a different speaker for the Context task. In a clinical setting, it is more likely that one judge will review both tasks. This sequence, however, provided the judge with two exposures to the test item when scoring the Context task. To determine the effect of multiple exposures to the Context test items, two graduate students from the Department of Speech and Hearing Sciences who had not served as judges were recruited. They completed the Context task only for speakers in this study. A Pearson product-moment correlation between the original judging format and the Context-only format was calculated. The coefficient was 0.97, indicating that repeated exposures during the original judging format probably did not confound the results for the Context task. Furthermore, this suggests that the same judges can score both tasks without affecting scores. The lack of significant benefit from previous exposure is probably related to the severity of the dysarthria and the difficulty of the No Context task.

Inter-judge reliability was examined by computing Pearson product-moment correlations between all possible judge pairs. Results presented in Figure 2 show that coefficients ranged from 0.95 to 0.98 for the No Context task, and from 0.96 to 0.98 for the Context task.

INDEX OF CONTEXTUAL INTELLIGIBILITY: RESULTS

The first question of interest was: Does semantic context affect speech intelligibility? The scores from the three judges for each judging task, No Context and Context, were averaged for each speaker. Figure 3 illustrates these results with speakers ranked by intelligibility scores without context.

The effect of context was strong and consistent. For all speakers, providing semantic context increased single-word intelligibility scores. This trend was exhibited even by Subject 21 who had a No Context score that was substantially higher than the majority. For this speaker, word intelligibility increased from 83% to 99% when semantic context was provided.

The next questions was: Does the effect vary as a function of severity? To answer this, data were grouped by level of severity into profound dysarthria (No Context task scores of less than 35%), severe dysarthria (No Context task scores between 35% and 50%), and moderate dysarthria (No Context task scores greater than 50%). Mean intelligibility scores for the No Context and Context tasks are presented in Figure 4.

Inter-judge Reliability

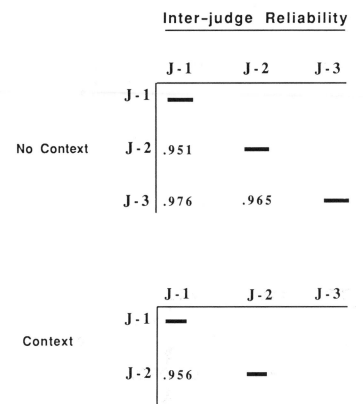

Figure 2. Pearson product-moment correlations between judge pairs for Context and No Context judging tasks.

All three severity groups showed improvement in speech intelligibility scores when semantic context was provided. The largest improvement was noted for the severe group, whose Context task scores increased by 40.2%. Scores from the moderate group increased by 29%, while the profound group showed an 18.5% increase in intelligibility with context. These trends were confirmed with a one-way repeated measures analysis of variance. The group by task interaction was found to be significant ($F = 4.753$, $p < 0.015$). Not surprisingly, the main effects for both group (profound, severe, and moderate) and task (Context and No Context) were also significant at the 0.01 level.

The final question was: Does the effect of semantic context vary also as a function of size of the semantic category? Category size was estab-

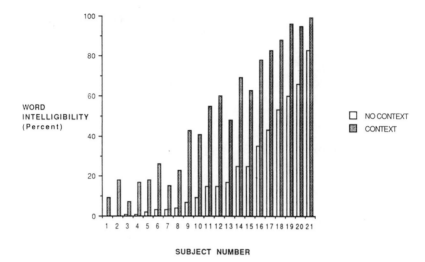

Figure 3. Single word intelligibility scores for No Context and Context tasks. Data represent the mean of three judges' scores. Subjects are rank ordered from least to most intelligible.

lished using a continuous scaling approach. Five individuals who did not participate in the generation of either the category or word lists served as raters. Figure 5 provides an example of the task used to generate category size estimates.

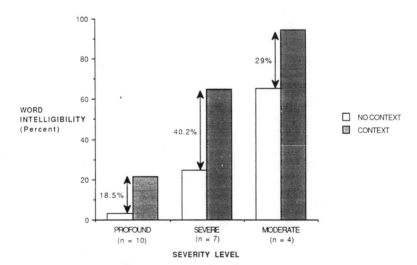

Figure 4. Single word intelligibility scores for the No Context and Context task when subjects were grouped according to dysarthria severity. (Severity was determined by the No Context score: profound = 0%–35%, severe = 35%–50%, moderate = >50%).

Type of sandwich:

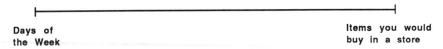

Days of
the Week

Items you would
buy in a store

Figure 5. Example of task used to determine category size.

The 60 categories were presented on a series of scoresheets with a 100 mm horizontal line drawn under each category. As illustrated, the ends of the scale were marked with a small category on the left and a large category on the right. Raters drew a line that bisected the scale at the point that represented their estimation of each category size relative to the end points. These distances are plotted in Figure 6, which ranks the 60 categories according to mean estimates of size.

As is evident, categories were distributed relatively evenly with respect to size. Because there was no bimodal distribution and therefore no

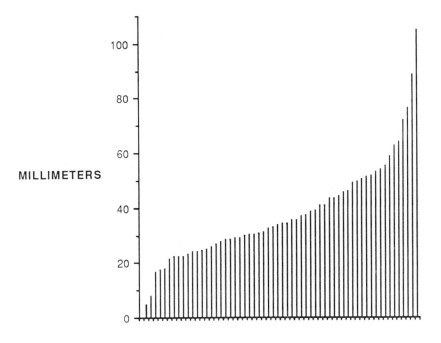

CATEGORY SIZE

Figure 6. Estimates of category size in millimeters, ordered from smallest to largest.

logical cutoff between large and small items, only the 20 smallest and 20 largest categories were used in subsequent analyses. The mean number of items analyzed for large and small categories were 16.7 and 16.9 items, respectively. Data from the original set were re-analyzed to determine intelligibility scores for the large and small category sizes. The results of this analysis are presented in Figure 7. The data were averaged across judges, and speakers were grouped into profound, severe, and moderate levels as in the earlier analysis. Also displayed in the figure, as a reference, is the mean No Context intelligibility score for each group. Note that semantic category size had the greatest effect for the profound group. The difference between the Context task scores for the large versus small category size was 12.2% for this group. The remaining groups also demonstrated a difference in word intelligibility scores based on category size, 9.9% and 2.1% for the severe and moderate groups, respectively. An analysis of variance indicated that size effect was not statistically significant. Since there were few speakers in some dysarthria categories, however, with additional speakers, this comparison might reach significance. There was no significant interaction between category size and dysarthria severity.

CONCLUSIONS

The results of this study indicate that the general effect of semantic context is consistent and powerful. In addition, the size of the effect varies

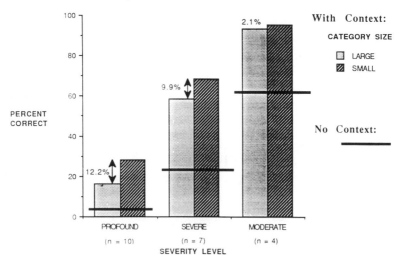

Figure 7. Percent correct for the two category sizes with data pooled by dysarthria severity. (Percentages imposed on the bars indicate difference in Context intelligibility between Large and Small category sizes, and the No Context scores are indicated by horizontal bars for comparison.)

with the severity of the dysarthria and, to a lesser extent, with the size of the semantic category. The implications of these data are quite important for persons with severe and profound dysarthria. Individuals in these groups usually come to our attention because they are being evaluated for an augmentative communication device. Clearly, their dysarthria is so severe that they are in need of these devices. Clinicians need to appreciate, however, the importance of using natural speech by severely or profoundly dysarthric individuals in some communicative situations. This project suggests that intelligibility measures derived from a task that provides semantic context may give a more accurate picture of the functional communication of these dysarthric individuals than other intelligibility tasks. In the following chapter, perceptual features that distinguish the best and worst productions of these severe and profoundly dysarthric speakers is examined with the long-term goal of improving behavioral intervention for these individuals.

REFERENCES

Berry, W., & Sanders, S. (1983). Environmental education: The universal management approach for adults with dysarthria. In W. Berry (Ed.), *Clinical dysarthria* (pp. 203–216). Boston: College-Hill Press.

Microsoft Corporation. (1988). *Excel* (version 1.5) [Computer program]. Seattle: Microsoft.

Yorkston, K.M., Beukelman, D.R., & Bell, K.R. (1988). *Clinical management of dysarthric speakers.* Boston: College-Hill Press.

Yorkston, K.M., Beukelman, D.R., & Traynor, C. (1984). *Computerized assessment of intelligibility of dysarthric speech.* Austin, TX: PRO-ED.

Dysarthria and Apraxia of Speech:
Perspectives on Management
edited by Christopher A. Moore, Ph.D., Kathryn M. Yorkston, Ph.D.,
and David R. Beukelman, Ph.D.
copyright © 1991   Paul H. Brookes Publishing Co., Inc.
Baltimore · London · Toronto · Sydney

Chapter 5

Index of Contextual
Intelligibility
A Perceptual Analysis of
Intelligible versus Unintelligible
Productions in Severe Dysarthria

Kathryn M. Yorkston,
Vicki L. Hammen, and Patricia Dowden

RESEARCH IN DYSARTHRIA has focused increasingly on factors associated with intelligibility. Kent, Weismer, and their colleagues (Kent, Kent, Weismer, & Martin, 1989; Kent et al., 1990; and Weismer, Kent, Hodge, & Martin, 1988) have explored acoustic correlates of speech intelligibility. Our group has identified some listener-related variables that may affect intelligibility. Results reported previously (Hammen, Yorkston, & Dowden, chap. 4, this volume) suggest that providing listeners with semantic context improves the intelligibility of dysarthric speakers. In this chapter, our attention turns to exploring perceptual characteristics of the productions of severely dysarthric speakers.

After listening to many samples of severely dysarthric speech, one is left with the subjective impression of consistency of productions by a given speaker. Although inter-speaker differences certainly exist, multiple productions of a single speaker tend to sound highly distorted and very similar. In some ways this consistency has led to speculation that these speakers can do little to modify their severely distorted productions. Vari-

This work was supported in part by Grant #H133B80081 from the National Institute of Disability and Rehabilitation Research, Department of Education, Washington, D.C. The authors wish to thank Kathleen Smith for her assistance.

ation in performance or ability to modify productions are factors that clinicians use to assess candidacy for behavioral intervention. This chapter attempts to identify perceptual correlates associated with the best and worst productions of severely dysarthric speakers. Specifically, the purpose is to examine the productions of severely dysarthric individuals to explore the extent and nature of perceptual variability. Our questions are: 1) What perceptual features distinguish intelligible from unintelligible productions?, and 2) Do severely dysarthric speakers use different patterns of perceptual features for most and least intelligible utterances?

METHODS OF PERCEPTUAL ANALYSIS

Subjects

Sixteen severely dysarthric adults were included in this project. A review of Table 1 indicates that the group consisted of 8 males and 8 females, ranging in age from 20 to 73 years. Although cerebral palsy was the most frequent diagnosis, other diagnoses included traumatic brain injury, my-

Table 1. Demographic characteristics and word intelligibility scores for subjects

Subject	Age/gender	Diagnosis	Word intelligibility (%)		Speech scale
			No context	Context	
1	36/F	Cerebral palsy	0	9	1
2	46/F	Cerebral palsy	0	18	1
3	30/M	Cerebral palsy	1	17	3
4	20/M	Traumatic brain injury	1	7	2
5	24/M	Traumatic brain injury	2	18	2
6	40/F	Cerebral palsy	4	23	2
7	29/M	Cerebral palsy	3	26	2
8	73/F	Myasthenia gravis	3	15	1
9	42/F	Cerebral palsy	7	43	2
10	33/M	Cerebral palsy	9	41	3
11	46/F	Cerebral palsy	15	60	3
12	38/M	Cerebral palsy	15	55	2
13	22/F	Cerebral palsy	17	48	3
14	34/M	Cerebral palsy	25	63	2
15	23/F	Traumatic brain injury	25	69	3
16	55/M	Amyotrophic lateral sclerosis	35	78	3

Speech function was scaled as 1 if speech was used only as a signal, as 2 if speech was functional at times, and as 3 if the subject depended entirely on natural speech.

asthenia gravis, and amyotrophic lateral sclerosis. Individuals were selected on the basis of dysarthria severity, and these were the least intelligible of the speakers described earlier (Hammen, Yorkston, & Dowden,
chap. 4, this volume). Word intelligibility scores with and without semantic context are presented to determine severity of dysarthria. Intelligibility
without context ranged from 0% to 35%, and intelligibility with semantic
context ranged from 10% to 78%. Also included in Table 1 is a rating of
speech function. All speakers could voluntarily initiate phonation. Three,
however, reported that they used speech only as a signal, that is, the only
function of their natural speech was to gain attention. Seven reported that
their speech was occasionally understandable, but that they depended on
augmentative communication systems at other times. Six reported that
they depended entirely on natural speech.

Speech Sample

Samples were drawn from those described in the previous study (Hammen, Yorkston, & Dowden, chap. 4, this volume). To review, samples were
recorded as speakers produced a series of 50 words. These samples were
scored by three judges who were naive to the target word. For each 50-
word sample, the 10 most intelligible and 10 least intelligible words were
identified. Data related to the intelligibility of the total sample, and to the
most and least intelligible words, are presented in Table 2. These data are
derived from conclusions reported previously (Hammen, Yorkston, &
Dowden, chap. 4, this volume). This information confirms that most and
least intelligible words differ markedly in intelligibility when measured
both with and without semantic context. Without context, the least intelligible words were not understood by any of our judges, while the most intelligible words were understood an average of 23%. When intelligibility
was measured with semantic context, the least intelligible words were
5.2% intelligible, while the most intelligible words were 80.6% intelligible. Data presented in a companion chapter suggest that when judges
were asked to guess, based on semantic context alone without hearing a
spoken sample, scores averaged 5.6%.

Table 2. Word intelligibility scores with and without semantic context for overall sample, most intelligible, and least intelligible words

Mean scores	Overall (%) (50 words)	Most intelligible (%) (10 words)	Least intelligible (%) (10 words)
Intelligibility (No Context)	10.0 (SD 10.8)	23.1 (SD 20.6)	0 (SD 0)
Intelligibility (With Context)	37.5 (SD 22.5)	80.6 (SD 19.7)	5.2 (SD 10.2)

Word Characteristics

An explanation for marked differences in word intelligibility might be ease of word production. One could speculate that the most intelligible word list contained a large proportion of "easy" words, and the least intelligible word list contained "difficult" words. In order to explore relative production ease of the target words, consonant difficulty and word length were examined. Consonant difficulty was based on data for dysarthric speakers from the work of Johns and Darley (1970), in which consonants were rank ordered by difficulty. The Johns and Darley list was divided into more and less difficult words. The consonant difficulty score for a particular word was a count of all the *more difficult* consonants. Word length in syllables was simply a count of the number of syllables in each target word.

The data from the most and least intelligible words were subjected to univariate F tests. Results of this analysis indicate that neither consonant difficulty or word length differentiate the least intelligible from the most intelligible words. Because these features relating to production ease were nonsignificant, word characteristics apparently did not contribute to intelligibility scores. That is, it can be argued that the most intelligible words were better productions than the least intelligible words, but not simply because they were easier words.

Adequacy of Word Production

Three perceptual measures of production adequacy were selected, based on review of the samples and on known characteristics of severely dysarthric speech. The perceptual measures were accuracy of syllable signaling, consonant approximation, and vowel approximation. These were gross measures, but more traditional measures, such as accuracy of phoneme production, could not be used because scores would have been near zero for many of our speakers. Procedures used for each perceptual judging task are outlined below.

Success of syllable signaling: The judge listened to each production without knowledge of the target word, and indicated the number of syllables. Scores for syllable signaling reflect the percentage of syllables produced that the judge correctly identified.

Vowel approximation: After samples were judged for adequacy of syllable signaling, the judge listened to all productions again, with knowledge of the target word. Each word was rated from 0% to 100%. This indicates the percentage of vowels that grossly approximated the target phonemes.

Consonant approximation: Consonant approximation judgments were made by the same method as vowel approximation judgments.

All perceptual judging was performed without knowledge of word placement in the most intelligible or least intelligible word lists. All judging was done by the first author. Half the sample were scored a second time with an interval of at least 2 months before the first and second scoring. Pearson product-moment correlations between the mean of the first and second judgments were 0.91, 0.97, and 0.93 for accuracy of syllable signaling, vowel approximation, and consonant approximation, respectively.

RESULTS OF PERCEPTUAL ANALYSIS

Two-Tier Analysis

Results of perceptual analysis of the characteristics of speech production are presented on two levels. The first is a group analysis in which the three perceptual measures (syllable signaling, consonant, and vowel approximation) were entered in discriminant analysis to identify those perceptual features that distinguish most intelligible words from least intelligible. The second level is individual, in which perceptual differences between most and least intelligible words are plotted by subject, and inter-subject differences examined.

Discriminant Analysis Two perceptual features, vowel approximation and consonant approximation, were found to discriminate between most and least intelligible words. Analysis of variance results indicated an F of 21.6 ($p < 0.001$) for vowel approximation, and an F of 15.3 ($p < 0.001$) for consonant approximation. There were no significant differences between most and least intelligible words for syllable signaling. When results from the discriminant analysis were used to generate a prediction table, 27 of 32 word lists (84%) would have been correctly placed, based on the two perceptual features measured in this study. In Figure 1, most and least intelligible word lists tend to fall into different areas of the graph, although there is some overlap.

The results of the group analysis are summarized in Figure 2. Although most intelligible word lists were judged more adequate on all perceptual features than least intelligible word lists, statistical analyses presented earlier indicate that the features of vowel and consonant approximation only were significantly different.

Individual Analysis An analysis was undertaken to determine how many individuals followed the overall trend identified in the group analysis. A review of all data suggested three distinct patterns of change in perceptual features from the least to the most intelligible word lists. Figure 3 illustrates the pattern typical for 3 of 16 speakers in which differences

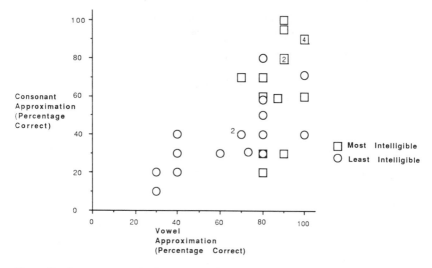

Figure 1. Consonant approximation versus vowel approximation scores for most and least intelligible words produced by 16 severely dysarthric speakers. (Numbers indicate multiple occurrences of a data point.)

are most pronounced for vowel approximation. Note that for Subject 4 there was a 50% change in vowel approximation from least to most intelligible words. The second pattern of performance was characterized by

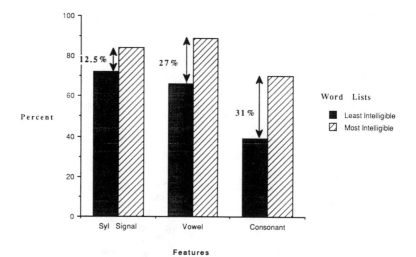

Figure 2. Mean percentages correct for syllable signaling, vowel approximation, and consonant approximation for the least and most intelligible words produced by 16 severely dysarthric speakers. (Differences are noted for each feature.)

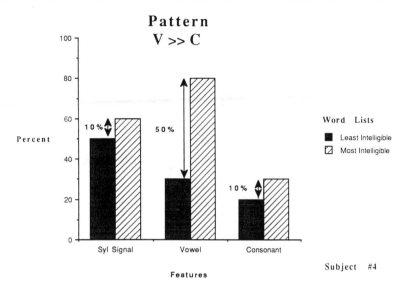

Figure 3. Percentage correct for syllable signaling, vowel approximation, and consonant approximation for least and most intelligible words produced by subject 4. (Data illustrate a pattern with the most change in vowel approximation.)

nearly equivalent differences in vowel and consonant approximation. This pattern was seen in 8 of 16 speakers (50%), and Figure 4 illustrates this pattern. The final pattern was one in which consonant approximation showed considerably more improvement than vowel approximation. This pattern was seen in 5 of 16 speakers (31%) and is illustrated in Figure 5.

To summarize the individual data, 3 speakers showed greater differences in vowel than consonant approximation (V>>C), eight showed nearly equivalent vowel and consonant approximation differences (V = C), and 5 showed greater performance differences in consonants than vowels (C>>V). This pattern of change may be related to overall severity of the dysarthria. When mean intelligibility scores with context were computed across speakers in the three groups, V >> C, V = C, and C >> V, an interesting severity-dependent relationship emerged. The mean intelligibility score for the V >> C group was 11.5%; for the V = C group, 35%, and for the C >> V group, 55.1%. Thus, the 3 individuals with differences greater in vowel than consonant approximation were the most severely dysarthric as measured by single-word intelligibility. The 8 speakers with nearly equivalent performance differences were in the mid-range of severity. The 5 individuals for whom consonant approximation showed greater differences than vowel approximation received the highest word intelligibility scores. One could speculate that the most severely dysarthric speakers do not have the ability to modify consonant produc-

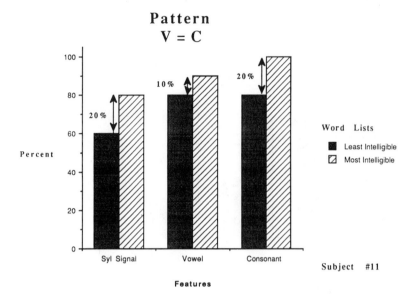

Figure 4. Percentage correct for syllable signaling, vowel approximation, and consonant approximation for the least and most intelligible words produced by subject 11. (Data illustrate a pattern with change nearly equivalent across all perceptual features.)

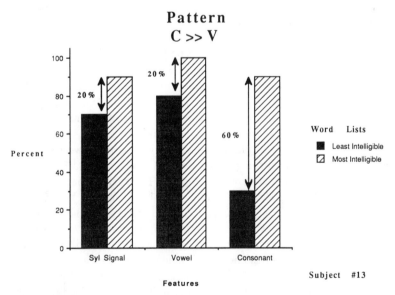

Figure 5. Percentage correct for syllable signaling, vowel approximation, and consonant approximation for least and most intelligible words produced by subject 13. (Data illustrate a pattern with most change in consonant approximation.)

tion in a significant way. Nevertheless, these severely dysarthric speakers may be able to change the quality of their vowel productions.

Despite nonsignificant results for the measure of syllable signaling, 8 of 16 speakers improved by 20% or more on this measure when the least intelligible were compared with the most intelligible words — in one case the difference was 40%. The lack of statistical significance is due in part to the nearly perfect scores of many speakers on this measure. The ability to signal syllables correctly may be an important contributor to intelligibility for some severely dysarthric speakers.

CONCLUSIONS

Findings reported in this chapter have clinical implications for the management of severe dysarthria. First, the most and least intelligible words produced by severely dysarthric individuals differ when adequacy is measured by ratings of gross perceptual features such as vowel or consonant approximation. Clinically, this is encouraging since most clinicians believe that the goal of behavioral intervention is to bring all performance to the level of pre-treatment "best" performance. A large gap between best and worst performance may signal potential for behavioral treatment.

A second noteworthy finding is that all severely dysarthric speakers do not necessarily exhibit similar changes when most intelligible and least intelligible word productions are compared. This finding may also have considerable clinical implication. Clinicians need to understand what contributes to lack of intelligibility in their clients, but perhaps more urgently, clinicians need to identify the factors that speakers are capable of modifying. These features should be initial targets of behavioral intervention for the severely dysarthric speaker.

Finally, in the beginning of this chapter we suggested that an impression of consistency is produced by listening to a long sequence of words spoken by severely dysarthric individuals. This perception of consistency exists despite measurable differences identified in the data presented. Thus, changes that distinguish best from worst productions are subtle ones and even the best productions are not normal. Changes are not dramatic, yet they may be very important functionally and should not be ignored in the clinical setting. Behavioral intervention with severe dysarthria has not received much research or clinical attention. This lack of attention may reflect a mistaken belief that these speakers can do nothing that will "make that much difference." These preliminary data suggest that this assumption may be incorrect when referring to the client's use of speech in natural communicative situations. In other words, differences need not be dramatic perceptually to be important functionally for the severely dysarthric speaker. The task of intervention in severe dysarthria does not involve finding a single factor that will make a large difference, but rather finding many small factors that will cumulatively make a large difference.

REFERENCES

Johns, D.F., & Darley, F.L. (1970). Phonemic variability in apraxia of speech. *Journal of Speech and Hearing Research, 13*, 556.

Kent, R.D., Kent, J.F., Weismer, G., & Martin, R.E. (1989). Relationship between speech intelligibility and the slope of second-formant transitions in dysarthric subjects. *Clinical Linguistics and Phonetics, 3*(4), 347–358.

Kent, R.D., Kent, J.F., Weismer, G., Sufit, R.L., Rosenbek, J.C., Martin, R.E., & Brooks, B.R. (1990). Impairment of speech intelligibility in amyotrophic lateral sclerosis. *Journal of Speech and Hearing Disorders, 55,* 721–728.

Weismer, G., Kent, R.D., Hodge, M., & Martin, R. (1988). The acoustic signature for intelligibility test words. *Journal of the Acoustic Society of America, 84*(4), 1281–1291.

Dysarthria and Apraxia of Speech:
Perspectives on Management
edited by Christopher A. Moore, Ph.D., Kathryn M. Yorkston, Ph.D.,
and David R. Beukelman, Ph.D.
copyright © 1991   Paul H. Brookes Publishing Co., Inc.
Baltimore · London · Toronto · Sydney

Chapter 6

Inexperienced Listener Ratings of Dysarthric Speaker Intelligibility and Physical Appearance

Julie Barkmeier, Linda S. Jordan,
Donald A. Robin, and Robert L. Schum

INTELLIGIBILITY REFERS TO how well a listener can understand the speech productions of a speaker. Research has demonstrated that measures of intelligibility may be influenced by factors inherent in the speaker (Massaro, 1987; Neely, 1956; O'Neill, 1954; Popelka & Berger, 1971); the message (Duffy & Giolas, 1974; Kalikow & Stevens, 1977; Leventhal, 1973; Miller, Heise, & Lichten, 1951; Tikofsky, 1970; Tikofsky & Tikofsky, 1964); the environment (Kalikow & Stevens, 1977); the method of measuring intelligibility (Beukelman & Yorkston, 1979; Yorkston & Beukelman, 1978; Yorkston & Beukelman, 1980); and the listener (Beukelman & Yorkston, 1980). A variety of methods are used for measuring intelligibility, and a variety of definitions of intelligibility have been used in research. This lack of consistency makes comparison across methods and studies difficult.

Dysarthric speakers commonly experience a loss of intelligibility resulting from impaired neuromuscular function. Measurements of intelligibility are used with dysarthric speakers to: 1) indicate speaking proficiency, 2) determine how the speaker compensates for structural or physical impairments that affect speech, 3) determine how effectively the speaker communicates in everyday situations, and 4) monitor the speaker through treatment or the course of a disease.

65

The Assessment of the Intelligibility of Dysarthric Speech was developed by Yorkston and Beukelman (1984) from investigations of factors influencing intelligibility. This instrument quantitatively measures intelligibility using audio stimuli but does not address the influence of visual cues. Studies of nondysarthric speakers with impaired intelligibility (e.g., speakers with laryngectomies and hearing impairments) suggest that visual cues improve intelligibility (Berry & Knight, 1975; Hubbard & Kuschner, 1980; Mencke, Ochsner, & Testut, 1983; Monsen, 1983; Neely, 1956; O'Neill, 1954; Popelka & Berger, 1971; Siegenthaler & Gruber, 1969; Sumby & Pollack, 1954).

The physical appearance of individuals also has been demonstrated to influence intelligibility scores (Clifford, 1975; Clifford & Walster, 1973; Guise, Pollans, & Turkat, 1982; Jones, Hannson, & Phillips, 1978; Landy & Sigall, 1974; Miller, 1970; Scherer, Scherer, Hall, & Rosenthal, 1977). Individuals with dysarthria may exhibit masked facies (e.g., parkinsonian patients), tremor, and involuntary movement of the oral structures (e.g., tardive dyskinesia), among other alterations in physical appearance and speaking behavior that can influence judgments of intelligibility.

Speech-language pathologists probably are accustomed to these alterations in appearance and have learned to attend to what the dysarthric speaker says rather than how the speaker appears. Listeners who are not experienced with dysarthric speakers, however, may become distracted by such visual cues, which results in reduced intelligibility. Therefore, presence or absence of visual cues and the physical appearance of speech behaviors of the dysarthric speaker may be important variables for intelligibility measurements.

As part of a larger study (Barkmeier, 1988), dysarthric speakers were videotaped while reading sentences randomly taken from the Assessment of Intelligibility of Dysarthric Speech (Yorkston & Beukelman, 1984). These recordings were presented individually to 10 experienced and to 10 inexperienced listeners on two separate occasions. Experienced listeners had clinical experience with dysarthric speakers ranging from 6 months to 14 years. Inexperienced listeners had no or limited exposure to dysarthric speakers. Speech recordings were presented at listening sessions in either audio or audiovisual form. The mode of presentation was balanced across listeners and sessions. Rating scale and transcription measures of intelligibility were obtained for each listening session. Visual cues were demonstrated to improve intelligibility transcription scores obtained from both experienced and inexperienced listeners. When listeners became familiar with speaking behaviors of the dysarthric speakers, however (i.e., during the second session), the addition of the visual cues did not facilitate intelligibility. Repeated presentations of speakers using a different random order resulted in improved intelligibility, regardless of presentation mode. Correlational analysis between rating scale and transcription measures of intelligibility indicate a relationship between those measures obtained using the two methods for experienced listeners ($r = -0.47$, $p < 0.05$). By contrast, no relationship was found between rating scale and transcription measures for inexperienced listeners ($r = -0.10$, $p < 0.69$).

Inexperienced listeners scored dysarthric speakers as less intelligible than experienced listeners (Barkmeier, Jordan, Robin, & Schum, 1990). This finding may be related to altered physical characteristics that distract inexperienced listeners and thus further reduce speech intelligibility. This investigation was undertaken to determine the relationship between the ratings of intelligibility that inexperienced listeners assigned and their judgments of physical appearance and personality attributes of dysarthric speakers. It was hypothesized that inexperienced listeners would focus on the physical appearance of dysarthric speakers. Thus, if physical appearance does influence intelligibility, inexperienced listeners should demonstrate the relationship more clearly than experienced listeners.

METHODS

The videotapes of 12 dysarthric speakers (Barkmeier et al., in press) were presented to listeners. The speakers were selected by the first author to represent a range of speech intelligibility. However, speakers were not selected to represent a range of physical attractiveness. One speaker exhibited severe facial rigidity, but no other speaker exhibited facial droop, involuntary articulatory movements, or other physical attributes or behaviors regarded as unattractive. For a description of the dysarthric speakers see Table 1. Stimuli were selected from a recording of dysarthric speakers reading 10 sentences chosen randomly (Yorkston & Beukelman, 1984). Two sentences were chosen from each of 6, 8, 10, 12, and 14 word–length pools. Five sentences from each speaker were randomly selected as stimuli.

Twenty inexperienced listeners, randomly selected from a pool of thirty, were presented with a videotape containing one set of five-sentence recordings from each speaker. A different videotape was used for each mode of presentation as a control for possible ordering effects. Listeners completed a Questionnaire for Attractiveness, consisting of: 1) rating of intelligibility on a 7-point interval scale, 2) six items highly correlated with physical appearance (Gough, 1960), and 3) 13 items from an adjective preference scale (Jackson & Minton, 1963). See Figure 1 for the Jackson and Minton (1963) questionnaire items, and Figure 2 for the Questionnaire for Attractiveness. The Jackson and Minton questionnaire is a standardized tool for obtaining measures of personality adjective ratings. The six items related to physical attractiveness were embedded within the

Table 1. Description of dysarthric speakers

Subject number and gender	Age	Etiology	Age at onset
1. F	65	Cerebral palsy	birth
2. M	63	Parkinson's disease	62
3. M	45	Cerebellar degeneration	41
4. F	25	Spinocerebellar degeneration, episodic brainstem dysfunction	6
5. F	62	Intracranial hematoma with subsequent frontoparietal craniotomy	62
6. M	75	Parkinson's disease	71
7. M	64	Parkinson's disease	38
8. M	46	Hodgkin's disease, cerebellar syndrome, brainstem CVA	42
9. M	63	Parkinson's disease	49
10. F	65	Parkinson's disease	55
11. F	60	Amyotrophic lateral sclerosis (ALS)	59
12. M	67	Parkinson's disease	63

1. Indifferent	1	2	3	4	5	6	7	Curious
2. Simple	1	2	3	4	5	6	7	Complex
3. Insensitive	1	2	3	4	5	6	7	Perceptive
4. Careless	1	2	3	4	5	6	7	Careful
5. Practical	1	2	3	4	5	6	7	Academic
6. Calm	1	2	3	4	5	6	7	Restless
7. Unsure	1	2	3	4	5	6	7	Confident
8. Submissive	1	2	3	4	5	6	7	Assertive
9. Happy	1	2	3	4	5	6	7	Sad
10. Passive	1	2	3	4	5	6	7	Active
11. Competitive	1	2	3	4	5	6	7	Cooperative
12. Aloof	1	2	3	4	5	6	7	Amiable
13. Candid	1	2	3	4	5	6	7	Guarded
14. Serious	1	2	3	4	5	6	7	Humorous
15. Self-controlled	1	2	3	4	5	6	7	Pleasure-seeking
16. Reserved	1	2	3	4	5	6	7	Outspoken
17. Rigid	1	2	3	4	5	6	7	Flexible

Figure 1. Attributes from Jackson and Minton. (From Jackson, D.N., & Minton, H.L. [1963]. A forced-choice adjective preference scale for personality assessment. *Psychological Reports, 12*, 515–520; reprinted by permission.)

1. Healthy	1	2	3	4	5	6	7	Sickly
2. Insensitive	1	2	3	4	5	6	7	Perceptive
3. Good-looking	1	2	3	4	5	6	7	Ugly
4. Restless	1	2	3	4	5	6	7	Calm
5. Confident	1	2	3	4	5	6	7	Unsure
6. Submissive	1	2	3	4	5	6	7	Assertive
7. Happy	1	2	3	4	5	6	7	Sad
8. Passive	1	2	3	4	5	6	7	Active
9. Attractive	1	2	3	4	5	6	7	Unattractive
10. Competitive	1	2	3	4	5	6	7	Cooperative
11. Desirable	1	2	3	4	5	6	7	Undesirable
12. Guarded	1	2	3	4	5	6	7	Candid
13. Humorous	1	2	3	4	5	6	7	Serious
14. Dirty	1	2	3	4	5	6	7	Clean
15. Intelligible	1	2	3	4	5	6	7	Unintelligible
16. Reserved	1	2	3	4	5	6	7	Outspoken
17. Flexible	1	2	3	4	5	6	7	Rigid
18. Aloof	1	2	3	4	5	6	7	Amiable
19. Pleasant	1	2	3	4	5	6	7	Unpleasant
20. Pleasure-seeking	1	2	3	4	5	6	7	Self-controlled

Figure 2. Questionnaire for Attractiveness. (For each pair of items, circle the number on the scale that best represents the speaker just presented.)

questionnaire to reduce suggestion of physical attractiveness as a focus of the study, with resulting bias.

Scores were obtained and tested for the 20 questionnaire items for the 12 speakers in each mode of presentation. These scores were tested for differences in ratings across all 20 questionnaire items under the three different modes of presentation. In addition, a one-way analysis of variance tested for effects of presentation form (e.g., audio, A; or audiovisual, V) and order of presentation (e.g., AV). Finally, the relationship between each of the 6 physical and 13 personality attributes and *intelligible/unintelligible* for all listeners was obtained using the Pearson product-moment correlation coefficient analysis.

RESULTS

A comparison of ratings by inexperienced listeners from the two modes of presentation was significantly different on four of six physical attributes and intelligibility. These items indicated that ratings from audiovisual presentations were more favorable than ratings from audio presentations (see Table 2). The mode of presentation was also significant on the ANOVA test on three physical attributes and one personality attribute, but

Table 2. Significant T-test values

T-test significant items	T values
Healthy/sickly	$t(38) = 4.23$
Good-looking/ugly	$t(38) = 2.54$
Dirty/clean	$t(38) = -4.07$
Pleasant/unpleasant	$t(28) = 2.92$
Intelligible/unintelligible	$t(38) = 2.33$

$p < .01.$

order of presentation was not significant. See Table 3 for significant ANOVA attributes.

The Studentized Neuman-Keul post hoc test was performed on each of the significant ANOVA items. Contrasted means were not significant at the $p < .05$ level. There was, however, a trend toward more favorable mean scores with audiovisual presentations.

Pearson product-moment correlation coefficient analysis indicated that 11 of the 19 bipolar items and five physical attributes were significantly related to intelligibility (see Table 4). The trend toward more positive traits to be correlated with intelligibility ratings, and for more negative or unattractive traits to be related to unintelligibility, can be seen in Table 5. For example, individuals rated as more intelligible were associated with the attributes of good-looking, attractive, desirable, clean, and healthy. By contrast, speakers rated as more unintelligible were more likely to be rated as appearing sickly, ugly, unattractive, undesirable, and dirty.

The remaining attributes from Jackson and Minton's (1963) adjective preference scale are shown in Table 6. Again, more positive personality traits were generally associated with ratings of intelligibility, while more negative traits were related to unintelligibility. For example, intelligibility was associated with happy, candid, flexible, confident, humorous, and amiable. By contrast, unintelligibility was associated with negative traits such as sad, guarded, rigid, unsure, serious, and aloof.

Table 3. Significant ANOVA attributes

Significant attributes	F ratio (F 3.36, p < .05)
Healthy/sickly	5.90
Dirty/clean	8.90
Pleasant/unpleasant	3.47
Flexible/rigid[a]	3.04

[a]Personality trait.

Table 4. Intelligibility and attribute correlations

Attribute	Correlation with intelligibility
1. Healthy/sickly	0.43 ($p < .01$)
2. Good-looking/ugly	0.40 ($p < .01$)
3. Happy/sad	0.45 ($p < .01$)
4. Attractive/unattractive	0.40 ($p < .01$)
5. Desirable/undesirable	0.39 ($p < .01$)
6. Guarded/candid	−0.45 ($p < .01$)
7. Flexible/rigid	0.44 ($p < .01$)
8. Confident/unsure	0.37 ($p < .05$)
9. Humorous/serious	0.34 ($p < .05$)
10. Dirty/clean	−0.34 ($p < .05$)
11. Aloof/amiable	−0.34 ($p < .05$)
12. Insensitive/perceptive	−0.28 (N.S.)
13. Restless/calm	−0.18 (N.S.)
14. Submissive/assertive	−0.04 (N.S.)
15. Passive/active	−0.23 (N.S.)
16. Competitive/cooperative	−0.16 (N.S.)
17. Reserved/outspoken	−0.21 (N.S.)
18. Pleasant/unpleasant	0.28 (N.S.)
19. Pleasure-seeking/self-controlled	−0.11 (N.S.)

N.S. = not significant.

CONCLUSIONS

Findings from the *attractiveness* rating appear to support the hypothesis that inexperienced listeners are influenced by the addition of a visual component in rating intelligibility. Regardless of mode presentation order, addition of the visual component resulted in more positive impressions for four of six physical attributes than occurred with audio presentation only.

Ratings of intelligibility and perceived physical attributes were so linked that speakers rated as more intelligible were also rated more

Table 5. Questionnaire for Attractiveness physical attributes

Significant	Nonsignificant
Healthy/sickly[a]	Pleasant/unpleasant
Good-looking/ugly[a]	
Attractive/unattractive[a]	
Desirable/undesirable[a]	
Clean/dirty[b]	

[a]$p < .01$.
[b]$P < .05$.

Table 6. Jackson and Minton (1963) attributes related to intelligibility

Significant	Nonsignificant
Happy/sad[a]	Perceptive/insensitive
Candid/guarded[a]	Assertive/submissive
Flexible/rigid[a]	Active/passive
Confident/unsure[b]	Cooperative/competitive
Humorous/serious[b]	Outspoken/reserved
Amiable/aloof[b]	Self-sufficient/pleasure-seeking

[a]$p < .01$.
[b]$p < .05$.

positively on physical and personality attributes, while speakers rated as less intelligible were rated higher negatively on physical and personality attributes. Since the audio presentation was linked to higher negative ratings than the audiovisual form, the auditory component of the dysarthric speaker may be more important in forming negative impressions.

It is possible that visual information reflected the "normality" of the appearance of the speakers. Dysarthric speakers exhibiting facial droop, involuntary articulator movements, or other physical appearances or behaviors judged as unattractive, may receive more negative ratings when an audiovisual presentation is used. Further investigations of this should be conducted with a wider range of physical appearance characteristics.

Another subject of interest is the effect, if any, of familiarity with dysarthria on ratings by speech-language pathologists, or experienced listeners, using the same task. This study could be repeated to clarify if experienced listener ratings demonstrate improved impressions of dysarthric speakers when a visual component is added to an audio presentation. Another area of inquiry is if intelligibility ratings by experienced listeners demonstrate a correlation with physical and/or personality attributes similar to that found with inexperienced listeners.

The significant correlations between intelligibility ratings and physical attractiveness and personality attributes were consistent with the hypothesis that inexperienced listeners were more likely to assign negative attributes to these speakers when presented with audio information alone. It is not clear why these personality attributes are related to ratings of intelligibility, but the more positive traits tended to be related to the more intelligible speakers, and the more negative traits were generally assigned to the less intelligible speakers. In addition to findings based on visual cues, informal comments by listeners were consistent with previous attractiveness research findings regarding the formation of impressions (Dailey, 1952; Landy & Sigall, 1974; Miller, 1970). Listeners presented with the audio mode for the first presentation indicated that they formed judgments of each speaker based upon voice characteristics. Raters consistently reported surprise that dysarthric speakers did not always appear "elderly" and "physically ill," or "ill in appearance." This suggests that rating intelligibility utilizing only the audio form is influenced by factors other than speaker intelligibility. A more comprehensive list of visual and audio features related to voice and appearance characteristics may provide more insight into important perceptual factors. Some characteristics mentioned by both experienced and inexperienced listeners, but not addressed by the Questionnaire for Attractiveness, include severity of dysarthria, vocal tremor, voice intensity, limb tremor, and other physical characteristics that might distract the listener from the speech stimulus.

More research is necessary to clarify the relation between positive personality attributes of speakers judged as intelligible and negative personality attributes of speakers judged as unintelligible when visual cues were both present and not present. In addition, the extent to which these attributes influence communication efficacy of dysarthric speakers is of interest.

In general, intelligibility assessments of dysarthric speakers by speech-language pathologists may not be representative of everyday communication situations that dysarthric speakers encounter with the general public. Though not clearly indicated in this study, it is possible that inexperienced listeners attend to "unattractive" visual qualities that detract from their comprehension of a person's dysarthric speech. As this study indicates, inexperienced listeners may have difficulty attending to *what* a dysarthric speaker is saying rather than *how* he or she is speaking. This component of communication interaction may contribute to the difficulty that dysarthric speakers have in being understood.

REFERENCES

Barkmeier, J., (1988). *Intelligibility of dysarthric speakers: Audio-only and audio-visual presentations.* University of Iowa.

Barkmeier, J., Jordan, L., Robin, D., & Schum, R. (in press). Intelligibility of dysarthric speakers using audio- versus audio-visual presentations. *Journal of Speech and Hearing Research.*

Berry, R.A., & Knight, R.E. (1975). Auditory versus audio-visual intelligibility measurements of alaryngeal speech: A preliminary report. *Perceptual and Motor Skills, 40,* 915–918.

Beukelman, D.R., & Yorkston, K.M. (1979). The relationship between information transfer and speech intelligibility of dysarthric speakers. *Journal of Communication Disorders, 12,* 189–196.

Beukelman, D.R., & Yorkston, K.M. (1980). Influence of passage familiarity on intelligibility estimates of dysarthric speech. *Journal of Communication Disorders, 13,* 33–41.

Clifford, M.M. (1975). Physical attractiveness and academic performance. *Child Study Journal, 5,* 201–209.

Clifford, M.M., & Walster, E. (1973). The effect of physical attractiveness on teacher expectations. *Sociology of Education, 46,* 248–258.

Dailey, C.A. (1952). The effects of premature conclusion upon the acquisition of understanding of a person. *Journal of Psychology, 33,* 133–152.

Duffy, J.R., & Giolas, T.G. (1974). Sentence intelligibility as a function of key word selection. *Journal of Speech and Hearing Research, 17,* 631–637.

Gough, H.G. (1960). The adjective check list as a personality assessment research technique. *Psychological Reports, 6,* 107–122.

Guise, B.J., Pollans, C.H., & Turkat, I.D. (1982). Effects of physical attractiveness on perception of social skills. *Perceptual & Motor Skills, 54,* 1039–1042.

Hubbard, D.J., & Kuschner, D. (1980). A comparison of speech intelligibility between esophageal and normal speakers via three modes of presentation. *Journal of Speech and Hearing Research, 23,* 909–916.

Jackson, D.N., & Minton, H.L. (1963). A forced-choice adjective preference scale for personality assessment. *Psychological Reports, 12,* 515–520.

Jones, W.H., Hannson, R.C., & Phillips, A.L. (1978). Physical attractiveness and judgments of psychopathology. *Journal of Social Psychology, 105,* 79–84.

Kalikow, D.N., & Stevens, K.N. (1977). Development of a test of speech intelligibility in noise using sentence materials with controlled word predictability. *Journal of the Acoustical Society of America, 61,* 1337–1351.

Keppel, G. (1973). *Design and analysis: A researcher's handbook.* Englewood Cliffs, NJ: Prentice Hall.

Landy, D., & Sigall, H. (1974). Beauty is talent: Task evaluation as a function of the performer's physical attractiveness. *Journal of Personality and Social Psychology, 29,* 299–304.

Leventhal, G. (1973). Effect of sentence context on word perception. *Journal of Experimental Psychology, 101,* 318–323.

Massaro, D.W. (1987). *Research perception by ear and eye: A paradigm for psychological inquiry.* Hillsdale, NJ: Lawrence Erlbaum Associates.

Mencke, E.O., Ochsner, G.J., & Testut, E.W. (1983). Listener judges and the speech intelligibility of deaf children. *Journal of Communication Disorders, 16,* 175–180.

Miller, A.G. (1970). Role of physical attractiveness in impression formation. *Journal of Psychometric Science, 19,* 241–243.

Miller, G.A., Heise, G.A., & Lichten, W. (1951). The intelligibility of speech as a function of the context of the test materials. *Journal of Experimental Psychology, 41,* 329–335.

Monsen, R.B. (1983). The oral speech intelligibility of hearing-impaired talkers. *Journal of Speech and Hearing Disorders, 48,* 286–296.

Neely, K.K. (1956). Effect of visual factors on the intelligibility of speech. *Journal of the Acoustical Society of America, 28,* 1275–1277.

O'Neill, J.J. (1954). Contributions of the visual components of oral symbols to speech comprehension. *Journal of Speech and Hearing Disorders, 19,* 429–439.

Popelka, G.R., & Berger, K.W. (1971). Gestures and visual speech reception. *American Annals of the Deaf, 116,* 434–436.

Scherer, K.R., Scherer, U., Hall, J.A., & Rosenthal, R. (1977). Differential attribution of personality based on multi-channel presentation of verbal and nonverbal cues. *Psychological Research, 39,* 221–247.

Siegenthaler, B.M., & Gruber, V. (1969). Combining vision and audition for speech reception. *Journal of Speech and Hearing Disorders, 34,* 58–60.

Sumby, W.H., & Pollack, I. (1954). Visual contribution to speech intelligibility in noise. *Journal of the Acoustical Society of America, 26,* 212–215.

Tikofsky, R.S. (1970). A revised list for the estimation of dysarthric single word intelligibility. *Journal of Speech and Hearing Research, 13,* 59–64.

Tikofsky, R.S., & Tikofsky, R.P. (1964). Intelligibility measures of dysarthric speech. *Journal of Speech and Hearing Research, 7,* 325–333.

Yorkston, K.M., & Beukelman, D.R. (1978). A comparison of techniques for measuring intelligibility of dysarthric speech. *Journal of Communication Disorders, 11,* 499–512.

Yorkston, K.M., & Beukelman, D.R. (1980). A clinician-judged technique for quantifying dysarthric speech based on single-word intelligibility. *Journal of Communication Disorders 13,* 15–31.

Yorkston, K.M., & Beukelman, D.R. (1984). *Assessment of intelligibility of dysarthric speech.* Austin, TX: PRO-ED.

Dysarthria and Apraxia of Speech:
Perspectives on Management
edited by Christopher A. Moore, Ph.D., Kathryn M. Yorkston, Ph.D.,
and David R. Beukelman, Ph.D.
copyright © 1991   Paul H. Brookes Publishing Co., Inc.
Baltimore · London · Toronto · Sydney

Chapter 7 _____

Use and Perceived Value of Perceptual and Instrumental Measures in Dysarthria Management

Bruce R. Gerratt, James A. Till, John C. Rosenbek, Robert T. Wertz, and Allen E. Boysen

THE COMPLEXITY OF dysfunction in dysarthria has spawned a number of methods for clinical management. Knowledge of the volume of clinical services provided to dysarthric patients, methods employed, instrumental resources, and attitudes of the clinicians about methods for speech assessment is important for dysarthria management. Such information may help to guide speech-language pathology training programs to meet the needs of clinical practice.

Since 1988, an advisory group of the Department of Veterans Affairs (DVA) has met to develop a training program in dysarthria management. The advisory group developed and distributed a questionnaire to each DVA Medical Center with a Speech Pathology Service to assess the level of service and methods and attitudes of providers. We attempted to determine what amount of clinical practice was devoted to the management of patients with dysarthria, and the availability and nature of computer resources for assessment and treatment. We wanted to know what assessment techniques clinicians use, how clinicians value them, and whether they would use additional techniques.

This chapter is in the public domain.

THE QUESTIONNAIRE

The questionnaire sent to clinicians is displayed in Appendix A. The questionnaire sent to speech pathology clinics regarding service and computer resources is presented in Appendix B. Respondents were instructed to use information from the last complete quarter to determine volume of service. The clinicians were asked to rate, on a 5-point scale, methods of speech evaluation for *clinical value, frequency of use,* and *if currently unavailable, predicted use.* The assessment methods in the following categories were selected to sample techniques from clinical practice. Techniques more often used in research than in clinical practice were included to examine how these methods are considered for clinical use.

Auditory Perceptual Measures

Methods included published measures, unpublished measures, and nonspeech maneuvers. All measures were assumed to be available to the clinicians.

Published methods include articulation tests, the Frenchay Dysarthria Assessment (Enderby, 1983), speech intelligibility tests such as the Assessment of Intelligibility of Dysarthria Speech (Yorkston & Beukelman, 1981), the Mayo Clinic classification system of dysarthric types (Darley, Aronson, & Brown, 1975), and the Mayo Clinic method of identifying dysarthric signs such as articulatory precision, loudness decay, and hypernasality. Unpublished methods may be particular to a clinic or clinician. The measures included unpublished tests of articulation, nasality, voice quality, prosody, speech naturalness, speech intelligibility, identification of dysarthric signs, and ability to modify speech deviation. Nonspeech maneuvers are commonly used in speech evaluation. The measures included vowel prolongation, pitch and loudness range, diadochokinesis, and strength, speed, range, and accuracy of movement of orofacial structures.

Acoustic Measures

These methods included oscilloscopic, spectrographic, and computer analysis for measurement of articulation, voice, and prosody, as well as special purpose devices, such as Visi-Pitch or the PM Pitch Analyzer for measures of voice, and nasalence measurement of nasal resonance.

Movement Transduction Methods

These included measurement of respiratory kinematics; electroglottographic and photoglottographic methods of measuring vocal fold movement; photodetection and accelerometric measurements of velopharyngeal function; palatographic, strain-gauge and microbeam radiologic methods for measuring orofacial movement; and electromyography.

Imaging Methods

These methods included laryngoscopy with and without stroboscopy, laryngeal radiology, laryngeal ultrasonography, velopharyngeal endoscopy, and velopharyngeal radiology.

Aerodynamic Methods

These included estimated subglottal air pressure and lung volume for respiratory function, estimated subglottal air pressure and oral air flow for laryngeal function, nasal airflow and intraoral air pressure for velopharyngeal function, and intraoral pressure for orofacial function.

RESULTS

Eighty-eight DVA speech pathologists responded to the questionnaire, and 66 clinics within the DVA responded to questions concerning volume of service and availability of computer resources.

Volume of Service

For the 66 clinics, a mean of 20% ($SD = 15\%$) of total treatment is provided to patients with dysarthria. Responses ranged from 0% to 90%. This represents a sizeable proportion of clinic resources in the DVA system.

Computer Resources

Two computers per clinic was the mean of 66 clinics responding. Most clinics had one, 15 had none, and 9 clinics had five or more. An analog-to-digital converter is typically necessary for computer processing of speech signals, and of the 66 clinics, only 6 had such a converter. Computer interfaces for Visi-Pitch, spectrographs, or other single purpose devices were not counted. Thus, 80% of the clinics had one or more computers, but only 9% had the hardware necessary to process speech signals.

Evaluation Methods Rated by Clinicians

Results are reported as the means of clinician ratings of each scale for each evaluation measure. Because auditory-perceptual measures were assumed to be available, clinicians did not rate these methods on the scale *if currently unavailable, predicted use.*

Published Auditory-Perceptual Measures Mean ratings for the five measures are shown in Figure 1. Methods most frequently used are the Mayo Clinic method for determining dysarthric signs, the Mayo Clinic method for classification of dysarthric types, and intelligibility tests, which all received mean ratings near 3.0. The Frenchay and articulation tests are used less frequently, receiving mean ratings closer to 2.0. The

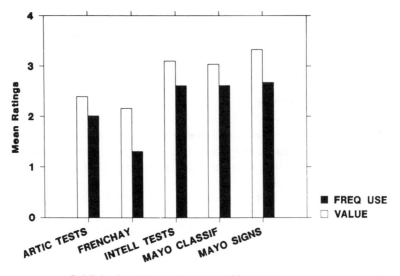

Published Auditory-Perceptual Measures

Figure 1. Mean ratings of *frequency of use* and *clinical value* for published auditory-perceptual measures. (Scale range: 0 = never used/no *clinical value*, 4 = used very frequently/extremely valuable. Artic tests = published articulation tests; Frenchay = Frenchay Dysarthria Assessment; Intell Tests = published intelligibility tests; Mayo Classif = Mayo Clinic dysarthria classification; Mayo Signs = Mayo Clinic identification of dysarthric signs.)

clinical value of the Mayo Clinic method for determining dysarthric signs, the Mayo Clinic method for classification of dysarthric types, and intelligibility tests was approximately 3.0, while mean ratings of Frenchay and articulation tests were slightly above 2.0.

Unpublished Auditory-Perceptual Methods Assessment of patient ability to modify deviant speech was used most frequently, with a mean rating slightly higher than 3.0 (Figure 2). All other methods received mean *frequency of use* ratings near 2.5. The mean *clinical value* of assessment of ability to modify deviant speech was approximately 3.25, while mean ratings of other methods were near 2.5.

Nonspeech Maneuvers Mean ratings of nonspeech maneuvers are shown in Figure 3. All measures were rated at or above 3.0 for both *frequency of use* and *clinical value* (Figure 3).

Acoustic Measures Mean ratings of measures of articulation and prosody are displayed in Figure 4, and those of nasal resonance and voice in Figure 5. The values for *frequency of use* were 1.0 or less for all acoustic measures except Visi-Pitch, with a value slightly greater than 2.0. Mean *clinical value* was approximately 2.0 or greater for all measures with the exception of Visi-Pitch, with a rating greater than 3.0. Mean ratings of *if currently available, predicted use* ranged from approximately 3.0 for Visi-

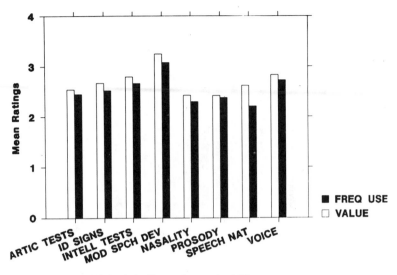

Unpublished Auditory-Perceptual Measures

Figure 2. Mean ratings of *frequency of use* and *clinical value* for unpublished auditory-perceptual measures. (Scale range: 0 = never used/no clinical value, 4 = used very frequently/extremely valuable. Artic Tests = unpublished articulatory tests; ID Signs = unpublished identification of dysarthric signs; Intell Tests = unpublished intelligibility tests; Mod Spch Dev = modification of speech deviation; Nasality = unpublished tests of nasal resonance; Prosody = unpublished tests of prosody; Speech Nat = unpublished test of speech naturalness; Voice = unpublished tests of vocal function.)

Pitch and measurement of voice by computer analysis, to approximately 1.0 for articulatory measurement by oscilloscopic display.

Movement Transduction Measures *Frequency of use* was near zero for the majority of measures, and respiratory kinematics received the highest mean rating, close to 0.5 (Figure 6). *Clinical value* varied between 1.5 and 2.25, and *if currently unavailable, predicted use* was approximately 1.5.

Aerodynamic Measures Mean ratings of the aerodynamic measures are shown in Figure 7. *Frequency of use* was approximately 1.0 or less for all seven measures; *clinical value* was 2.0 or above; and *if currently unavailable, predicted use* was approximately 2.0.

Imaging Measures Mean ratings of the six imaging measures are displayed in Figure 8. *Frequency of use* ranged from near zero for ultrasound to 2.0 for laryngoscopy without stroboscopy (Figure 8). *Clinical value* was approximately 3.0 for both laryngoscopy with and without stroboscopy, while other measures were near 2.0. *If currently unavailable, predicted use* ranged from 1.0 for laryngeal radiology to approximately 2.5 for laryngoscopy with stroboscopy.

Table 1 summarizes *clinical value, frequency of use,* and *if currently unavailable, predicted use.* Auditory-perceptual methods were more fre-

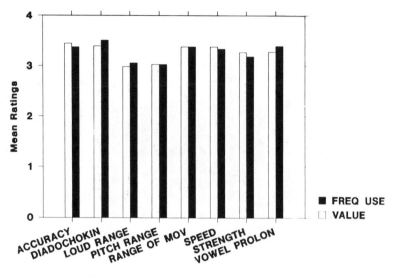

Measures of Nonspeech Maneuvers

Figure 3. Mean ratings of *frequency of use* and *clinical value* for nonspeech maneuvers. (Scale range: 0 = never used/no clinical value, 4 = used very frequently/extremely valuable. Accuracy = accuracy of movement of orofacial structures; Diadochokin = diadochokinesis; Loud Range = vocal loudness range; Pitch range = vocal pitch range; Range of Mov = range of movement of orofacial structures; Speed = speed of movement of orofacial structures; Strength = strength of movement of orofacial structures; Vowel Prolon = vowel prolongation.)

quently used and judged to have higher clinical value than instrumental methods. Of auditory-perceptual methods, nonspeech maneuvers were used most frequently and considered to have the most clinical value. Acoustic, aerodynamic, and imaging measures were used less than auditory-perceptual measures, and movement transduction measures were seldom used. Instrumental measures were judged lower in clinical value than auditory-perceptual measures. Clinicians predicted that they would use acoustic, aerodynamic, and imaging measures about equally if instrumentation were available, but rating values, which ranged from 2.2 for aerodynamic measures to 1.5 for movement transduction measures, demonstrated only limited prediction of their use.

CONCLUSIONS

As an advisory group of the DVA working to develop training for dysarthria management, we wanted to assess service provision, availability of resources, and use and opinions of assessment methods. How representative are these data? The DVA provides services for adult patients, and that population is aging — mean age for veterans is approximately 63 years.

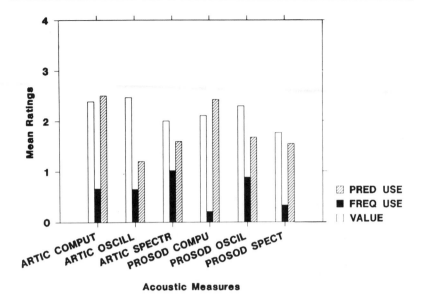

Figure 4. Mean ratings of *predicted use if available, frequency of use,* and *clinical value* for the first six acoustic measures. (Scale range: 0 = never used/no clinical value, 4 = used very frequently/extremely valuable. Artic Comput = computer analysis of articulation; Artic Oscill = oscilloscopic analysis of articulation; Artic Spectr = spectrographic analysis of articulation; Prosod Compu = computer analysis of prosody; Prosod Oscil = oscilloscopic analysis of prosody; Prosod Spect = spectrographic analysis of prosody.)

Our questionnaire sampled programs nationwide that differed in size, patients served (acute, chronic, inpatient, and outpatient), and available resources. Similarly, respondents varied in their training, experience with dysarthric patients, and primary professional interests.

Amount of Service

It may be that more dysarthric patients are seen in DVA clinics than in other clinical settings. The average total clinical activity devoted to management of dysarthria was 20%. This volume of service is considerable and represents a sizeable expenditure of resources. The extent of clinical service documents the need to examine the management of dysarthric patients and to improve this management through research and training.

Instrumental Resources

Availability of instrumentation varied among clinics. Although 88% of DVA clinics had one or more computers available, only six had an analog-to-digital converter to process speech signals from dysarthric patients. This, of course, limited *frequency of use* for computer-based evaluation, and

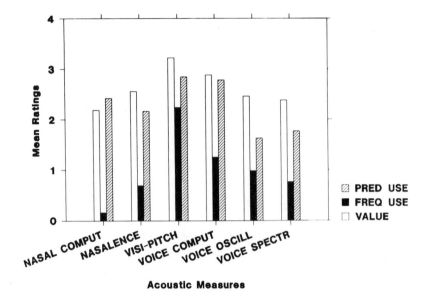

Figure 5. Mean ratings of *predicted use if available, frequency of use,* and *clinical value* for the second six acoustic measures. (Scale range: 0 = never used/no clinical value, 4 = used very frequently/extremely valuable. Nasal Comput = computer analysis of nasal resonance; Nasalence = nasometer analysis of nasal resonance; Visi-Pitch = voice analysis using Visi-Pitch; Voice Comput = computer analysis of vocal function; Voice Oscill = oscilloscopic analysis of vocal function; Voice Spectr = spectrographic analysis of vocal function.)

probably influenced responses to the other rating scales, *clinical value,* and *if currently unavailable, predicted use.* Obviously, clinicians who have no experience with a method have difficulty rating clinical value or predicting use.

Clinical Use, Value, and Predicted Use of Evaluation Methods

We suspect that clinicians use what they are familiar with, whether from coursework or clinical literature. Thus, it is not surprising that published and unpublished auditory-perceptual measures and nonspeech maneuvers are used more frequently than instrumental measures. Furthermore, we reason that clinicians use methods that they value. Consequently, auditory-perceptual measures and nonspeech maneuvers receive clinical value ratings that correspond to their frequency of use. Preference for nonspeech maneuvers over other auditory-perceptual measures, both in clinical value and frequency of use, is surprising, since little research exists of the relation of these measures to speech. Nevertheless, preference for these measures may be influenced by the clinician's purpose in evaluating a dysarthric patient. If the diagnostic purpose of evaluation is to distinguish sites of lesion, the clinician may rely on this type of measure more than on articulation or intelligibility tests. If, however, dysarthria is de-

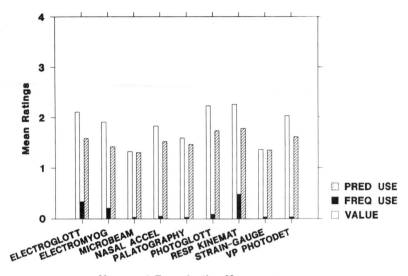

Movement Transduction Measures

Figure 6. Mean ratings of *predicted use if available, frequency of use,* and *clinical value* for movement transduction measures. (Scale range: 0 = never used/no clinical value, 4 = used very frequently/extremely valuable. Electroglott = electroglottography (EGG) of vocal fold movement; Electromyog = electromyography (EMG); Microbeam = microbeam radiology of orofacial movement; Nasal Accel = accelerometry of nasal tissue vibration; Palatography = display of tongue to palate contact; Photoglott = photoglottography (PGG)of vocal fold movement; Resp Kinemat = transduction of respiratory kinematics; Strain-Gauge = transduction of orofacial movement; VP Photodet = photodetection of velopharyngeal movement.)

fined as a reduction in intelligibility and naturalness of speech, and the diagnostic purpose of evaluation is the description of signs of the speech disorder, then the use and validity of nonspeech maneuvers might be questioned.

Instrumental methods are not used frequently, with the exception of Visi-Pitch and laryngoscopy. This results from a scarcity of instrumentation, inability to use the instrument, or clinician preference. We suspect it is probably a combination of all three. Because ratings of *clinical value* and *if currently unavailable, predicted use* exceed *frequency of use* in most cases, it appears that lack of instrumentation is the most important reason for the infrequent use of these measures. Nevertheless, these ratings of *clinical value* and *if currently unavailable, predicted use* for the majority of instrumental measures do not approach those for nonspeech maneuvers. Generally, clinicians demonstrate only a mild enthusiasm for most of the instrumental techniques. On the other hand, several of the *clinical value* and *if currently unavailable, predicted use* ratings for acoustic, aerodynamic, and imaging measures do approach those for published and unpublished auditory-perceptual measures. Thus, clinicians perceive some instrumental

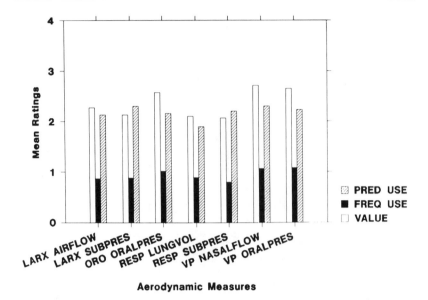

Figure 7. Mean ratings of *predicted use if available, frequency of use,* and *clinical value* for aerodynamic measures (Scale range: 0 = never used/no clinical value, 4 = used very frequently/extremely valuable. Larx Airflow = oral airflow as an index of laryngeal airflow; Larx Subpres = estimated subglottal air pressure to measure laryngeal function; Oro Oralpres = intraoral pressure to measure orofacial function; Resp Lungvol = lung volume; Resp Subpres = estimated subglottal air pressure to measure respiratory function; VP Nasalflow = nasal airflow to measure velopharyngeal function; VP Oralpres = intraoral pressure to measure velopharyngeal function.)

measures to be as valuable as some auditory-perceptual measures. Furthermore, clinicians would use, if available, some instrumental measures as often as they use some auditory-perceptual measures.

McNeil (1986) argued that instrumental measures had not been justified in management of patients with dysarthria, because they are indirect measures and their predictive value has not been established. Some clinicians who judged instrumental measures to be of low clinical value may share this opinion. Although dysarthria is a perceptual phenomenon, we think that instrumental measures can complement the clinician's ear and provide information about speech physiology to describe the breakdown in speech subsystems and to guide dysarthria management.

Data from our questionnaire suggest that DVA speech pathologists devote a large portion of their work to managing dysarthric patients, and they rely on readily available auditory-perceptual and nonspeech measures. Clinicians indicate that a few instrumental measures would improve their efforts, and they would use them if available. Generally, however, clinicians' reluctance to use instrumentation may result from a lack of

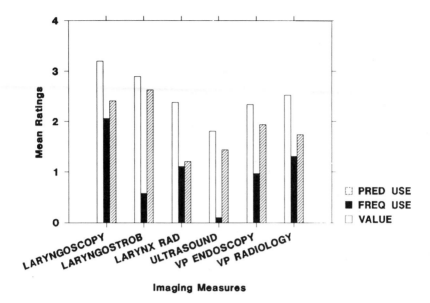

Figure 8. Mean ratings of *predicted use if available, frequency of use,* and *clinical value* imaging measures. (Scale range: from 0 = never used/no clinical value, 4 = used very frequently/extremely valuable. Laryngoscopy = laryngoscopy without a stroboscopic light source; Laryngostrob = laryngoscopy with a stroboscopic light source; Larynx Rad = laryngeal radiology; Ultrasound = laryngeal ultrasonography; VP Endoscopy = velopharyngeal endoscopy; VP Radiology = velopharyngeal radiology.)

knowledge and a lack of evidence to support the contributions of instrumentation in dysarthria management. The former requires the attention of training programs; the latter demands the attention of clinical research.

Table 1. Means and standard deviations of ratings on the 5-point scale for judged clinical value, frequency of use, and predicted use

Method	Clinical value		Frequency of use		Predicted use	
	X̄	SD	X̄	SD	X̄	SD
Published auditory-perceptual measures	2.8	0.5	2.2	0.6	—	—
Unpublished auditory-perceptual measures	2.7	0.3	2.5	0.3	—	—
Nonspeech maneuvers	3.3	0.2	3.3	0.2	—	—
Acoustic measures	2.4	0.4	0.8	0.6	2.0	0.5
Aerodynamic measures	2.4	0.3	0.9	0.1	2.2	0.5
Imaging measures	2.5	0.5	1.0	0.7	1.9	0.5
Movement transduction measures	1.9	0.4	0.1	0.2	1.5	0.2

REFERENCES

Darley, F.L., Aronson, A.E., & Brown, J.R. (1975). *Motor speech disorders.* Philadelphia: W.B. Saunders.

Enderby, P. (1983). *Frenchay Dysarthria Assessment.* San Diego: College-Hill Press.

McNeil, M.R. (1986, February). *A critical appraisal of instrumentation methods in the evaluation and management of dysarthria.* Paper presented at the Clinical Dysarthria Conference, Tucson, AZ.

Yorkston, K.M., & Beukelman, D.R. (1981). *Assessment of intelligibility of dysarthric speech.* Austin, TX: PRO-ED.

Dysarthria and Apraxia of Speech:
Perspectives on Management
edited by Christopher A. Moore, Ph.D., Kathryn M. Yorkston, Ph.D.,
and David R. Beukelman, Ph.D.
Paul H. Brookes Publishing Co., Inc.
Baltimore · London · Toronto · Sydney

Clinician's Questionnaire

Techniques of evaluation	Clinical value (0–4; none to extremely valuable)	Frequency of use (0–4; never to very frequently)	If currently unavailable, predict use (0–4; never to very frequently)
Auditory-perceptual methods			
Mayo Clinic method for identifying dysarthric signs			
Unpublished methods for identifying dysarthric signs	——	——	——
Mayo Clinic method for classifying types of dysarthria	——	——	——
Frenchay test of dysarthria	——	——	——
Published intelligibility tests	——	——	——
Unpublished methods for assessing intelligibility	——	——	——
Unpublished methods for assessing speech naturalness	——	——	——
Published articulation tests	——	——	——
Unpublished methods for assessing articulation	——	——	——
Unpublished methods for assessing nasality	——	——	——
Unpublished methods for assessing prosody	——	——	——
GRBAS voice scale (Japan Society of Logopedics)	——	——	——
Unpublished methods for assessing vocal quality	——	——	——
Assessment of ability to modify speech deviation	——	——	——

(continued)

89

Clinician's Questionnaire
(continued)

Techniques of evaluation	Clinical value (0–4; none to extremely valuable)	Frequency of use (0–4; never to very frequently)	If currently unavailable, predict use (0–4; never to very frequently)
Nonspeech maneuvers:	——	——	——
a. Vowel prolongation	——	——	——
b. Pitch range	——	——	——
c. Loudness range	——	——	——
d. Diadochokinesis	——	——	——
e. Strength of movement of orofacial structures	——	——	——
f. Speed of movement of orofacial structures	——	——	——
g. Range of movement of orofacial structures	——	——	——
h. Accuracy of movement of orofacial structures	——	——	——
Other methods (Please specify below:)			
_____	——	——	——
_____	——	——	——
_____	——	——	——
_____	——	——	——
_____	——	——	——

Acoustic methods
Articulatory

a. Oscilloscope	——	——	——
b. Spectrograph	——	——	——
c. Computer analysis Name of software used: _____	——	——	——

Velopharyngeal

a. Endoscopy	——	——	——
b. Radiology	——	——	——

Aerodynamic methods
Respiratory

a. Estimate of subglottal air pressure	——	——	——
b. Lung volume	——	——	——

(continued)

Clinician's Questionnaire
(continued)

Techniques of evaluation	Clinical value (0−4; none to extremely valuable)	Frequency of use (0−4; never to very frequently)	If currently unavailable, predict use (0−4; never to very frequently)
Laryngeal			
a. Estimate of subglottal air pressure	___	___	___
b. Oral air flow	___	___	___
Velopharyngeal			
a. Nasal air flow	___	___	___
b. Intraoral air pressure	___	___	___
Orofacial			
a. Intraoral pressure	___	___	___
Voice			
a. Oscilloscope	___	___	___
b. Spectrograph	___	___	___
c. Visi-Pitch or PM Pitch Analyzer	___	___	___
d. Computer analysis Name of software used:			
Resonance			
a. Nasalence	___	___	___
b. Computer analysis Name of software used:			
	___	___	___
Prosody			
a. Oscilloscope	___	___	___
b. Spectrograph	___	___	___
c. Computer analysis Name of software used:			
	___	___	___

Movement transduction methods

Respiratory			
a. Respiratory kinematics	___	___	___
Laryngeal			
a. Electroglottography	___	___	___
b. Photoglottography	___	___	___

(continued)

Clinician's Questionnaire
(continued)

Techniques of evaluation	Clinical value (0–4; none to extremely valuable)	Frequency of use (0–4; never to very frequently)	If currently unavailable, predict use (0–4; never to very frequently)
Velopharyngeal			
a. Photodetection	——	——	——
b. Accelerometry	——	——	——
Orofacial			
a. Palatography	——	——	——
b. Strain-gauge	——	——	——
c. Microbeam radiology	——	——	——
Electromyography	——	——	——
Imaging methods			
Laryngeal			
a. Radiology	——	——	——
b. Laryngoscopy	——	——	——
c. Strobolaryngoscopy	——	——	——
d. Ultrasonography	——	——	——

If any instruments or techniques were not included in the list above, please name them, and discuss their clinical value and frequency of use in your evaluation of speech disorders:

_____

_____

_____

_____

_____

_____

_____

_____

_____

Name of respondent: _____

Name of medical center: _____

City: _____

Questionnaire for
the Service Chief

Please provide information from the last complete quarter.

Incoming Referrals
Number of dysarthric patients evaluated: _____

Treatment
Number of dysarthric patients treated: _____
Estimated percent of total therapy accounted for by dysarthria therapy: ___

Instrumental Resources
Computers: Please indicate name and model for each one: _____
_____
_____
_____

Analog-to-digital converters: Please indicate name and model for each
one: _____
_____
_____
_____

Name of respondent: _____
Name of medical center: _____
City: _____

SPECIFIC DISORDERS

DESCRIPTIVE STUDIES OF specific patient populations are of special value for at least two basic reasons. Clinically, these studies serve to characterize a disorder generally so that treatment principles can be developed and applied to other patients. More basically, descriptive studies catalog "Nature's experiments," and describe the responses of speech sensorimotor systems to pathology. For example, neuropathologies with known physiologic consequences may suggest the control structures that underlie normal speech. This section includes four valuable descriptions of narrowly defined neuropathologies and their consequent speech effects. These chapters include case studies of rarely studied disorders (Chapters 8, 10, and 11) and a careful refinement of established diagnostic categories (Chapter 9).

Chapter 8

Dysarthria Following Reye's Syndrome
A Case Report

Sheela L. Stuart,
David R. Beukelman, Karen K. Kenyon,
E. Charles Healey, and John E. Bernthal

INDIVIDUALS WHO HAVE recovered from Reye's syndrome may exhibit a variety of residual impairments, including motor speech disorders. Abkarian, Dworkin, and Brown (1980) have provided the only published description of dysarthria in Reye's syndrome. They describe a 6-year-old who recovered from Reye's with mixed spastic and hypokinetic dysarthria in addition to a language disorder. In this chapter we describe the motor speech disorder of a teenager who recovered from Reye's syndrome.

The disease now known as Reye's syndrome was first identified in 1963 by Reye, Morgan, and Baral as they described clinical and pathologic features of 21 Australian children who demonstrated similar symptoms and progression of the disease. Almost simultaneously, Johnson, Scurelitis, and Carrol (1963) described the same clinicopathologic findings in 16 children from North Carolina. In both reports, high mortality rates were associated with vomiting, progressive coma, and fatty infiltration of the viscera. Since identification, over 2,000 cases of Reye's syndrome have been reported to the Centers for Disease Control in Atlanta, Georgia. Reye's syndrome usually affects infants, children, and adolescents. There have been few cases reported among adults.

The number of reports of Reye's syndrome in the United States has declined during the 1980s. According to the Centers for Disease Control (D. Wells, personal communication, 1989), the incidence of Reye's syndrome in the United States during 1986 was 99 cases. In 1987, this number was 36, and only 13 cases were reported in the United States in 1988.

The clinical presentation of Reye's syndrome is fairly typical and specific. Epidemiologic studies in Ohio, Michigan, and Arizona (Halpin et al., 1982; Starko, Ray, Dominguez, Stromberg, & Woodall, 1980; Waldman, Hall, McGee, & VanAmburg, 1982) suggest an etiologic link between aspirin usage and Reye's syndrome. Low-grade fever may be present, but is usually absent.

The progression of the disease has been charted into a five-stage sequence. Typically, the child initially has an uncomplicated upper respiratory illness, varicella, or, less frequently, diarrhea. As the child begins to improve (usually 3–5 days after onset), persistent vomiting begins. It has been suggested (Crocker, Ozere, Safe, Rozee, & Hutzinger, 1976) that there may be a synergistic relationship between exogenous toxins, viral infections, and the development of Reye's syndrome. Patients may be well-oriented, though irritable and/or lethargic, when vomiting begins. A progression of sensorial changes may occur. Some individuals have no change in consciousness and remain lethargic in varying degrees with no progression to unconsciousness (level I and level II). When the disease plateaus at this level, recovery is usually uneventful. Persons with level III symptoms enter a hyperexcitable state (agitated delirium) and frequently become disoriented and have screaming episodes. Further progression into deeper comatose states is characterized by decerebrate and decorticate posturing with hyperventilation and hyperpyrexia (level IV) and finally, by flaccid paralysis with loss of involuntary ventilatory control (level V). The encephalopathy typically persists for 24–96 hours with gradual improvement in neurologic function. For a small number of patients, return to consciousness may require weeks.

The outcome of individuals with Reye's syndrome is the subject of considerable investigation (Benjamin, Levinsohn, Drotar, & Hanson, 1982; Brunner, O'Grady, Partin, Partin, & Schubert, 1979; Shaywitz et al., 1982). Although these authors have investigated different aspects of surviving patients, they all report evidence that severe encephalopathy is associated with severe residual deficits. Benjamin et al. (1982) reported significant emotional problems observed in 9 of 16 patients. Brunner et al. (1979) reported unspecified school problems occurring in 85% of children who had been comatose. Shaywitz et al. (1982) noted a stereotypic pattern of behavior, including irritability, agitation, inattention, impulsiveness, and exacerbation of existing speech and learning problems. With the exception of the work by Abkarian et al. (1980), there have been no detailed descriptions of the communication disorders associated with this disease. In this case study we describe the dysarthria of a 16-year-old girl who survived Reye's syndrome and her response to some initial intervention approaches.

During the summer of 1988, the second author was asked to evaluate the dysarthria of a teenager who had survived the onset of Reye's syndrome 2 years previously. This case study describes her habitual speech performance and reports the effects of a diagnostic intervention strategy to control her speaking rate and improve her speech intelligibility.

METHODS
Subject

The client, R.K., was an active, competent, 16-year-old female who successfully participated in music, sports, and academics prior to the onset of Reye's syndrome at 14 years of age. Following a brief illness, she was admitted to the emergency room of a local hospital with symptoms of violent nausea and vomiting. A diagnosis of Reye's syndrome was made, and the patient was transferred to a regional medical center where she received aggressive treatment appropriate for Reye's syndrome. She stabilized at a level IV coma for 21 days. As she regained consciousness, she initially had difficulty in maintaining respiration without ventilator support. This resulted in the placement of a tracheostomy tube that was removed after 10 days. After removal of the tube, she was able to produce single words in a whisper only. Her speech performance remained at this level for approximately 2 weeks.

Thirty-seven days post-onset, the young woman was admitted to an acute rehabilitation facility. A review of those records reveal a diagnosis of Reye's syndrome level IV, with pseudobulbar palsy. She began a regimen of daily therapy, involving physical therapy, occupational therapy, speech-language therapy, and psychological counseling.

Her initial speech and language assessment in the acute rehabilitation facility revealed no expressive or receptive aphasia. Reading comprehension and graphic skills were moderately impaired as were her cognitive skills. Speech intelligibility was moderately to severely decreased due to rapid speaking rate, imprecise articulation, periodic aphonia, and breathy voice quality. She received speech and language therapy for 2½ months until she left the facility. Records indicate that she made mild gains in speech and language abilities, but her overall functioning remained similar to that described upon admission. Twenty-nine months after diagnosis, she was referred to the second author for a motor speech evaluation.

Data Collection

Speech samples were recorded as R. K. read an abbreviated Rainbow Passage (72 words) (Fairbanks, 1960). Her performance was recorded in a quiet recording environment using a Sony ECM-44B microphone positioned approximately 6 inches anterior to the lips, and a TEAC model EE X-300 audio recorder. The first speaking condition was "habitual" in that R.K. was instructed to read the passage in a natural way. The second speaking condition involved supplemented (paced) speech in which R. K. pointed to the first letter of each word on an alphabet board as she spoke the word (Beukelman & Yorkston, 1978).

Due to cognitive limitations, R.K. was unable to use the supplemented technique efficiently in her spontaneous speech during the assessment session. Therefore, communication samples were recorded during the reading task rather than during spontaneous speech.

An attempt was made to have R.K. control her speaking rate by using several clinical strategies in addition to the supplemented speech approach. Nevertheless, she was unable to modify her habitual speech rate either with verbal instruction by the examiner to speak more slowly or with a computerized pacing program (Beukelman, Yorkston, & Tice, 1988).

Measurement and Analysis

Perceptual Rating of Transition Passage Speech Dimensions The patient's habitual and paced speech samples were judged by three speech-language pathologists according to the 38 speech dimensions described by Darley, Aronson, and Brown (1969). These speech-language pathologists, who routinely serve persons with neurogenic communication disorders, were unfamiliar with R.K. and her speaking patterns. Each perceptual dimension was rated on a 7-point interval scale with *1* representing normal performance and 7 representing severely deviant performance.

Speech Intelligibility and Overall Speaking Rate Intelligibility of recorded samples (habitual and paced) of the Rainbow Passage was transcribed by graduate students in speech-language pathology who were unfamiliar with the Rainbow Passage. Each sample was transcribed by a group of three different judges, so that passage familiarity would not influence their transcriptions. Speech intelligibility scores were reported as the mean number of correctly transcribed words divided by total words in the sample.

Overall speaking rate (words per minute) was measured using the Microspeech Lab computer program hosted in an IBM XT computer (SRC Software Research Corporation). Duration and overall speaking rate (words per minute) of the abbreviated passage were measured.

Word-Level Analysis To document differences in speech performance in speaking conditions, articulatory performance of the habitual and paced speech samples was analyzed by a jury of four experienced speech-language pathologists. The samples were transcribed using a modified IPA approach. Judgments about individual words and sounds reflected the majority opinion of the judges. At times, the judges used wide band spectrograms to segment the speaker's utterances. Three measures of articulatory performance were completed by the judges: 1) number of words omitted (deleted) from the passage; 2) number of words spoken that contained sound omissions, distortions, or substitutions; and 3) number of words correctly produced. Finally, the characteristics of the sound distortions and substitutions were described.

Reliability To obtain intra-judge reliability data, the abbreviated Rainbow Passage was transcribed a second time by three judges. The second transcription was conducted 1 month after the first. The index of intelligibility was within 4% for all judges for both transcriptions of the paced sample and within 10% for the habitual sample.

Speaking rate data for habitual and paced speech samples were measured and calculated a second time by the first author. The second measures for both samples were within two words per minute of the initial measures.

RESULTS

Perceptual Ratings of Habitual Speech Characteristics

In order to describe R.K.'s natural speech, her production of the abbreviated Rainbow Passage was rated by three judges using the 7-point scale for the 38 speech dimensions defined by Darley et al. (1969). The responses of the judges to each dimension were averaged and are reported in Table 1. In this table dimensions have been clustered according to mean severity ratings of habitual speech. Twelve dimensions received a mean rating of four or higher. The extent of her speech disability was reflected by the high overall ratings of bizarreness (6.0) and (un)intelligibility (5.0). Several articulatory, prosodic, and velopharyngeal dimensions were rated as severely disordered. Both irregular articulatory breakdown and imprecision of consonant production were reported as severely disordered with a rating of 5. Several dimensions related to prosody, including monoloudness (5), monopitch (4.6), reduced stress (4.6), rate (4.6), and short rushes of speech (5.0) received high ratings. Several additional dimensions related to prosody were rated as somewhat less deviant. These included increase of rate in segments (3.1), increase of rate overall (2.6), and variable rate (2.1). Two dimensions related to velopharyngeal dysfunction, nasal emission (4) and hypernasality (4.6), were rated as disordered.

Table 1. Mean ratings of 38 speech dimensions during habitual and paced speaking conditions

Habitual	Paced	Dimension
6	3.3	Bizarreness
5	2.0	Monoloudness
5	2.3	Imprecise consonants
5	3.0	Short rushes of speech
5	2.5	Irregular artic. breakdown
5	2.0	Intelligibility
4.6	4.0	Monopitch
4.6	1.3	Hypernasality
4.6	5.0	Rate
4.6	1.6	Reduced stress
4.6	2.0	Breathy voice
4	1.0	Nasal emission
3.6	2.0	Phonemes repeated
3.1	3.0	Audible inspiration
3.1	3.3	Phrases short
3.1	3.0	Increase of rate in segments
2.6	1.0	Increase of rate overall
2.3	1.0	Voice tremor
2.3	1.0	Harsh voice
2.1	2.0	Variable rate
2.1	1.3	Vowels distorted
2	3.3	Inappropriate silences
2	1.0	Loudness
1.7	2.0	Excess-equal stress
1.6	1.3	Forced inspiration-expiration
1.5	1.3	Breathy voice (transient)
1.3	1.0	Pitch level
1.3	1.0	Voice stoppages
1.0	1.0	Pitch breaks
1.0	1.0	Excess loudness variation
1.0	1.0	Loudness decay
1.0	1.0	Alternating loudness
1.0	1.0	Hoarse wet
1.0	1.0	Strained/strangled
1.0	1.0	Grunt at end of expiration
1.0	1.0	Intervals prolonged
1.0	1.0	Phonemes prolonged
1.0	1.0	Hyponasality

Fifteen dimensions received mean ratings of less than 2. These dimensions reflected respiratory and phonatory functions and prolongation of intervals or phonemes.

The impact of Reye's syndrome on the speech performance of this previously normally functioning teenager was profound. According to her parents and speech-language pathologist, she experienced substantial communication disability and was frequently unintelligible communicating with persons who knew her well, and she had very limited ability to communicate independently with strangers. Two years following the onset of Reye's syndrome, the intelligibility of her habitual speech was rated as severely impaired. In addition to reduced intelligibility, her speech was rated as very bizarre (unnatural). Certainly the unnatural quality of her speech contributed to the communication disability that she experienced.

Perceptual Ratings of Paced Speech Characteristics

A comparison of perceptual ratings for the habitual sample and paced sample (Table 1) reveals improvement on a number of dimensions and deterioration on only three. Specifically, each dimension rated 6, 5, 4, or 3.6 for habitual speech, with the exception of speaking rate, showed marked improvement in performance. Speaking rate was rated as 4.6 for habitual speech, and 5 for the paced speech. Perhaps during habitual speech, the judges reacted to a speaking rate that was excessively fast given the speaker's intelligibility; however, slow speaking rate was also rated as deviant in habitual speech. Those dimensions rated as more deviant for paced speech included inappropriate silences and excess and equal stress. Apparently, the "word-by-word" speaking approach resulting from the paced speech technique contributed to these ratings of deviancy.

Speech Rate and Intelligibility

In addition to perceptual assessment, the duration of the subject's reading of the abbreviated Rainbow Passage was measured using the Microspeech Lab program. Overall speaking rate for habitual speech was 159 words per minute (Table 2). Because R.K. omitted 11 words from the stimulus passage as she read, her actual speaking rate was 180 words per minute. As reported earlier, the judges perceived rushes of speech. The overall speaking rate does not reflect the observation that R.K. produced some utterances at very rapid rates and then paused for extended periods. During habitual speech, R.K.'s mean speech intelligibility as transcribed by three judges was 40% (Table 2). During paced speech, R.K.'s overall rate was 29 words per minute, and her mean speech intelligibility score was 98%.

Table 2. Mean speaking rate (words per minute) and speech intelligibility (percent of words correctly transcribed) for habitual and paced conditions

Condition	Rate (wpm)	Intelligibility (%)
Habitual	159	40
Paced	29	98

Obviously, speaking rate was reduced in paced speech. This reduction in speaking rate was accompanied by a 58% increase in speech intelligibility.

Sound Production Analysis

Results of the word-level analysis (Table 3) reveal that 41% of the words in the abbreviated Rainbow Passage were produced correctly during habitual speech, while 79% of the words were produced without error during paced speech.

Articulatory error patterns also differed for the two conditions (Table 3). During habitual speech, the subject deleted 14% of the words in the passage, and no words were omitted in paced speech. In habitual speech, 26% of the words in the passage (33% of the words actually produced by R.K.) contained sound omissions, with half the omissions occurring in the initial and final positions of words and half in the medial position. During paced speech, 7% of the words contained sound omissions, with nearly half in the initial and final positions and half in the medial position. The reduction in speaking rate associated with paced speech allowed the speaker to include all words in the passage and to omit fewer sounds in words.

Table 3 also reveals that during habitual speech, 23% of the words spoken by R.K. contained sound substitutions or distortions. During paced speech, 14% of the words contained substitution or distortion errors. Although articulatory errors persisted in paced speech, errors occurred less frequently.

A further analysis of the distortion errors reveals that two types predominated in habitual speech. The liquids /r/ and /l/ accounted for half the distortions, and frication during the stop phase of voiceless plosive sounds accounted for 30% of distortion errors. Vowel distortions and a single nasal distortion accounted for the remainder of errors. In paced

Table 3. Word-level analysis of the Rainbow Passage in habitual and paced conditions

Condition	Percent of words				
	Omitted	Sounds omitted (initial/final)	Sounds omitted (medial)	Sounds in error	Correct
Habitual	14	13	13	19	41
Paced	0	3	4	14	79

speech there were no distortions of liquids or fricated distortions during the stop phase of voiceless plosives. Instead, three of the four distortion errors involved a partial devoicing of the release of a final voiced plosive. Only two substitution errors occurred in habitual speech. These involved a place error (/d/ for /g/ substitution in the word "legend") and a manner error (/d/ for voiced /ð/ substitution in the word "the"). During paced speech, two voiceless for voiced substitutions occurred. In summary, the number of articulatory errors was reduced in the paced speech. In addition, the type of errors also differed in the two conditions. Voicing errors predominated in paced speech, while word omissions, sound omissions, and liquid and frication distortions were the most common errors in habitual speech.

CLINICAL COMMENT

The combination of articulatory imprecision and extensive prosodic deficits are indicative of a speaker who has substantial disorders of speech timing and coordination. The improvement in intelligibility accompanying a reduction in speaking rate is consistent with successful rate control intervention with discoordinated speakers reported by other researchers (Crow & Enderby, 1989; Schumacher & Rosenbek, 1986; Yorkston & Beukelman, 1981).

Diagnostic intervention revealed that R.K. was unable to reduce her speaking rate voluntarily in response to verbal instruction, or even to choral reading with the speech-language pathologist. Furthermore, she was unable to comply with the software program pacing cursor (Beukelman, Yorkston, & Tice, 1988), which cues the speaker to read at a prescribed rate. She was unable to modify her speaking rate to correspond to a cursor that underlined words, though she could describe the task accurately to the examiner. Although the speaker was experiencing extensive communication failure in her habitual speech, she appeared unable to adopt compensatory strategies to increase speech intelligibility. Results of this study showed that she habitually read aloud at an overall communication rate of 180 words per minute, a rate within the upper end of the normal range. Thus, she spoke at a normal rate, even though she was aware that she was not being understood by her listeners. She mastered the supplemental speech method with just a few minutes of instruction. Although additional practice with the technique would be necessary to achieve conversational speech, a marked improvement in her speech performance was noted.

Unfortunately, from a clinical perspective, the reduction of R.K.'s speaking rate from 180 to 29 words per minute with supplemental speaking was drastic. The authors expected that she would be able to speak more rapidly and still produce intelligible speech, but from the evidence, there appears to be no additional way to increase her speaking rate at this time. Because the supplemental speaking technique was new to her and because of her cognitive limitations, she worked deliberately to locate the first letter of each word on an alphabet board as she spoke. We can speculate that her pacing rate would increase as she became more familiar with the task.

The incidence of Reye's syndrome in the United States appears to be decreasing steadily. However, individuals who recover from this condition can experience multiple sequelae, including cognitive, emotional, motor control, and communication disorders. This case study is presented to document the motor speech disorder of a teenager who had Reye's syndrome. During a diagnostic intervention session she was introduced to the paced speech technique of pointing to the first letter of each word as that word was spoken. In response to this intervention strategy, her speaking rate was reduced from 159 to 29 words per minute, and her speech intelligibility improved from 40% to 98%.

REFERENCES

Abkarian, G.G., Dworkin, J.P., & Brown, S.R. (1980). Signed English as a transitional step in the treatment of a child with Reye's Syndrome. *Human Communication*, Spring, 23–28.

Benjamin, P.Y., Levinsohn, M., Drotar, D., & Hanson, E. (1982). Intellectual and emotional sequelae of Reye's Syndrome. *Critical Care Medicine*, *10*(9), 583–587.

Beukelman, D.R., & Yorkston, K. (1978). Communication options for patients with brain stem lesions. *Archives of Physical Medicine and Rehabilitation*, *59*, 337–340.

Beukelman, D.R., Yorkston, K., & Tice, R. (1988). *Pacer/tally*. [Computer program]. Tucson: Communication Skill Builders.

Brunner, R.L., O'Grady, D.J., Partin, J.C., Partin, J.S., & Schubert, W.K. (1979). Neuropsychologic consequences of Reye's Syndrome. *Journal of Pediatrics*, *95*, 5(1), 706–711.

Crocker, J.F.S., Ozere, R.L., Safe, S.H., Rozee, K.R., & Hutzinger, O. (1976). Lethal interaction of ubiquitous insecticide carriers with virus. *Science*, *192*, 1352–1353.

Crow, E., & Enderby, P. (1989). The effect of an alphabet chart on the speaking rate and intelligibility of speakers with dysarthria. In D. Beukelman, & K. Yorkston (Eds.), *Recent advances in dysarthria*. Boston: Little, Brown.

Darley, F., Aronson, A., & Brown, J. (1969). Differential diagnostic patterns of dysarthria. *Journal of Speech and Hearing Research*, *12*, 246–269.

Fairbanks, G. (1960). *Voice and articulation drill book*. (2nd ed.). New York: Harper and Brothers.

Halpin, T.J., Holtzhauer, F.J., Campbell, R.J., Hall, L.J., Correa-Villasenor, A., Lanese, R., Rice, J., & Hurwitz, E.S. (1982). Reye's Syndrome and medication use. *Journal of the American Medical Association*, *138*, 687–691.

Johnson, G.M., Scurelitis, T.D., & Carrol, N.B. (1963). A study of sixteen fatal cases of encephalitis-like disease in North Carolina children. *North Carolina Medical Journal, 24,* 464–473.

Reye, R.D.K., Morgan, G., & Baral, J. (1963). Encephalopathy and fatty degeneration of the viscera: A disease entity in childhood. *Lancet, 2,* 749–752.

Schumacher, J., & Rosenbek, J. (1986). Behavioral treatment of hypokinetic dysarthria: Further investigation of aided speech. *Asha, 28,* 145.

Shaywitz, S.E., Cohen, P.M., Cohen, D.J., Mikkelson, E., Morowitz, G., & Shaywitz, B.A. (1982). Long term consequences of Reye's Syndrome: A sibling matched, controlled study of neurologic, cognitive, academic, and psychiatric function. *Journal of Pediatrics, 100*(1), 41–46.

Starko, K.M., Ray, G., Dominguez, L.B., Stromberg, W.L., & Woodall, D.F. (1980). Reye's Syndrome and salicylate use. *Pediatrics, 66,* 859–864.

Waldman, R.J., Hall, W.N., McGee, H., & Van Amburg, G. (1982). Aspirin as a risk factor in Reye's Syndrome. (1982). *Journal of American Medical Association, 247,* 3089–3094.

Yorkston, K.M., & Beukelman, D.R. (1981). Ataxic dysarthria: Treatment sequences based on intelligibility and prosodic considerations. *Journal of Speech and Hearing Disorders, 46,* 398–404.

Dysarthria and Apraxia of Speech:
Perspectives on Management
edited by Christopher A. Moore, Ph.D., Kathryn M. Yorkston, Ph.D.,
and David R. Beukelman, Ph.D.
copyright © 1991   Paul H. Brookes Publishing Co., Inc.
Baltimore · London · Toronto · Sydney

Chapter 9

Perceptual Analysis of the Dysarthrias in Children with Athetoid and Spastic Cerebral Palsy

Marilyn Seif Workinger and Raymond D. Kent

CEREBRAL PALSY IS one of the most devastating disorders of childhood, affecting two people of every thousand (Paneth & Kiely, 1984). Cerebral palsy was defined by Bax (1964) as "a disorder of movement and posture due to a defect or lesion of the immature brain" (p. 295). Bobath (1980) describes the condition further by stating that:

> The brain lesion is nonprogressive and causes variable impairment of the coordination of muscle action, with resulting inability of the child to maintain normal postures and perform normal movements. This central motor handicap is frequently associated with affected speech, vision and hearing, with various types of perceptual disturbances, some degree of mental retardation, and/or epilepsy. (p. 1)

The identification of subtypes of cerebral palsy has evolved over time. W.J. Little, in 1843, was among the first to describe the condition(s) now labeled cerebral palsy. He described a condition of infants, "spastic rigidity," which became known as "Little's disease." He viewed neuromotor disorders of infants as a common occurrence, resulting primarily from prematurity. By the late 1800s, the term cerebral palsy came into use. Freud, in 1897, argued that Little's "spastic rigidity" was only one subtype of cerebral palsy and that other types of neuromotor involvement, including involuntary motion disorders, also should be included as subtypes (Hardy, 1983). Crothers and Paine (1959) studied a large population of children with cerebral palsy and concluded that most could be classified by three major subgroups: spasticity, involuntary motion disorders, or mixed signs.

Bobath (1980) described movement patterns of the two major groups. In describing the spastic group, he states:

> The spastic child shows hypertonia of a permanent character, even at rest. The degree of spasticity varies with the child's general condition, that is, his excitability and the strength of stimulation to which he is subjected at any moment. If the spasticity is severe the child is more or less fixed in a few typical patterns due to the severe degree of co-contraction of the involved parts, especially around the proximal joints — shoulders and hips. Some muscles may appear 'weak' as a result of tonic reciprocal inhibition by their spastic antagonists. . . . However, true weakness may develop in some muscle groups because of disuse in cases of long standing, and after prolonged immobilization in plaster casts or apparatus. Spasticity is of typical distribution and changes initially in a predictable manner, owing to tonic reflex activity. Movements are restricted in range and require excessive effort. (pp. 45–46)

The athetoid group is described (Bobath, 1980) as follows:

> All athetoid children show an unsteady and fluctuating type of postural tone. In the pure cases, basic postural tone is below normal and the amplitude of the fluctuation varies widely in the individual child, depending on the severity of the condition, and the degree of stimulation and effort. These children lack a sustained postural tone and ability to fixate. . . . They lack proximal co-contraction and are therefore unable to maintain a stable position against gravity. Their inability to control their movements and give postural fixation to the moving part interferes with the performance of manual skills. They are in many ways the counterpart of the spastic child in whom permanent hypertonus and exaggerated co-contraction produce an exaggerated static attitude at the expense of mobility. The athetoid child, unless his condition is complicated by spasticity, lacks grading of antagonistic and synergistic activity during a movement. Contraction of one group of muscles leads to an almost complete inhibition of the antagonists. . . . Movements are therefore jerky, uncontrolled and extreme in range, with poor control of the mid-ranges.
>
> Head control is poor and the upper limbs are usually more involved than the lower limbs. In pure cases the lower extremities are usually primitive rather than abnormal. Because of the lack of co-contraction and the extreme ranges of movement combined with low postural tone, there is hypermobility of all joints with a tendency to subluxation, especially of the mandibles, shoulder and hip joints and the fingers. (pp. 59–60)

Dysarthria is the speech disorder seen most commonly in individuals with cerebral palsy. In their classic perceptual study, Darley, Aronson, and Brown (1969) demonstrated that the speech and voice characteristics associated with various types of neurologic movement disorders differ. Netsell (1975) calls on clinicians and researchers to view dysarthrias as a set of movement disorders.

Normal patterns of muscle contraction depend upon proper levels of background tension (or tonus), adequate strength or contractile force, and accurate timing (i.e. the activation and deactivation of all the muscles at the proper time). Disturbances in the peripheral nervous system (PNS) or central nervous system (CNS) control of these muscle actions are responsible for abnormalities in the range, velocity, and/or direction of speech movements. The crux of the research problem is to determine the exact nature of these PNS and CNS controls and the joint study of neurologically normal and abnormal speakers represents one important and viable approach in this area. The crux of the clinical problem obviously is to improve or maintain current levels of speech intelligibility for the individual client, and the thesis proposed here is better treatment plans will be developed with greater knowledge of the precise character of the speech movement disorder and the underlying neural control problem. (pp. 1–2)

In a perceptual study describing differences in the speech of children with athetoid and spastic cerebral palsy, Rutherford (1944) determined that "there is no speech which is characteristic of all children handicapped by cerebral palsy; . . . there is a difference with respect to some speech trends between the two main groups of cerebral palsy; and . . . a difference in therapy for . . . [these] groups is indicated" (p. 271). Results of a perceptual study by Seif, Netsell, and Kent (1981) are in agreement with Rutherford's determination. They found that experienced listeners can differentiate with 80% accuracy between the speech of individuals with spastic and athetoid cerebral palsy. Perceptual dimensions of their speech samples were rated and a subset of dimensions was used to predict the neurologic diagnosis for 90% of the cases. *Breathy voice quality, monopitch,* and *monoloudness* were most characteristic of the spastic group, whereas *inappropriate voice stoppage or release, slow rate,* and *dysrhythmia* were most characteristic of the speakers with athetosis. This is in contrast to previous reports by Hedges (1955) and Shapiro (1960), who found that inexperienced listeners could not judge, at a rate greater than chance, whether youngsters were diagnosed as athetoid or spastic on the basis of a taped speech sample. In addition, descriptive or phonetic studies have not found consistent differences between the two groups (Byrne, 1959; Irwin, 1955; Leith, 1954; Rutherford, 1939), and research describing the two groups has provided contradictory results. A brief review of literature describing various parameters of speech production in youngsters with athetoid and spastic cerebral palsy follows.

SPEECH PRODUCTION PARAMETERS

Respiration

Wolfe (1950) reported that all youngsters with athetosis in his sample had respiratory involvement. Blumberg (1955) and Achilles (1955) confirmed this finding, and added that although youngsters with spasticity may show respiratory involvement, it is more severe in those with athetosis. Blumberg speculated that the poorer speech quality in children with athetosis probably is directly related to their problems of respiratory control.

Clement and Twitchell (1959) described the respiratory pattern of youngsters with spasticity as shallow inspiration and forced expiration. In youngsters with athetosis, they found shallow inspiration with variable and uncontrolled expiration, resulting in "sudden bursts of breath." Hardy (1964) examined pulmonary function of youngsters with athetosis, with spasticity, and in normal children. He found performances of the three groups to be essentially the same for rest breathing rate, minute ventilation, tidal volume, expiratory reserve, inspiratory capacity, and vital capacity. He noted, however, that the respiratory patterns of youngsters with cerebral palsy seemed "less flexible" than those of normal children.

Phonation

Rutherford (1944) described children with athetosis as having voices that are louder, lower pitched, more monotonous, and breathier than voices of children with spasticity. Leith (1954) found no differences between the two groups regarding deviations of pitch level, but more children with athetosis were judged to have "monotonous pitch" and "uncontrolled variability of pitch." Ingram and Barn (1961) describe "transient arrest of speech" in patients with dyskinesia (athetosis) and attribute this to obstruction of the airway at the larynx. Farmer and Lencione (1977) identified by spectrographic analysis a pattern of extraneous vocalization (prevocalization) in the speech of individuals with spastic and athetoid cerebral palsy. They reported that this feature occurs more frequently and with longer mean duration in speakers with athetosis than in those with spasticity.

Velopharyngeal Adequacy

Ingram and Barn (1961) described youngsters with spasticity as having slight to moderate nasal escape due to palatal paresis with resulting hypernasality and wastage of breath. Netsell (1969) described several types of velopharyngeal dysfunction found in youngsters with cerebral palsy, including gradual opening, gradual closing, anticipatory opening, retentive opening, and premature opening. He did not, however, attribute these to any specific subgroup. Kent and Netsell (1978) and Hardy (1961) described children with athetosis as having intermittent velopharyngeal closure caused by instability of velar elevation.

Articulation

Rutherford (1939) found that children with both athetoid and spastic cerebral palsy showed definite and persistent sound substitutions, and the order of frequency is essentially the same for both groups. Wolfe (1950) determined that 100% of youngsters with athetosis in his study had inadequate articulation, but only 59% of children with spasticity had this deficit. Lencione (1953) reported that individuals with spasticity were superior to individuals with athetosis their ability to produce speech sounds independent of word position, in their ability to produce sounds in all physiologic categories, and their ability to produce voiced and voiceless cognates. The individuals with spasticity made fewer omission and substitution errors, and their speech was significantly more intelligible than that of individuals with athetosis. Achilles (1955) reported that children with athetosis produced more than twice as many consonant errors for sentences and words than did children with spasticity.

In contrast to these findings, Irwin (1955) found no statistical difference in mastery of speech sounds (vowel type, consonant type, vowel frequency, and consonant frequency) between groups of youngsters diagnosed as having athetosis, spasticity, or tension athetosis. This supported the findings of a previous study by Leith (1954). Byrne (1959) agreed with these authors and reported that the sequence of sound development in youngsters with cerebral palsy followed that of normal children but was delayed.

A more recent study by Platt, Andrews, Young, and Quinn (1980) of the speech of adults with cerebral palsy indicates that "spastic dysarthric speech is more intelligible and less articulatorily impaired than athetoid dysarthric speech" (p. 37). Adults with athetosis were found to produce twice as many incomprehensible words as those with spasticity. However, the study reported that, "with regard to specific phonemic factors, spastics and athetoids appeared to differ only in terms of amount of accuracy and not in terms of any distinctive phonetic differences" (p. 38).

Physiologic evidence that would lead to an understanding of articulatory problems is scarce. Kent and Netsell (1978) and Kent, Netsell, and Bauer (1975) described adults with athetoid cerebral palsy as having large ranges of jaw movement, inappropriate tongue positioning, and prolonged transition times. They also reported intermittent velopharyngeal inadequacy for speakers with athetosis, as did Hardy (1961). Netsell (1978) reported differences between adults with spasticity and those with athetosis in lip opening and closing gestures. Adults with spasticity showed difficulty with antagonist co-contraction of the depressor labii inferior and orbicularis oris superior, and in bringing movement velocity to a rapid peak. In contrast, adults with athetosis showed reciprocal activity of these muscles and nearly normal peak velocities, but they showed variability in time of peak velocity and abnormal duration. Neilson and O'Dwyer (1981, 1984) report abnormal patterns of muscle activity (by electromyography) but found no variability in patterns over repeated trials.

Thus, much of the information regarding the speech of individuals with cerebral palsy has been obtained from perceptual studies or from descriptive, anecdotal reports. Physiologic and acoustic studies are beginning to appear, but a great need exists for more information before we can point to definite differences between the groups, identify physiologic reasons for those differences, and provide appropriate treatment for speech problems, as suggested by Rutherford in 1944.

This study expands the study by Seif et al. (1981). Goals of the present study were: 1) to determine the ability of experienced listeners to identify perceptual differences in the speech of children with spastic and those with athetoid cerebral palsy, and 2) to develop a perceptual profile of the groups and compare the results with previous findings.

METHODS OF PROCEDURE

Subjects

Eighteen children with cerebral palsy between the ages of 7 and 14 who had been diagnosed as having spastic diplegia or quadriplegia or athetosis (quadriplegia) were studied. The children had been diagnosed by a physician specializing in treatment of cerebral palsy, and children with mixed signs were excluded. Nine children in each diagnostic category were chosen from populations available at the Marshfield Clinic, Marshfield, Wisconsin; Southern Wisconsin Cerebral Palsy Clinic, Madison, Wisconsin; the DuPage Easter Seal Treatment Center, Villa Park, Illinois; and the University of Iowa Hospital School, Iowa City, Iowa. All children but one were of normal intelligence (70 IQ and above) as determined by an individually administered standardized test of intelligence. (Subject S_2 was accepted with below average intelligence since spastic speakers with severe dysarthria were difficult to locate.) This criterion for normal intelligence is stated in the *Diagnostic and Statistical Manual of Mental Disorders (DSM — III* 1980). All passed at least a puretone screening test for hearing that determined they had bilateral hearing thresholds less than 30 dB at 4, 6, and 8 kHz. The Peabody Picture Vocabulary Test — Revised (PPVT-R) (Dunn & Dunn, 1981) was administered as a language screening device. There was wide variation in PPVT scores as Table 1 reveals. It is hypothesized that these speakers may show reduced recognition vocabulary, in spite of documented normal intelligence, because of their inability to explore and experience their environment. Therefore, individuals were not rejected on the basis of PPVT scores. Speakers were matched for age and severity of dysarthria, which was judged on a 7-point interval scale.

Table 1. Subject age, severity of dysarthria, and Peabody Picture Vocabulary Test—Revised (PPVT) score.

	Spastic diagnosis				Athetoid diagnosis		
Subject	Age (years, months)	PPVT[a] score	Overall severity[b]	Subject	Age (years, months)	PPVT[a] score	Overall severity[b]
S_1	13-3	NT[c]	6	A_1	10-9	(−) 4-3	6
S_2	14-9	(−) 6-7	6	A_2	11-0	equal	5.5
S_3	10-0	(−) 0-10	5	A_3	9-5	(−) 1-4	5.5
S_4	10-3	(−) 4-5	3.5	A_4	11-7	(−) 4-4	4.5
S_5	11-11	(+) 0-3	2.5	A_5	10-4	(−) 0-11	3.5
S_6	6-11	(+) 0-3	2.5	A_6	7-6	(−) 1-0	3
S_7	12-2	(+) 1-10	2	A_7	9-2	(+) 0-5	3
S_8	12-6	(−) 2-10	2	A_8	12-10	(−) 1-6	2.5
S_9	13-6	(+) 2-1	2	A_9	12-9	equal	2.5
Mean	11-8		3.5		10-7		4

[a]Difference between chronological age and score on the Peabody Picture Vocabulary Test—Revised.
[b]Judged by the first author at the time of data collection.
[c]Measure was omitted for this speaker since it could be assumed from school placement that receptive vocabulary was within normal limits.

Listeners

Two certified speech pathologists, each with more than 15 years of experience in treatment of children with cerebral palsy, served as listeners for the perceptual section of the study. Transcription of speech samples was completed by a third certified speech pathologist with similar experience and by a speech scientist with more than 15 years experience in the study of dysarthric speech.

Speech Sample Components

1. Sustained vowels: Speakers were instructed to take in as much air as they could and to sustain each vowel as long as possible. Speakers were encouraged by gestures from the investigator to continue production of the desired sound. Three repetitions of each of the following vowels were recorded in random order: /i/, /ɑ/, /u/, and /æ/.
2. Sentence repetition: Speakers repeated each of the following sentences five times:

   I saw you hit the cat.
   I took a spoon and a dish.
   The box is blue and red.

   Again, a different order was presented to each speaker.
3. Automatic speech: Each speaker counted from 1 to 20 at a comfortable rate.
4. Spontaneous speech sample: Each subject described his or her home.

Procedure

Each speech sample was recorded in a sound-treated room or in a quiet environment. Individuals practiced portions of the speech sample at least once. Stimuli were presented by way of audio tape to standardize the presentation. Recordings were made on a Nagra IV L tape recorder with a high quality, unidirectional microphone. The microphone was placed 15 cm from the speaker's mouth. Samples of vowel production, counting, sentence repetition, and spontaneous speech were transferred to a master tape. Three speakers' recordings were recorded on the master tape twice to provide reliability information. A 1 kHz tone at 90 db SPL was recorded at the beginning of the tape so that listeners standardized their machines at a fixed playback level. The sentence repetition subtest for each speaker was transcribed twice by the author using broad transcription. Ten percent of these sentences were transcribed by a second listener.

Perceptual Analysis

Listeners rated each speaker on 22 perceptual dimensions (see Table 2) chosen from the study by Seif et al. (1981) or added as expanded dimensions. Definitions of dimensions were given to each listener. A 7-point interval scale was used with *1* indicating performance within normal limits and *7* indicating extremely severe involvement (Darley et al., 1969). Listeners were asked to make initial ratings of *type* and *severity of dysarthria* and loudness dimensions with their recorders at fixed playback gain. After making these initial ratings, listeners were allowed to vary the loudness level to help determine other judgments, such as articulation. Listeners were allowed to listen to each subject as many times as necessary to make their ratings. After rating the 22 dimensions, listeners again rated *type* and *severity of dysarthria*.

Inter-listener reliability was assessed by having each listener rate the 22 dimensions twice for three speakers. Listener 1 rated 92% of the twice-rated dimensions within one scale value and 100% within two scale values. Listener 2 rated 92% within one scale value and 97% within two scale values. The reliability of each listener across speakers was determined by having each listener also scale *type of dysarthria* and overall *severity of dysarthria* twice. Listener 1 rated 97% of the repeated measures within one scale value and 100% within two scale values. Listener 2 rated 100% of the repeated measures within one scale value.

Results

The arithmetic mean of ratings for each dimension was calculated for each speaker group. These means were rank ordered and are displayed in Table 3. The highest ranked characteristic dimensions for the speakers with spasticity were *consistent hypernasality, breathy voice quality,* and *voice quality*

Table 2. Perceptual dimensions used in study

Overall severity of dysarthria	Vowel errors
Intelligibility of speech	Monoloudness
Inappropriate voice stoppage or release	Excessive loudness
Inappropriate voice onset	Reduced stress
Intrusive sounds	Continuous voicing
Slow rate	Voice quality change within an
Dysrhythmia	utterance
Inappropriate phrasing	Breathy voice quality
Consonant omission	Harsh voice quality
Consonant distortion	Strained/strangled voice quality
Consonant substitutions	Consistent hypernasality
	Nasal emission

Table 3. Means for perceptual dimensions in spastic and athetoid speaker groups.

Group	Rank	Dimension	Mean
Spastic	1	Consistent hypernasality	4.28ᵃ
	2	Breathy voice quality	3.89ᵃ
	3	Inappropriate phrasing	3.78
	4	Voice quality change	3.78ᵃ
	5	Dysrhythmia	3.72
	6	Monoloudness	3.61
	7	Reduced stress	3.61
	8	Inappropriate voice stoppage/release	3.44
	9	Slow rate	3.44
	10	Consonant distortions	3.39
	11	Consonant omissions	3.28
	12	Vowel errors	3.22
	13	Continuous voicing	3.11
	14	Harsh voice quality	3.11
	15	Inappropriate voice onset	2.94
	16	Strained/strangled voice quality	2.94
	17	Nasal emission	2.83
	18	Consonant substitutions	2.76
	19	Excessive loudness	2.61
	20	Intrusive sounds	2.41
Athetoid	1	Inappropriate phrasing	4.65
	2	Dysrhythmia	4.50
	3	Reduced stress	4.33ᵃ
	4	Inappropriate voice stoppage/release	4.28ᵃ
	5	Slow rate	4.28ᵃ
	6	Consonant omission	4.22
	7	Voice quality change	4.22
	8	Continuous voicing	4.17
	9	Vowel errors	4.11
	10	Breathy voice	4.11
	11	Inappropriate voice onset	4.06
	12	Consonant distortion	4.06
	13	Monoloudness	4.00
	14	Consistent hypernasality	4.00
	15	Intrusive sounds	3.89
	16	Excessive loudness	3.72
	17	Consonant substitution	3.61
	18	Harsh voice	3.06
	19	Strained/strangled voice quality	2.83
	20	Nasal emission	2.50

ᵃThree highest ranked/most characteristic dimensions.

change. Highest-ranking dimensions for speakers with athetosis were *reduced stress, inappropriate voice stoppage or release,* and *slow rate.*

Standard deviations were calculated for each dimension. Most standard deviations overlapped the mean for the opposite group. For the *inappropriate voice stoppage or release* dimension, the standard deviation for the group of speakers with athetosis did not overlap the mean of the group of speakers with spasticity. For the *intrusive sounds* dimension, neither standard deviation overlapped the mean of the opposite group.

Rankings for each dimension are compared by group in Figure 1. The group with athetosis was ranked as being more severely involved on all dimensions, except those assessing laryngeal and resonant voice quality. For measures of *voice quality change, breathy voice, harsh voice, strained/strangled voice quality, consistent hypernasality,* and *nasal emission,* scores for the group with spasticity were equal to, or greater than, those for the group with athetosis.

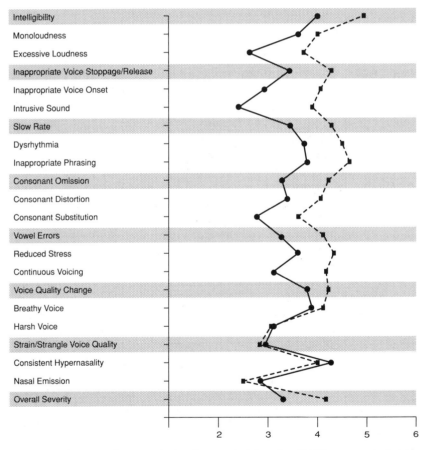

Figure 1. Comparison by group of ratings for perceptual dimensions. Solid line represents athetoid group, dotted line represents the spastic group.

Both listeners were able to identify speakers with spasticity or with athetosis with 78% accuracy. Four speakers were incorrectly judged by both listeners. These were S_1, S_2, A_5, and A_8.

Phonetic transcriptions were made of the five sentence repetitions. Error patterns for each speaker are displayed in Table 4. Speakers with athetosis produced more errors, in general, than speakers with spasticity. For both groups, the primary error was omission, with vowel errors and substitutions following. For the group with athetosis, the next most frequent errors were voicing errors and additions. These errors were not common among speakers with spasticity but nasalization was, and this error was not common for the group with athetosis. Developmental articulation errors were infrequent in either group.

CONCLUSIONS

Perceptual Analysis

Perceptual data gathered in this study are in agreement with a previous study by Seif et al. (1981), which showed that experienced listeners are able to differentiate speakers with cerebral palsy. This result contrasts with reports by Hedges (1955) and Shapiro (1960). Analysis of perceptual dimensions rated in this study suggests that speakers with athetosis and those with spasticity show some deficit in all areas examined. Those with athetosis tended to have more severe deficits in all areas, with the exception of dimensions assessing laryngeal and resonant voice quality. As mentioned, involvement for individuals with spasticity was equal to or greater than that of the group with athetosis for those dimensions. The similarity in perceptual profiles of the groups (see Figure 1) may account for difficulty in identifying the two types by inexperienced listeners (Shapiro, 1960), or when severity is not controlled.

Profiles of the two groups show similarities and differences. Speakers with athetosis were judged to be more severely involved for all measures of articulation and coordination of articulatory movement, or timing. Greatest perceptual differences between the two groups occurred in the dimensions of *excessive loudness* and *intrusive sounds*, where scores for the group with spasticity approached the normal to mild range. Scores for the two groups were nearly equivalent for several measures of phonation including *monoloudness, voice quality change, breathy voice, harsh voice, strained/strangled voice quality, consistent hypernasality,* and *nasal emission*. Individuals whose speech patterns were misidentified tended to show profiles attributed to the given diagnosis. Speakers with spasticity, whose speech patterns were misidentified as athetoid, showed greater involvement of articulation skills and were generally scored more severe overall than other subjects diag-

Table 4. Frequency of articulation errors in sentences for speakers by diagnostic category

	Type of error										
	Vowel error	Substitution	Omission	Addition	Pharyngeal fricative	Nasal emission	Dysfluency	Distortion	Voicing	Nasalization	Total
Spastic											
S_1	9	2	14	0	0	0	0	1	0	15	41
S_2	16	13	32	7	3	0	4	6	6	0	87
S_3	4	19	15	0	0	28	0	7	0	10	83
S_4	9	1	3	0	0	0	0	0	0	0	13
S_5	1	1	5	1	0	1	0	0	2	6	17
S_6	11	3	2	0	0	0	1	0	0	0	17
S_7	0	0	0	0	0	0	0	0	0	0	0
S_8	8	0	7	0	0	0	0	0	2	1	18
S_9	9	2	14	0	0	0	0	1	0	15	41
Group total	59	39	79	15	3	29	5	14	12	32	287
Percentage of total errors	20.6%	13.6%	27.5%	5.2%	1%	10.1%	1.7%	4.9%	4.2%	11.1%	
Athetoid											
A_1	30	21	26	3	0	0	4	0	9	1	94
A_2	3	9	23	2	0	2	0	5	7	0	51
A_3	18	2	9	9	0	0	0	1	10	5	54
A_4	9	6	2	18	0	0	8	0	29	2	74
A_5	9	1	28	1	2	0	0	0	0	0	41
A_6	8	6	23	1	0	1	1	4	3	0	47
A_7	7	8	10	1	0	0	0	0	6	0	32
A_8	5	2	2	6	0	0	0	0	0	1	16
A_9	25	15	5	13	0	0	0	0	5	0	63
Group total	114	70	128	54	2	3	13	10	69	9	472
Percentage of total errors	24.2%	14.8%	27.1%	11.4%	0.4%	0.6%	0.3%	0.2%	14.6%	1.9%	

nosed as spastic. Speakers with athetosis misdiagnosed as spastic showed less involvement of articulation skills than did most other speakers with athetosis.

Nevertheless, there seem to be clusters of dimensions that typify each group. The three highest-ranked and most characteristic dimensions for the group with spasticity related to resonant and laryngeal voice quality: *consistent hypernasality, breathy voice quality,* and *voice quality change.* Equivalents for the group with athetosis reflect difficulty with timing and coordination: *reduced stress, inappropriate voice stoppage or release,* and *slow rate.* Darley, Aronson, and Brown (1969, 1975) did not include individuals with congenital dysarthria in their subject pool. They did speculate, however, that speakers diagnosed with spastic cerebral palsy would evidence a spastic dysarthria, and those with athetoid cerebral palsy would evidence slow hyperkinetic dysarthria. Some individuals with spastic and hyperkinetic dysarthria in the Mayo Clinic study were diagnosed as having pseudobulbar palsy and dystonia (slow hyperkinesia). Comparison of the deviant dimensions that were uniquely characteristic of each group are listed:

Spastic
  Low pitch
  Hypernasality
  Pitch breaks
  Breathy voice
  Excess and equal stress
Slow Hyperkinesia
  Irregular articulatory breakdowns
  Inappropriate silences
  Prolonged intervals
  Prolonged phonemes
  Excessive loudness variation
  Voice stoppage

As with the present study, the majority of deviant dimensions characteristic of the group with spasticity in the Darley et al. (1969, 1975) study related to resonant and laryngeal voice production. Deviant dimensions most characteristic of the group with slow hyperkinesia reflected difficulty with timing and coordination, as was the case for the group with athetosis in this study.

Considering results of perceptual analysis in relation to a subsystems evaluation of speech mechanism suggests a different distribution of involvement for each group. Children diagnosed as having spastic diplegia or quadriplegia show primary involvement of functions implicating the respiratory, laryngeal, and velopharyngeal systems, with less involvement of the lips, tongue, and jaw. In contrast, children diagnosed as having athetosis show significant involvement of all speech subsystems, with articulatory dysfunction the most severe.

Clinical Observations

Bobath and Bobath (1975) describe very different developmental profiles for children with spasticity and those with athetosis regarding patterns of movement and achievement of motor milestones. They also advocate distinct approaches for therapeutic management of these two different groups. Clinical observation by the authors confirms perceptual findings of this study, which indicate differences between the dysarthrias of the two groups. The youngsters with spasticity tend to develop speech relatively early and have comparatively good articulation skills. As they grow, they spend increasing amounts of time in fixed positions, and tend to develop contractures that lead to flexed postures. Respiratory support for speech becomes increasingly impaired, and they experience increased difficulty with voice quality and intensity. Youngsters with athetosis experience considerable difficulty with control of the oral mechanism from birth. They are late to speak and are frequently unintelligible. Communication boards are frequently used to augment communication. As they grow and gain stability their speech improves, and may become intelligible in their teens or early adulthood.

Although perceptual differences have been demonstrated to exist between the two groups in this study, they are subtle. This may lead to the conclusion that because the differences are not major, children with either spastic or athetoid cerebral palsy and dysarthria can be treated as a homogeneous group. On the contrary, we suggest that the most important reason for distinguishing these groups is that different treatment approaches are needed for speech as they are for management of fine and gross motor deficits. The clinician working with this population of children with dysarthria should, of course, evaluate each youngster as an individual and design a program of treatment to fit that child's needs. With information confirming differences in nature of the dysarthrias in children with spastic and with athetoid cerebral palsy, appropriate treatment goals and long- and short-term objectives can be planned.

Implications for Clinical Research

On the basis of this data and previous reports, it seems that medical diagnosis of athetosis or spasticity can be made with greater ease and certainty than can differentiation of speech patterns in each group. Perhaps this disparity relates to the fact that, for the most part, we as speech pathologists measure the end product of movement, the speech signal, rather than the physical findings (e.g., reflexes and range of movement), that physicians use in diagnosis.

Results of the present study establish: 1) that experienced listeners are able to differentiate speakers with spasticity from those with athetosis, and 2) that perceptual differences exist between these groups. Since the group consisted of only 18 speakers, and there were only 4 listeners, it seems important to corroborate these results. Because a large number of variables were included, work with a smaller set of the more sensitive dimensions might better delineate the groups. Dimensions included in this study were based on previous research, and consideration could be given to dimensions not used in this study. Longitudinal acoustic and perceptual and physiologic studies of both groups are warranted to document the development of speech production. Physiologic measures are needed to corroborate the findings of acoustic analysis and to reveal differences in spastic and athetoid speakers. Treatment techniques must be evaluated systematically and objectively to determine their effectiveness.

REFERENCES

Achilles, R. (1955). Communicative anomalies of individuals with cerebral palsy. *Cerebral Palsy Review, 16*(5), 15–24.

American Psychiatric Association. (1980). *Diagnostic and statistical manual of mental disorders.* (3rd ed.). Washington, DC: Author.

Bax, M.C.O. (1964). Terminology and classification of cerebral palsy. *Developmental Medicine and Child Neurology. 6*, 295–297.

Blumberg, M. (1955). Respiration and speech in the cerebral palsied child. *American Journal of Disorders of Childhood, 89*, 48–53.

Bobath, B., & Bobath, K. (1975). *Motor development in the different types of cerebral palsy.* London: William Heinemann Medical Books Limited.

Bobath, K. (1980). *A neurophysiological basis for the treatment of cerebral palsy.* Lavenham, Suffolk, England: The Lavenham Press, Ltd.

Byrne, M. (1959). Speech and language development of athetoid and spastic children. *Journal of Speech and Hearing Research, 24*, 231–240.

Clement, M., & Twitchell, T. (1959). Dysarthria in cerebral palsy. *Journal of Speech and Hearing Disorders, 24*, 118–122.

Crothers, B., & Paine, R.J. (1959). *The natural history of cerebral palsy.* Cambridge, MA: Harvard University Press.

Darley, F.L., Aronson, A.E., & Brown, J.R. (1969). Differential diagnostic patterns of dysarthria. *Journal of Speech and Hearing Research, 12*, 246–269.

Darley, F.L., Aronson, A.E., & Brown, J.R. (1975). *Motor speech disorders.* Philadelphia: W.B. Saunders.

Dunn, L.M., and Dunn, L.M. (1981). *Peabody Picture Vocabulary Test — Revised.* Circle Pines, MN: American Guidance Service.

Farmer, A., & Lencione, R. (1977). An extraneous vocal behavior in cerebral palsied speakers. *British Journal of Disorders of Communication, 12,* 109–118.

Hardy, J.C. (1961). Intraoral breath pressure in cerebral palsy. *Journal of Speech and Hearing Disorders, 26,* 309–319.

Hardy, J.C. (1964). Lung function of athetoid and spastic quadriplegic children. *Developmental Medicine and Child Neurology, 6,* 378–388.

Hardy, J.C. (1983). *Cerebral palsy.* Englewood Cliffs, NJ: Prentice Hall.

Hedges, T.A. (1955). *The relationship between speech understandability and the diadochokinetic rates of certain speech musculatures among individuals with cerebral palsy.* Unpublished doctoral dissertation, Ohio State University, Columbus, OH.

Ingram, T.T.S., & Barn, J. (1961). A description and classification of common speech disorders associated with cerebral palsy. *Cerebral Palsy Bulletin, 3*(1), 57–69.

Irwin, O.C. (1955). Phonetic equipment of spastic and athetoid children. *Journal of Speech and Hearing Disorders, 20,* 54–57.

Kent, R., & Netsell, R. (1978). Articulatory abnormalities in athetoid cerebral palsy. *Journal of Speech and Hearing Disorders, 43,* 353–373.

Kent, R.D., Netsell, R., & Bauer, L.L. (1975). Cineradiographic assessment of articulatory mobility in the dysarthrias. *Journal of Speech and Hearing Disorders, 40,* 467–480.

Leith, W.R. (1954). *A comparison of judged speech characteristics of athetoids and spastics.* Unpublished master's thesis, Purdue University, West Lafayette, IN.

Lencione, R.M. (1953). *A study of the speech sound ability of a group of educable cerebral palsied children.* Unpublished doctoral dissertation, Northwestern University, Evanston, IL.

Neilson, P.D., & O'Dwyer, N.J. (1981). Pathophysiology of dysarthria in cerebral palsy. *Journal of Neurology, Neurosurgery and Psychiatry, 44,* 1013–1019.

Neilson, P.D., & O'Dwyer, N.J. (1984). Reproducibility and variability of speech muscle activity in athetoid dysarthria of cerebral palsy. *Journal of Speech and Hearing Research, 27,* 502–517.

Netsell, R. (1969). Evaluation of velopharyngeal function of dysarthria. *Journal of Speech and Hearing Disorders, 34,* 113–122.

Netsell, R. (1975). Kinesiologic observations of the dysarthrias. Paper presented to the Workshop on Speech Production and Perception, Stockholm, Sweden.

Netsell, R. (1978). *Speech motor control research in cerebral palsy.* Paper presented at the annual convention of the American Speech and Hearing Association, San Francisco, CA.

Paneth, N. & Kiely, J. (1984). The frequency of cerebral palsy: A review of population studies in industrialised nations since 1950. *Clinics in Developmental Medicine (87),* 46–56.

Platt, L.J., Andrews, G., Young, M., & Quinn, P.T. (1980). Dysarthria of adult cerebral palsy: I. Intelligibility and articulatory impairment. *Journal of Speech and Hearing Research, 23,* 28–40.

Rutherford, B.R. (1939). Frequency of articulation substitutions in children handicapped by cerebral palsy. *Journal of Speech and Hearing Disorders, 4,* 285–287.

Rutherford, B. (1944). A comparative study of loudness, pitch, rate, rhythm and quality of the speech of children handicapped by cerebral palsy. *Journal of Speech and Hearing Disorders, 9,* 263–271.

Seif, M., Netsell, R., & Kent, R. (1981). *Differences in the speech of children with spastic and athetoid cerebral palsy.* Unpublished manuscript, University of Wisconsin-Madison, Madison.

Shapiro, J. (1960). *An investigation of the ability of auditors to assess athetoid and spastic cerebral palsy by listening to speech samples.* Unpublished master's thesis, Syracuse University, Syracuse, NY.

Wolfe, W.G. (1950). A comprehensive evaluation of 50 cases of cerebral palsy. *Journal of Speech and Hearing Disorders, 15,* 234–251.

Dysarthria and Apraxia of Speech:
Perspectives on Management
edited by Christopher A. Moore, Ph.D., Kathryn M. Yorkston, Ph.D.,
and David R. Beukelman, Ph.D.
copyright © 1991   Paul H. Brookes Publishing Co., Inc.
Baltimore · London · Toronto · Sydney

Chapter 10

Dysarthria
in Progressive
Supranuclear Palsy

E. Jeffrey Metter and Wayne R. Hanson

PROGRESSIVE SUPRANUCLEAR PALSY (PSP) is a degenerative neurological disease in which speech disturbances are among the most common findings. A review of the literature, however, reveals that of the pertinent clinical signs, speech pathology is the least well described. PSP was first delineated as a clinicopathologic entity by Steele, Richardson, and Olszewski (1964). Main clinical features of this disease include supranuclear ophthalmoplegia, chiefly affecting vertical gaze, dystonic rigidity of the neck and upper trunk, and pseudobulbar palsy (Dix, Harrison, & Lewis, 1971). Patients with PSP often have parkinsonian manifestations such as bradykinesia, lack of facial expression, and poor postural reflexes (Hanson & Metter, 1980; Metter & Hanson, 1986; Steele, 1972). Unlike patients with Parkinson's disease, those with PSP tend to stand straight rather than stooped, may have a retroflexion of the neck, and may have a tendency to fall backward. Also, as a group PSP patients do not respond well to parkinsonian medications. Histologically, neuronal cell loss, gliosis, and neurofibrillary tangles are present in the brain stem, basal ganglia, and cerebellar nuclei. Marked atrophy of the midbrain and pontine tegmentum usually exist. These are not the pathologic findings in Parkinson's disease.

METHODS

Subjects

Fifteen consecutive patients who had complete neurologic examinations and were confirmed to have PSP were selected for study. All the PSP patients presented with movement disorders, including abnormalities in conjugate eye movements. In addition, each had a moderate to severe motor speech disturbance. The 15 PSP patients were male and had a mean age of 63 with a range from 54 to 76 years. The neurologic status of each patient was graded by a neurologist (EJM), and these findings are shown in Table 1. A number of patients showed positive signs of rigidity, spasticity, bradykinesia, and ataxia, with rigidity and bradykinesia the most prominent findings. These last two features are characteristic of parkinsonism.

Table 1. Description of patients with progressive supranuclear palsy (PSP)

Patient number	Age in years	Months duration	Dysarthria	Dysarthria severity rating[a]	Dysarthria prominent early	Early diagnosis
1	73	30	Spastic	7	Yes	Cerebellar degeneration
2	50	160	Hypokinetic	7	Yes	Parkinson's disease
3	59	24	Hypokinetic	7	—	Parkinson's disease
4	70	48	Spastic	5	—	—
5	63		Hypokinetic	4	No	Parkinson's disease
6	60	180	Hypokinetic	5	Yes	Parkinson's disease
7	62	36	Hypokinetic	6	No	Parkinson's disease
8	67	36	Hypokinetic	5	No	None
9	60	36	Spastic	7	Yes	—
10	69	170	Hypokinetic	7	Yes	Parkinson's disease
11	66	2	Spastic-ataxic	4	Yes	None
12	65	150	Hypokinetic	4	Yes	Parkinson's disease, stroke
13	63	110	Hypokinetic	7	Yes	Cerebellar degeneration
14	61	70	Hypokinetic	6	Yes	Parkinson's disease
15	67		Spastic	6		

— = not applicable; 0 = normal; 1 = mild; 2 = moderate; 3 = severe.
[a] 7-point interval scale in which 1 represents least severe and 7 represents most severe dysarthria.

Note the absence of tremor, the third characteristic feature of parkinsonism. Signs of spasticity indicate upper motor neuron involvement, seen with pseudobulbar palsy, and ataxia is the primary diagnostic indicator in patients with cerebellar disease. All patients had a dysarthria.

Speech Recordings

Perceptual speech measurements were made from recorded speech samples. Each audio sample was recorded with the speaker seated in a sound treated test room (IAC Model 403A) directly in front of a microphone (Electrovoice Model RE-15) that was coupled to an Ampex tape recorder (AE600B) located in an adjacent control room. The microphone-to-mouth distance was 20 cm. Prior to recording, a 1000 Hz calibration tone was read at the face of this microphone to provide a constant VU setting

Medications	Ataxia	Dyskinesia	Rigidity	Spasticity	Tremor	Bradykinesia
None	0	—	2	1	0	2
None	0	—	2	0	0	1
Phenobarbitol	—	—	3	—	0	2
—	—	—	2	—	—	—
—	0	0	1	0	0	1
Bromocriptine, amantadine	0	0	1	0	0	0
Sinemet, amantadine	0	0	2	0	0	2
None	0	0	2	1	0	—
None	1	0	1	1	0	—
Sinemet, Symmetrel	0	0	2	0	0	—
None	2	0	1	0	0	0
Sinemet	0	0	0	3	0	1
None	1	—	2	0	0	2
None	0	1	2	2	—	—

for both recording and playback of speech stimuli. Speech samples consisted of 3 minutes of conversation to the Job Task (Williams, Darley, & Spriestersbach, 1978). The first minute of each sample was used to make a listening tape.

Perceptual Assessment

Using procedures similar to those described by Darley, Aronson, and Brown (1975), the recorded speech samples of the PSP patients were played separately to 3 expert listeners (2 speech pathologists and a neurologist) who rated each of 38 speech dimensions (Darley et al., 1975) using a 7-point interval scale in which *1* represented normal speech and 7, extreme abnormality. A mean of the 3 ratings was determined as an index of the impairment of each speech attribute. Fifteen samples of connected speech, with 3 repeated for reliability measurement, were played in random order to each judge. Listeners were seated in a sound isolated test room 3 feet in front of an Ampex speaker (model 150G). When percentages of intra-judge agreement (+ or − 1 scale value) for two ratings of the 3 reliability samples were obtained, the lowest intra-judge agreement was 92%. When inter-judge agreement in the original 15 samples was similarly evaluated, the lowest agreement between judges was 86%. A Pearson *r* of 0.97 was obtained when the mean of the first and second ratings of each sample in the reliability group was studied. The intra-judge and inter-judge reliability indicated by these data appeared to be adequate for this investigation.

PERCEPTUAL RESULTS

The mean severity ratings of prominent speech dimensions in the 15 patients with PSP are ranked in Table 2. Speech dimensions with an average rating greater than 1.50 have been included. Table 2 shows prominence of the imprecise consonants dimension in dysarthria associated with PSP. Darley et al. (1975) found similarly high rankings for this dimension in other patient groups, including pseudobulbar palsy and cerebellar disorders. This dimension is not as prominent in patients with Parkinson's disease. The next dimensions are reduced stress, monopitch, and monoloudness, which together contribute substantially to the dysprosody heard in the speech of patients with PSP. The next set of features includes rate, phrases short, and intervals prolonged, which further indicate abnormalities in speech timing. These are followed by loudness overall, breathy voice, pitch level, and harsh voice, which are evidence of the extent of phonatory impairments in this group of patients.

In the present study, listener judges were asked to classify (Darley et al., 1975) the dysarthria of each speaker. Speakers were identified as hav-

Table 2. Speech dimensions prominent in patients with supranuclear palsy (PSP)

Rank	Dimension	Mean rating
1	Imprecise consonants	4.50
2	Reduced stress	4.10
3	Monopitch	3.78
4	Monoloudness	3.75
5	Rate	3.40
6	Phrases short	3.35
7	Intervals prolonged	3.27
8	Loudness overall	3.24
9	Breathy voice (continuous)	3.21
10	Pitch level	2.93
11	Harsh voice	2.75
12	Inappropriate silences	2.59
13	Phonemes prolonged	2.34
14	Hoarse (wet) voice	1.90
15	Short rushes of speech	1.88
16	Hypernasality	1.84
17	Strained/strangled voice	1.71
18	Loudness decay	1.61
19	Variable rate	1.60

ing predominantly hypokinetic dysarthria ($n = 10$), or predominantly spastic dysarthria ($n = 5$). Ataxic speech features were reported occasionally among patients in both the hypokinetic and spastic dysarthria groups. Tables 3 and 4 give the dimensions of speech judged to be most deviant in the two PSP subgroups. The most striking phenomena in the PSP hypokinetic subgroup (Table 3) are the prominence of 3 speech dimensions constituting prosodic abnormality or hypoprosody: reduced stress, monopitch, and monoloudness. In the PSP spastic subgroup, the most deviant speech dimensions are imprecise consonants and harsh voice. Perhaps the most characteristic perceptual change that occurs in the PSP spastic subgroup is hyperphonation. While not restricted to spastic dysarthria, hyperphonation is characteristic of this disorder. Although hypoprosody and hyperphonation are seen in both PSP subgroups, these categories serve to distinguish patients with predominant parkinsonian features from those who appear to be more pseudobulbar. Comparing speech characteristics of the two groups of PSP patients to speech characteristics of speakers with other dysarthrias as described by Darley et al. (1975), we see (Table 5) that hypokinetic PSP patients are similar to parkinsonian dysarthric patients for the first 3 dimensions (prosodic insufficiency) and for imprecise consonants. They differ in dimensions of timing. The spastic PSP group was similar to the pseudobulbar palsy group with the exception of phrases

Table 3. Speech dimensions prominent in patients with PSP and hypokinetic dysarthria

Rank	Dimension	Mean rating
1	Reduced stress	4.54
2	Monopitch	4.26
3	Monoloudness	4.26
4	Imprecise consonants	4.23
5	Rate	3.80
6	Loudness overall	3.67
7	Breathy voice (continuous)	3.54
8	Intervals prolonged	3.28
9	Phrases short	3.22
10	Pitch level	3.07
11	Inappropriate silence	2.52
12	Phonemes prolonged	2.41
13	Harsh voice	2.19
14	Short rushes of speech	2.09
15	Hypernasality	1.90
16	Loudness decay	1.82
17	Variable rate	1.68
18	Hoarse (wet) voice	1.66
19	Phonemes repeated	1.66

Table 4. Speech dimensions prominent in patients with PSP and spastic dysarthria

Rank	Dimension	Mean rating
1	Imprecise consonants	4.94
2	Harsh voice	3.88
3	Phrases short	3.62
4	Intervals prolonged	3.26
5	Reduced stress	3.06
6	Monopitch	2.82
7	Monoloudness	2.74
8	Inappropriate silence	2.74
9	Pitch level	2.66
10	Rate	2.60
11	Breathy voice (continuous)	2.54
12	Loudness overall	2.38
13	Hoarse (wet) voice	2.32
14	Strained/strangled	2.26
15	Phonemes prolonged	2.20
16	Hypernasality	1.72
17	Alternating loudness	1.54

Table 5. Ranked speech dimensions common to four neurological disorders

Dimensions	Disorders				
	PSP hypokinetic (N = 10)	PSP spastic (N = 5)	Parkinson's disease (N = 32)[a]	Pseudobulbar palsy (N = 30)	Cerebellar disorders (N = 30)
Reduced stress	1	5	2	3	8
Monopitch	2	6	1	2	9
Monoloudness	3	7	3	5	1
Imprecise consonants	4	1	4	1	
Rate	5	10		7	10
Loudness overall	6	12			
Breathy voice (continuous)	7	11	8	13	7
Intervals prolonged	8	4			
Phrases short	9	3		10	
Pitch level	10	9	9	6	
Inappropriate silence	11	8	5		
Phonemes prolonged	12	15			6
Harsh voice	13	2	7	4	5
Short rushes of speech	14		6		
Hypernasality	15	16		8	
Loudness decay	16				
Variable rate	17		10		
Hoarse (wet) voice	18	13			
Phonemes repeated	19				
Strained/strangled	20	14		9	

[a]Data for subject groups other than PSP are from the study of Darley, Aronson, and Brown (1975).

133

short, intervals prolonged, and inappropriate silences, which appear to be involved with timing and pause length. This suggests much longer pauses in the spastic PSP group than in the spastic dysarthria group.

CONCLUSIONS

As was expected from the neurologic findings, the dysarthria in patients with PSP contains components that resemble the dysarthria of patients with parkinsonism (hypokinetic), pseudobulbar palsy (spastic), and, to a lesser extent, cerebellar disorders (ataxic). Dysarthria in PSP apparently originates from multiple-system involvement within the nervous system with a mix of neurologic as well as speech symptoms. Thus it might be logical to call dysarthria in PSP a "mixed dysarthria" with two prominent components, hypokinetic and spastic, with ataxic dysarthria a less common feature. The combination and severity of symptoms vary, of course, from patient to patient.

Of the 10 PSP patients with prominent hypokinetic dysarthria, 8 had been diagnosed previously as having Parkinson's disease. In 5 of these 8, a prominent early feature of the illness was severe dysarthria. When dysarthria is a severe, early symptom in a parkinsonian illness, the likelihood that the illness is PSP may be increased. Another abnormal speech feature noted in PSP patients with predominant hypokinetic dysarthria was the frequent occurrence of palilalia. Cortical stuttering, or palilalia, has been described in other individuals, but in our population of PSP patients, this seemed to be a particularly prevalent symptom. It was not observed, however, in any of our PSP patients with primarily spastic dysarthria.

Rate of speech also distinguished spastic and hypokinetic PSP speakers. The hallmark of the spastic PSP speaker was a slow speaking rate, prolonged intervals, and rough, harsh voice. With hypokinetic speakers the hallmark was prosodic insufficiency with variable rate, high pitch, and some breathiness, and they may have a normal speaking rate, slower than normal rate, or faster than normal rate. In PSP patients with spastic dysarthria, vocal roughness tended to have a more pronounced strained/strangled quality. PSP patients with hypokinetic dysarthria had less severe roughness that tended toward breathiness in connected speech. Occasional swells in vocal loudness were heard in the spastic PSP speakers but not in those with hypokinetic dysarthria. Prominence of the dysphonia can be explained neurophysiologically by the presence of positive spastic findings in PSP. These findings indicate involvement of cortical bulbar pathways (upper motor neuron) in this disease that result in laryngeal hypertonus and spastic dysarthria symptoms.

The severity of dysarthria in PSP patients appears to be influenced more by prosodic changes than by other speech differences. Our results indicate that lesions in various portions of the central nervous system will have different and definable effects on speech, particularly the prosodic features of speech. Particular centers and pathways in the human motor system appear to be responsible for particular components of prosody. Prosodic patterns that are markedly abnormal contribute significantly to the bizarreness of PSP speakers. Because normal prosody requires precise coordination of all speech processes, PSP dysarthric speakers are particularly susceptible to deficits in this area. These abnormalities, however, have not been described previously. Normal stress patterns are thought to be achieved by a combination of fundamental frequency shifts, loudness variations, and durational adjustments. A normal speaker may use any or all of these strategies, probably relying most heavily on fundamental frequency adjustments (Lehiste, 1970). One can speculate that, because of the extent of ataxia in cerebellar disorders and PSP, these patients would attempt to compensate for articulatory incoordination by slowing their speech to produce each syllabic unit in a controlled pattern of prosodic excess.

The dimensions of reduced stress, monopitch, and monoloudness are the three dominant speech characteristics in both Parkinson's disease and pseudobulbar palsy. Because of rigidity and akinesia in Parkinson's disease, and spastic weakness in pseudobulbar palsy, patients with these diseases are apparently unable to alter pitch and loudness to produce normal stress and intonation patterns, resulting in insufficient prosody. Since both spasticity and rigidity are part of the clinical description of PSP, it stands to reason that prosodic insufficiency would be prominent in PSP.

In the process of rating the severity of the dysarthria in each PSP subject, the listener judges heard sound intrusions that were difficult to describe. Sounds resembling throat clearing, tongue clicking, and other extraneous noises were heard frequently in most of the speakers with PSP. These inappropriate sound additions in the ongoing speech of PSP speakers may have diagnostic importance in separating these patients from those with other neurologic diseases such as Parkinson's disease.

Characterizing the speech of PSP patients differentiates them from normal speakers and from other dysarthric groups. Study of patterns of speech impairment in individual PSP patients leads to awareness of the variability between speakers. Variable patterns of impairment in individuals, and perhaps, in subgroups of individuals, are important to consider in planning treatment or in establishing baselines from which to measure change. The extent of individual variation in speech parameters suggests that either PSP motoric speech abnormalities differ or individuals use different compensatory strategies. It may be that our search for the sources of individual variation among PSP speakers may lead us to a more complete understanding of the neuropathology that underlies this disorder.

REFERENCES

Darley, F.L., Aronson, A.E., & Brown, J.R. (1975). *Motor speech disorders.* Philadelphia: W.B. Saunders.

Dix, M.R., Harrison, M.S.G., & Lewis, P.D. (1971). Progressive supranuclear palsy (the Steele-Richardson-Olszewski syndrome): A report of nine cases with particular reference to the mechanism of the oculomotor disorder. *Journal of the Neurologic Sciences, 13,* 237–256.

Hanson, W.R., & Metter, E.J. (1980). DAF as instrumental treatment for dysarthria in progressive supranuclear palsy: A case report. *Journal of Speech and Hearing Disorders, 45,* 268–275.

Lehiste, I. (1970). *Suprasegmentals* (p. 194). Cambridge, MA: MET Press.

Metter, E.J., & Hanson, W.R. (1986). Clinical and acoustical variability in hypokinetic dysarthria. *Journal of Communication Disorders, 19,* 347–366.

Steele, J.C., (1972). Progressive supranuclear palsy. *Brain, 95,* 693–704.

Steele, J.C., Richardson, J.C., & Olszewski, J. (1964). Progressive supranuclear palsy. *Archives of Neurology, 10,* 333–359.

Williams, D. Darley, F., & Spriestersbach, D. (1978). Appraisal of rate and fluency. In F. Darley & D. Spriesterbach (Eds.), *Diagnostic methods in speech pathology* (2nd ed.). New York: Harper & Row.

Dysarthria and Apraxia of Speech:
Perspectives on Management
edited by Christopher A. Moore, Ph.D., Kathryn M. Yorkston, Ph.D.,
and David R. Beukelman, Ph.D.
Paul H. Brookes Publishing Co., Inc.
Baltimore · London · Toronto · Sydney

Chapter 11

Speech and Prosodic Problems in Children with Neurofibromatosis

Donald A. Robin and Michele J. Eliason

NEUROFIBROMATOSIS (NF) IS a relatively common disorder, affecting 1 in 3,000 individuals (Riccardi & Eichner, 1986). There are multiple forms of NF, but the focus of this chapter is von Recklinghausen's or NF1, which is the most common. NF1 is a chronic progressive disorder with highly variable physical manifestations that include multiple café-au-lait spots (flat, hyperpigmented skin lesions with no associated morbidity), neurofibromas (benign tumors arising from nerve tissue that can occur anywhere in or on the body), and plexiform lesions (benign tumors with vascular and nervous tissue involvement). These three manifestations of NF1 can be quite disfiguring as well as producing functional consequences, such as limited joint mobility.

Central nervous system lesions occur in 15% of individuals with NF1. The central nervous system manifestation of tumors is variable. Neurofibromas can occur in the brain or spinal cord. Optic gliomas represent the most common CNS tumor and affect 10%–15% of individuals with NF1. Most optic gliomas are asymptomatic and slow growing. Other CNS tumor types have been found in individuals with NF1 and include schwannomas, astrocytomas, and meningiomas. Seizure disorders occur in 5% of the NF1 population.

The diagnosis of NF1 is based on family history and the presence of neurocutaneous lesions: café-au-lait spots (Figure 1), and neurofibromas (Figure 2). Café-au-lait spots are often present at birth and may increase in

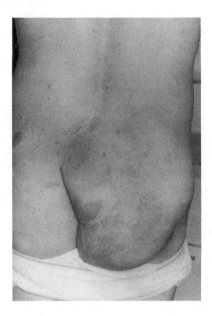

Figure 1. Patient with café-au-lait spots and a large plexiform lesion on the right buttock.

size and number, but neurofibromas are more likely to develop later in life. Often neurofibromas first appear at adolescence triggered by pubertal changes, and continue to increase in size and number through adulthood. Plexiform lesions (Figure 1) are benign tumors with considerable underlying tissue and vascular involvement. Like other neurofibromas, they can occur anywhere on the body.

The presence of nonverbal learning disability may signal central nervous system involvement. Riccardi (1984) reported that 30% of the Baylor University NF1 patient sample presented with learning disability characterized by distractibility, impulsivity, and poor visual-motor coordination. Eliason (1986) found that performance scores were poorer than verbal scores in a group of children with NF1. In a follow-up study, Eliason (1988) found that NF1 children scored particularly poorly on visual perception tests. Comparison of the NF1 group to a group of children with developmental learning disability (DLD) suggested that the DLD group was impaired on verbal/language-based tasks, while the NF1 group was impaired primarily on nonverbal tasks (Eliason, 1988). These findings of poor nonverbal and spatial skills have been replicated by Eldridge et al. (1989), and Varnhagen et al. (1988).

There has been little examination of speech production abilities of individuals with NF1. Pollack and Shprintzan (1981) reported that patients with NF1 were hypernasal, but did not have structural aberrations

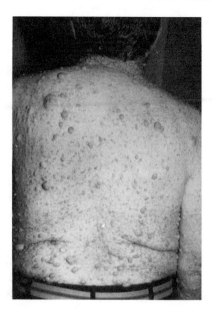

Figure 2. Patient with multiple neurofibromas.

to account for this attribute. Accordingly, they suggested that the hypernasal speech was neural in origin.

Other reports of NF1 speech are anecdotal. Riccardi (1982) noted that NF1 patients often have speech problems, in particular, a lack of affect. Individuals who encounter NF1 patients in the clinic often comment on the lack of emotion in their speech and their "flat" speaking style. Clinic nurses and staff often comment that the individual with NF1 is "hard to understand." We are aware of no studies on the prosodic characteristics of the speech of these individuals, although their abnormal prosody has been noted clinically.

This chapter represents a preliminary description of speech production and prosodic characteristics of children diagnosed as having NF1. It was hypothesized that speech characteristics would be consistent with a diagnosis of dysarthria, and prosodic abnormalities would be characteristic of these speakers. This prediction was based on the anecdotal reports of "flat speech" by professionals with many years of experience.

METHOD

Subjects

Four male and three female children (5–16 years old) with NF1 agreed to undergo speech and prosodic evaluations. Six control speakers ages 6–11 were also tested. Individuals were diagnosed as having NF1 by a clinical geneticist based on the presence of multiple café-au-lait spots, neurofibromas, and other clinical features of NF1. Some children also had a familial history of NF1. All the children with NF1 had received neuropsychological evaluations prior to the study, and all had symptoms of nonverbal learning disability (see Eliason, 1988) with verbal scores higher than performance scores. Full scale IQ scores ranged from 85 to 102.

Clinical Speech Evaluation

Clinical evaluation included assessment of the structure and movement of speech mechanisms. We also administered the Templin-Darley Test of Articulation (1969) and made informal ratings of intelligibility. All testing was conducted by two certified speech-language pathologists with experience in neurogenic speech disorders. Judgments of intelligibility and nasality during conversational speech were also made by the clinicians. In addition, diadochokinetic rates were obtained for the syllable /p ʌ/, /t ʌ/, /k ʌ/, and /p ʌ t ʌ k ʌ/. Data on fundamental frequency (Fo), Fo range, and vocal tremor were obtained using the Kay Visi-Pitch.

Prosodic Evaluation

Prosodic evaluation followed our previously described method (Klouda, Robin, Graff-Radford, & Cooper, 1987; Robin, Klouda, & Hug, in press). This method has been used in testing prosodic ability in children with normal speech and in those with speech disorders (Robin, Hall, & Jordan, 1987).

The assessment examines the ability to produce sentences using a variety of intonation and stress patterns. The first test elicits intonation patterns by asking subjects to speak with happy, sad, angry, questioning, and neutral intonation patterns. The first three intonations are considered emotive, and the others, linguistic. Four sentences were used, so that 20 utterances per subject were evaluated on this portion of the prosodic test. Sentences used for this intonation test were:

1. The bird flew away.
2. Tomorrow I'm leaving for Chicago.
3. My horse jumped over the fence.
4. We sold our cottage last month.

These were chosen because of their affective neutrality and because they could be rendered with different affective tones. Subjects were asked to read the sentence aloud and then in one of the intonations. Younger children imitated the clinician's model of the sentence in a neutral pattern and then repeated it in a given intonation pattern.

The second test was designed to produce stress patterns, specifically in the initial and final positions and a neutral version as well. Stress patterns were elicited by having subjects read the following sentences:

1. Don shot the puck to Kent.
2. Sheila took the money from Chip.
3. Stan paid the check for Peg.
4. The salesman sold the couch to my father.
5. Mary typed the paper for Kate.
6. Chuck ate supper with George.

A set of three primary questions were used to elicit stress patterns. For example, questions used with Sentence 1 were:

1. What happened? (neutral pattern)
2. Who shot the puck to Kent? (word initial stress)
3. Who did Don shoot the puck to? (word final stress)

Younger subjects were asked to imitate a sentence in a neutral tone and then repeat the sentence following a stimulus question. A priming question was asked to elicit initial stress (Who shot the puck to Kent?), final stress (Who did Don shoot the puck to?), or neutral stress (What happened?). Thus this test included three patterns per sentence and a total of 18 utterances per subject.

All utterances were recorded with a high-quality cassette recorder using an electrostatic microphone on a head mount to ensure a 15 cm microphone-to-mouth distance. Utterances for each test were obtained in random order.

Each subject's responses were combined in random order on tapes. Intonational utterances were on one tape and stress utterances on another. A group of five listeners judged the recorded stimuli using a forced-choice paradigm. Listeners noted if sentence intonation was happy, sad, angry, questioning, or neutral. Listeners also noted stress as initial, medial, final, or neutral.

RESULTS

Speech Production

The speech mechanism examination revealed symptoms consistent with a diagnosis of dysarthria. There were three major findings in the articulatory system. First, all children produced imprecise consonants. Inaccurate production of consonants were largely distortions, although there were also substitutions. Distortions occurred in word-initial positions on /br/,

/tr/, /fr/, and /str/. Substitutions occurred in all word positions. Initial position substitutions included w/r, f/θ, d/ð, and θ/z. Medial position substitutions were the same, with the inclusion of ʤ/z. Final position substitutions included f/θ, v/ð, and ʧ/ʃ. Consonant errors occurred approximately 20% in single words elicited from the articulation test. This imprecision did not have a major effect on intelligibility since all 7 subjects with NF1 were rated as 80% intelligible or better with context known. No structural anomalies could account for the consonant imprecision. All 7 NF1 children had a visible tremor of the tongue at rest and during movement. The mean rate of repetitions for single syllables was 2.8 per second for /pʌ/ (normal, 3.7 per second), 1.2 per second for /tʌ/ (normal, 3.9 per second, and 1.1 per second for /kʌ/. Mean repetition rate for the trisyllable /pʌtʌkʌ/ was 0.87 per second (normal, 3.2 per second).

Three of the seven children had mild hypernasal speech, particularly in conversation. All 7 had visible tremor of the soft palate. No structural anomalies of the palate were noted to account for hypernasality.

All 7 also had pronounced vocal tremor. When analyzed on the Visi-Pitch, the tremor in all occurred at 4Hz–5Hz. Six had decreased pitch range (<1.25 octaves), and four had a hoarse vocal quality. Two had decreased loudness levels in conversation.

Prosody

Listeners correctly identified more than 90% of the intonational utterances and more than 80% of the stress sentences of the normal speakers. By contrast, only 55% of intonational sentences of NF1 children were correctly identified. Neutral intonation was identified correctly 89% of the time, questioning, 62%, and emotive utterances fell far below this: happy, 35%; sad, 48%; angry, 38%. Intonations were most often perceived by listeners as neutral intonation. Thus, normal production of neutral utterances by the NF1 group was due to their generally monotone intonation.

Results for stress production show that listeners perceived the NF1 group correctly only 49%. As with normal speakers, the NF1 children were most accurate in producing sentence initial stress and least accurate at final and neutral versions. For the NF1 children, listeners correctly identified 61% of initial stress patterns, 45% of final stress patterns, and 42% of the neutral patterns.

Error analyses reveal that when initial stress was intended, listeners perceived final stress more often than neutral or medial, although neutral and medial forms were also heard in NF1 speakers. When final stress was intended, listeners heard neutral forms, although initial and medial stress were noted occasionally. When neutral stress was intended, listener errors were equally distributed, and the NF1 group produced initial, final, and medial stress patterns.

CONCLUSIONS

NF1 is a common neurogenetic disorder, but its behavioral aspects have not been well studied, and the impact of the disorder on speech has never been studied. This preliminary description of speech and prosodic ability of seven children with NF1 suggest that systematic study is needed. The prominence of tremor in the speech production mechanisms of all 7 NF1 children is indicative of nervous system involvement. Moreover, all children had articulation errors, primarily distortions. Some of the children were hypernasal, and most had abnormal vocal qualities and reduced pitch ranges. These findings suggest that individuals with NF1 are at risk for dysarthria, which may affect one or more of the speech production subsystems.

Performances of NF1 children on the prosodic tests are also noteworthy. The NF1 children were quite impaired in their ability to convey emotional (e.g., happy) or linguistic (e.g., interrogative, stressed) information by changes in prosodic patterns to adult listeners. On intonation tests, listeners perceived that NF1 children produced neutral speech patterns. This supports frequent anecdotal reports that the speech of individuals with NF1 seems "flat and lacks melody." On the stress test, however, errors did not always involve neutral stress patterns. In fact, these children frequently placed stress on the wrong word in a sentence, making communicative intent difficult to understand or adding a strange quality to speech.

The data, with those on nonverbal learning in NF1 children (Eliason, 1988), show a constellation of cognitive and speech patterns characterized by spatial difficulties, neuromotor speech production problems, and an impaired ability to accurately convey prosodic intent in both linguistic and emotive contexts. Thus, children with NF1 appear to have difficulty conveying and interpreting nonverbal social cues. Unlike verbal/language disabilities, this may have a greater impact on social relationships than on academic achievement. For instance, a study by Eliason (1988) found that children with NF1 had nearly normal reading and spelling achievements, but had poor study skills and independent work habits in the classroom. Parents of children with NF1 report that their children are impulsive, do not interpret or convey moods accurately, stand too close, and have difficulty making and keeping friends (Eliason, 1988).

In summary, our data suggest that more research is needed on the speech and language capabilities of individuals with NF1. It is our experience that the prosodic problems in these children are often undiagnosed and untreated. We would urge clinicians to evaluate carefully speech production and prosody in individuals with NF1 and to initiate treatment. We hypothesize that speech-language intervention might lessen the social problems these children experience.

REFERENCES

Eldridge, R., Denckla, M.B., Bien, E., Myers, S., Kaiser-Kupfer, M.I., Pikus, A., Schlesinger, S.L., Parry, D.M., Danbrosia, J.M., Zasloff, M.A., & Mulvihill, J.J. (1989). Neurofibromatosis type 1. *American Journal of Diseases of Children, 143,* 833–837.

Eliason, M.J. (1986). Neurofibromatosis: Implications for learning and behavior. *Journal of Developmental and Behavioral Pediatrics, 7,* 175–181.

Eliason, M.J. (1988). Neuropsychological profiles: Neurofibromatosis compared to developmental learning disability. *Neurofibromatosis, 1,* 17–25.

Klouda, G.V., Robin, D.A., Graff-Radford, N.R., & Cooper, W.E. (1987). The role of callosal connections in speech prosody. *Brain and Language, 35,* 154–171.

Pollack, M.A., & Shprintzan, R.J. (1981). Velopharyngeal insufficiency in neurofibromatosis. *International Journal of Pediatric Otorhinolaryngology, 3,* 257.

Riccardi, V.M. (1982). The multiple form of neurofibromatosis. *Pediatrics in Review, 3,* 293–298.

Riccardi, V.M. (1984). Neurofibromatosis as a model for investigating hereditary versus environmental factors in learning disabilities. In M. Arima, Y. Suzuki, & M. Yabuuchi (Eds.), *The developing brain and its disorders.* Tokyo: University of Tokyo Press.

Riccardi, V.M., & Eichner, J.E. (1986). *Neurofibromatosis: Phenotype, natural history, and pathogenesis.* Baltimore: Johns Hopkins University Press.

Robin, D.A., Hall, P.K., & Jordan, L.S. (1987, November). *Prosodic impairment in developmental verbal apraxia.* Paper presented at the annual meeting of the American Speech, Language, and Hearing Association, New Orleans.

Robin, D.A., Klouda, G.V., & Hug, L.N. (in press). Neurogenic disorders of prosody. In M.P. Cannito & D. Vogel (Eds.), *Treating disordered speech motor control: For clinicians by clinicians.* Austin, TX: PRO-ED.

Templin, M., & Darley, F.L. (1969). *The Templin-Darley Test of Articulation* (2nd ed.). Iowa City: University of Iowa Bureau of Educational Research and Service.

Varnhagen, C.K., Lewin, S., Das, J.P., Bowen, P., Ma, K., & Klinak, M. (1988). Neurofibromatosis and psychological processes. *Developmental Medicine and Child Neurology, 9,* 257–265.

Dysarthria and Apraxia of Speech:
Perspectives on Management
edited by Christopher A. Moore, Ph.D., Kathryn M. Yorkston, Ph.D.,
and David R. Beukelman, Ph.D.
copyright © 1991   Paul H. Brookes Publishing Co., Inc.
Baltimore · London · Toronto · Sydney

SECTION IV

PHYSIOLOGY

A WIDE ARRAY of physiologic measures and treatment are used to describe disorders of speech motor control. This battery of electromyographic, kinematic, acoustic, aerodynamic, and perceptual techniques is applied in differential diagnosis, treatment, clinical trials, and basic description. Because of the adaptability of speech systems, and sometimes contrary to perceptual clinical judgment, dysarthric or apraxic speakers may demonstrate coordinative behavior that is remarkably inconsistent with their speech signs. For example, mildly dysarthric speakers may manifest severely limited control of speech subsystems during continuous speech, or they may exhibit marked deficiencies in nonspeech strength and endurance. Physiologic symptoms can occur with varying speech effects and may be apparent only through specific observations and analytic methods. Nevertheless, measurements such as those in this section provide the foundation for understanding the mechanisms underlying motor speech disorders, as well as a distinct frame of reference for understanding treatment effects and diagnostic decisions.

Chapter 12

Kinematic, Electromyographic, and Perceptual Evaluation of Speech Apraxia, Conduction Aphasia, Ataxic Dysarthria, and Normal Speech Production

Karen Forrest, Scott Adams,
Malcolm R. McNeil, and Helen Southwood

APRAXIA OF SPEECH (AOS) is described clinically by phoneme distortions (Odell, McNeil, Hunter, & Rosenbek, 1990) and substitutions (La Pointe & Johns, 1975), groping articulatory behavior (Johns & Darley, 1970), difficulty in utterance initiation (Kent & Rosenbek, 1983; Robin, Bean, & Folkins, 1989), and inconsistent production errors, especially during extended or complex sequences (Kent & Rosenbek, 1983). To some theorists, these error patterns suggest an impairment in speech motor control (Rosenbek, Kent, & LaPointe, 1984), while others interpret these

This research was supported by NINCDS Grant NS18797, NINCDS Core Grant 5030 HD03352, and NIDCD DC00783. We wish to express our appreciation to Dr. Claudia Blair, Dr. Michael Caligiuri, Ann Fennell, Dr. Linda Hunter, Ruth Martin, Dr. E. Jeffrey Metter, Dr. John C. Rosenbek, and Dr. Gary Weismer for assistance with this study.

clinical descriptions as manifestations of a phoneme selection or sequencing disorder (Martin, 1974). It is difficult to resolve this disparity in theoretical perspectives of AOS because the divergence may represent a philosophical, not empirical, schism and because of the paucity of empirical data on which to base a motor control interpretation. Few common features emerge from the available data on articulatory control in AOS. For example, Itoh et al. (Itoh & Sasanuma, 1987; Itoh, Sasanuma, Hirose, Yoshioka, & Ushijima, 1980; Itoh, Sasanuma, & Ushijima, 1979) found reduced articulatory velocity among apraxic subjects, whereas McNeil et al. (McNeil & Adams, 1990; McNeil, Caliguiri, & Rosenbek, 1989) and Robin, Bean, and Folkins (1989) found no such velocity differences between normal and apraxic speakers. McNeil and Adams (1990) found differences in the slope of the function relating peak velocity to peak amplitude in apraxic versus normal subjects, but Robin et al. (1989) report no differences between groups in this respect.

Researchers agree that interarticulator coordination is aberrant in apraxic speakers (e.g., Kent & Rosenbek, 1983), although not all investigations have provided data to substantiate this claim (Robin et al., 1989). Disturbances in coordination of the sub-systems involved in speech production have been identified in apraxic speakers. For example, voicing errors are a common feature of apraxic speech. Several researchers have shown distortions of voice onset time (VOT) in apraxic speakers (Blumstein, Cooper, Goodglass, Statlender, & Gottlieb, 1980; Blumstein, Cooper, Zurif, & Caramazza, 1977; Itoh et al., 1980; Kent & Rosenbek, 1983). Word-final voicing, as indexed by duration of the preceding vowel, has been investigated to a lesser extent in AOS (Blumstein & Baum, 1987; Duffy & Gawle, 1984), but appears to be controlled much like that in normal speakers. The relation between voicing and movement initiation and termination may provide insight into the coordination between phonatory and articulatory control, but this has not been explored.

Generalization to other apraxic speakers from existing data on articulatory and phonatory control may be inappropriate for reasons beyond variations in investigative findings. In general, studies of AOS have relied on small numbers of subjects (e.g., a single subject in the work of Itoh et al.). This is surprising given the variability both within and across apraxic speakers (Kent & Rosenbek, 1983; Munhall, 1989). However, the incidence of AOS without accompanying aphasia or dysarthria appears low, so that ideal subjects are difficult to identify. For this reason, some investigations have included speakers with aphasia (e.g., Itoh & Sasanuma, 1987), which complicates interpretation because the basis for separating aphasia from AOS is unclear. Although apraxia of speech is viewed by many as distinct from aphasia, few direct comparisons of articulatory behavior have been made between the two groups (Itoh & Sasanuma, 1987; McNeil & Adams, 1990). Similarly, AOS is distinct from dysarthria in that apraxic speakers do not demonstrate maximum force deficits commonly associated with dysarthria, but comparisons of articulatory behavior of these speakers are few (but see McNeil & Adams, 1990). In short, existing data do not permit clear statements as to whether the articulatory disturbances noted in AOS are: 1) unique to individual apraxic speakers and/or 2) uniquely related to AOS and not related to general neurological impairment.[1]

In addition, no data have been reported on the relation between physiologic abnormalities in AOS and apraxic qualities perceived in speech, and so it is difficult to ascribe meaning to movement or muscle abnormalities. Speakers vary widely in producing articulatory gestures for any given sequence (Munhall, 1989). Unless it can be shown that certain types of movements or muscle activity patterns lead to perceived abnormalities in a person's speech, the importance of physiologic data in understanding speech pathologies is limited.

We investigated patterns of lip movement and associated muscle activity for apraxic, conduction aphasic, ataxic dysarthric, and normal adults. Because previous research has shown that AOS (Kent & Rosenbek, 1983) and limb apraxia (Poizner, Mack, Verfaellie, Rothi, & Heilman, 1990) are characterized by disturbances in the production of transitions, we chose to investigate some time-varying aspects of movement. Likewise, on the basis of previous research (Fromm, Abbs, McNeil, & Rosenbek, 1982) we have indexed muscle coordination by patterns of contraction: reciprocal, antagonistic cocontraction, and incidental co-contraction. This index of muscle activity was chosen because differences in these patterns found by previous research have been suggested to: "illustrate very powerfully the neurophysiological calculation errors which are at the basis of the articulatory errors of [apraxic] patients" (Keller, 1987, p. 153). Finally, the relation between kinematic and electromyographic findings and perceived AOS was investigated to determine whether physiologic differences between groups and/or speakers had perceptual consequences.

---

[1]Although Fromm, Abbs, McNeil, and Rosenbek (1982) state that their data were compared to ataxic dysarthrics, it is difficult to assess these comparisons. Of the papers cited to have data on ataxic dysarthria, only one is available and presents data from only one ataxic speaker. Further, the most notable feature of those data (Abbs, Hunker, & Barlow, 1983, Figures 2–15) is the clear co-contraction of OOI and DLI, a pattern that Fromm et al. claim is a causal feature of apraxic speech disturbances ("This apraxic subject began to lose control during the third bilabial stop due to antagonist cocontraction. . . " p. 166).

METHODS

Subjects

Sixteen adults, fourteen males and two females, served as subjects in this investigation (see McNeil & Adams, 1990; McNeil, Weismer, et al.,1990). All spoke English as their primary language and had speech discrimination of at least 70% in one ear with live voice presentation of a PB 50 word list presented at 40 dB HL. Prior to participation in this investigation, a battery of tests was administered to each potential subject to determine if he or she met inclusion criteria for one of the four groups: speech apraxic, conduction aphasic, ataxic dysarthric, or neurologically normal. Tests administered to individuals included a structural-function evaluation, Coloured Progressive Matrices (Raven, 1962), Word Fluency Measure (Borkowski, Benton, & Spreen, 1967), Porch Index of Communicative Ability (Porch, 1967), Revised Token Test (McNeil & Prescott, 1978), Boston Diagnostic Aphasia Examination (Goodglass & Kaplan, 1972) for speech and auditory comprehension, and Apraxia Battery for Adults (Dabul, 1979).

Apraxic Speakers Four men, 54–72 years of age who had speech characteristics consistent with AOS (Kent & Rosenbek, 1983) without concomitant dysarthria or aphasia (Darley, 1982) as judged by two certified speech-language pathologists constituted the apraxic group. Performance on the assessment battery revealed no weakness or incoordination of speech musculature for nonspeech activities, articulatory agility, melodic line and phrase length, and ratings of 1–4 on the Boston Diagnostic Aphasia exam, scores at or above the first percentile for normal subjects on the average of subtests II, III, V, VI, VII, VIII, X, and XI on the Porch Index, and a score of at least 22 on the Coloured Progressive Matrices.

Conduction Aphasic Speakers The conduction aphasic speakers were four men between the ages of 48 and 66 who did not present signs of accompanying dysarthria or apraxia as defined above. In addition to frequent sound substitutions in repeated, compared with spontaneous, speech, speakers were diagnosed as conduction aphasic if they had articulatory agility, and phrase length and melodic line ratings between 4 and 7 on the Boston Diagnostic Aphasia exam. (The data for three speakers only is included because the fourth speaker did not produce any on-target utterances for the test phrases and condition presented in the current report data.)

Ataxic Dysarthric Speakers Two men and two women between 32 and 55 years, with neurologic histories consistent with cerebellar lesion or disease and speech consistent with ataxic dysarthria (Darley, Aronson, & Brown, 1975), served as subjects. In addition to a neurologic examination, the dysarthric speakers were assessed by two speech-language pathologists and met the linguistic and cognitive criteria described for the apraxic speakers.

Normal Control Speakers Four neurologically normal men between 57 and 69 years served as control speakers. They had no histories of speech, language, or neurologic disorders and scored within normal limits on all the speech, language, cognitive, and neurologic screening tests.

Speech Sample

The speech sample included 40 sentences and phrases. Each utterance was presented from tape through loudspeaker, and the speaker repeated the utterance at his or her normal rate. Utterances were presented five times each in random order. In this chapter, only the data from the utterance, "Buy Bobby a poppy," were used.

Procedure

Kinematic and Electromyographic Data Inferior-superior movement of the upper and lower lips and jaw were transduced by strain gauges attached to the articulatory structures by cantilever beams. The beams were bonded to the speakers' lips at the midline of the vermilion border and posterior to the mental symphysis at a placement that was influenced minimally by tongue or labial movement. The strain gauge system was attached to an aluminum headmount (Barlow, Cole, & Abbs, 1983).

Bipolar hook-wire electrodes were used to record activity of orbicularis oris superior (OOS), orbicularis oris inferior (OOI), depressor labii inferior (DLI), and anterior belly of digastric (ABD).[2] Electrode placements were consistent with the procedures outlined in Kennedy and Abbs (1979) and a series of speech and nonspeech movements were elicited to verify placement in the targeted muscles.

Speech was transduced with a Sony unidirectional microphone, which was placed approximately 6 cm from the speaker's mouth. This signal, along with the kinematic and electromyographic data, were recorded (Honeywell 5600C FM recorder) and subsequently low-pass filtered and digitized on a desktop computer using a CSpeech and waveform

---

[2]In this study, OOI and DLI were studied as antagonists, as in Fromm et al., 1982. This seemed appropriate because the data indicated that lower lip elevation occurred subsequent to OOI activation, and labial depression followed DLI activity. It should be noted, however, that McClean, Goldsmith, and Cerf (1984) have provided data to suggest that OOI may be more involved in lip protruding than in elevation and, as such, OOI and DLI may not be the best choices for investigating antagonist co-contraction. As an additional caveat to the present data, Blair and Smith (1986) demonstrated a clear interdigitation of OOI and DLI fibers. It is therefore possible that activity from these antagonist muscles was recorded by the same electrode. Although this possibility exists, neither the electrode placement maneuvers prior to the experiment or the resulting data suggest that activity from antagonist muscles was recorded by a single electrode.

editing program. Sampling rates were 1.5 kHz for each movement and EMG channel, as well as for the acoustic speech signal. Anti-aliasing filters were set at half the sampling rate.

Perceptual Data A metric of the perceived magnitude of each speaker's apraxia was obtained to relate movement and muscle activity patterns to the apraxic "quality" of each speaker. Although only four speakers had AOS, the identifying characteristics of this disorder in terms of movement and muscle activity were the focus of this investigation. It is for this reason that information on the perceived magnitude of AOS was desired. A direct magnitude estimate was chosen to evaluate the degree of AOS. Two stimulus tapes were prepared with all repetitions of each apraxic, dysarthric, and normal speaker's utterances. Adequate recordings were available for one conduction aphasic only, and his utterances were included in the perception tape. A modulus was chosen for each tape and assigned an arbitrary value of 100. In an effort to minimize bias associated with modulus selection, one tape used a moderately apraxic speaker as the modulus, and the second tape used a dysarthric speaker. Twenty-five percent of the tokens were repeated for estimates of intra-listener reliability. All tokens were used for calculation of Cronbach's alpha, a measure used to determine inter-listener reliability.

Six speech-language pathologists experienced with neurologically impaired speakers served as listeners. Their task was to scale the magnitude of apraxic speech for each utterance relative to the modulus. Listeners were free to use their own definitions of AOS, but were informed that speakers included apraxic, conduction aphasic, ataxic dysarthric, and neurologically normal adults. Numbers greater than the modulus were used to denote an apraxic quality of speech greater than the modulus and lower numbers indicated that the listener perceived a quality less apraxic than the modulus.

Data Analysis

Figure 1 presents a graphic representation of data for an apraxic subject. The EMG signals were rectified, down-sampled at 500 Hz, and smoothed with a 40 Hz low-pass filter. Point-by-point correlation coefficients were then computed between the muscle pairs OOI-OOS, OOI-DLI and OOS-DLI (Loeb, Pratt, Chanaud, & Richmond, 1986). Muscle pairs with a correlation of greater than +.15 were considered to be co-contracted, correlations of less than −.15, reciprocally contracted, and correlations between −.15 and +.15, ambiguous. The cutoff of ±.15 was determined from perceptual judgments of EMG signals by two judges (the first two authors), who viewed a random sampling of signals. Both identified muscle activity patterns as co-contracted when the correlation exceeded +.15.

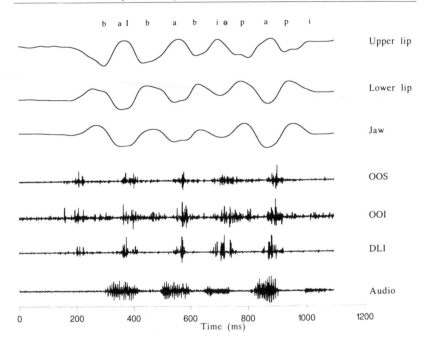

Figure 1. Acoustic, kinematic, and electromyographic record of one apraxic speaker's sentence, "Buy Bobby a poppy," at normal rate.

Consistent judgments of reciprocally contracted muscle pairs were made for correlations below −.15, and between these no unanimity was reached. Figures 2 and 3 present patterns of co-contracted and reciprocally contracted muscle pairs, respectively. As a second step, muscle pairs were examined to determine if a positive correlation was epiphenomenal of one muscle maintaining continuous activity throughout the utterance. The pattern of co-contraction termed incidental coactivation by Moore and Scudder (1989) is shown in Figure 4.

Kinematic data from the lower lip + jaw (noted as lower lip) were displayed as phase planes relating movement amplitude to movement velocity and compared across speaker groups for opening and closing gestures. An example of a phase plane trajectory is presented in Figure 5 along with associated time histories of movement amplitude and velocity. Phase plane trajectories were chosen because they describe the dynamics of articulatory movement, a feature of apraxic speech that may be disturbed (Kent & Rosenbek, 1983). Description of opening and closing gestures focused on movement from /b/ in /baɪ/ to the initial /b/ in /babi/. This sequence is the most complex utterance in the test utterance, and clinical and research findings (e.g., Kent & Rosenbek, 1983; Shewan,

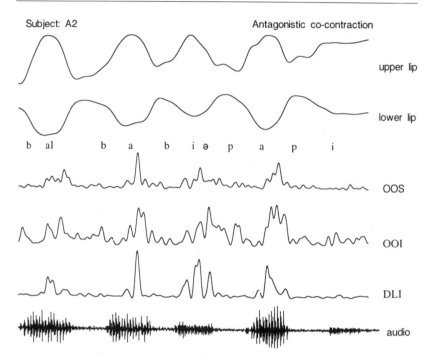

Figure 2. Kinematic, rectified electromyographic, and acoustic records of one apraxic speaker's sentence. Note antagonistic co-contraction of OOI and DLI. (Time base is 1.5 seconds.)

1980) suggest that complex strings are more impaired in apraxic speakers than single phonemes. Therefore, if movement differences did exist between groups, they would most likely be evident in these gestures.

Average phase plane trajectories were determined from time-normalized amplitude and velocity profiles. Averages of amplitude versus velocity were calculated across repetitions for opening (/b/ to /aɪ/ in /baɪ/) and closing (/aɪ/ to the first /b/ in /babi/) gestures produced by each speaker. These averages were plotted on x–y coordinates for each subject. Variability around the average phase planes was also investigated qualitatively. Although the magnitude of variability was constant for any subject independent of the point of alignment, the pattern of variability changed with the chosen reference point. Because phase planes are portrayed relative to a single point (i.e., movement onset), no quantitative statements are made about the relative magnitude of variability through these movements.

RESULTS

Perceptual Analysis

A single scale is presented in Table 1 because the rankings of the speakers were the same for both tapes. Correlation coefficients for intra-listener

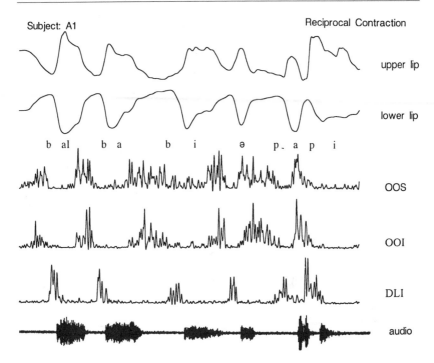

Figure 3. Kinematic, rectified EMG, and acoustic traces for the sentence "Buy Bobby a poppy" by an apraxic speaker. Antagonist muscles (OOI and DLI) were reciprocally activated. (Time base is 4.2 seconds.)

reliability ranged from .79 to .99 with no apparent differences in reliability for the two tapes. Inter-listener reliability measured by Cronbach's alpha, was approximately .9 for each tape. In general, apraxic speakers were judged more apraxic than other speaker groups and the normal speakers were judged free of any apraxic quality. All normal speakers were rated less apraxic than any neurologically impaired subject.

EMG Analysis

Figure 6 presents the range of correlation coefficients for the muscle pairs and speaker groups. All groups evidenced co-contraction between antagonist muscles (OOI-DLI) as well as reciprocal activity between antagonists. Mean values of each distribution of correlation coefficients suggest that there were no differences between groups. This is further substantiated by the summary in Table 2. Observation of the agonist muscle pair (OOI-OOS) also suggests no difference in coordination for disordered versus normal speakers or between any pairs of disordered speaker groups.

When the activation patterns of OOI versus DLI were judged qualitatively, the dominant relation between muscles was incidental co-

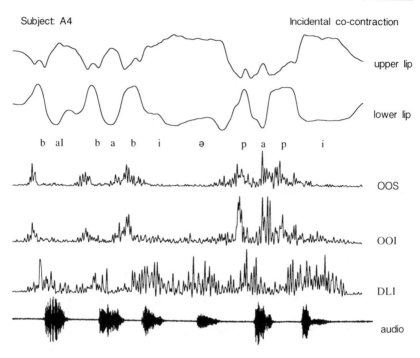

Subject: A4   Incidental co-contraction

upper lip

lower lip

b al   b a b   i   ə   p a p   i

OOS

OOI

DLI

audio

Figure 4. Kinematic, rectified EMG, and acoustic traces of an apraxic speaker's "Buy Bobby a poppy" with EMG pattern of incidental co-contraction between antagonistic muscles. (Time base is 4.3 seconds.)

contraction. Figure 7 shows that approximately 60%–70% of OOI-DLI activation patterns were incidental in ataxic dysarthric, conduction aphasic, and normal groups. All patterns (incidental, antagonistic co-contraction, and reciprocal activation) occurred equally in the group of apraxic speakers, although patterns seemed idiosyncratic. One speaker always demonstrated reciprocal activation between OOI and DLI (A1), one had both reciprocal and incidental co-contraction (A4); for one apraxic speaker, all repetitions were characterized by incidental co-contraction between OOI and DLI (A3), and another (A2) evidenced antagonistic co-contraction in all repetitions of the test utterance. These differences in activation patterns did not correspond to the perceived apraxia of these speakers (Table 1) in a way that might be predicted by the results of Fromm et al. (1982).

Kinematic Analysis

Average phase plane trajectories for the opening gesture from consonant to vowel in /baɪ/ are presented in Figures 8–11 for each group. Figures are aligned at the onset of the gesture (upper right), and display the relationship between movement amplitude on the abscissa, and movement velocity through the gesture. Time is not an explicit variable in these

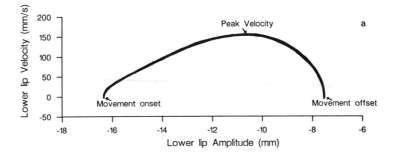

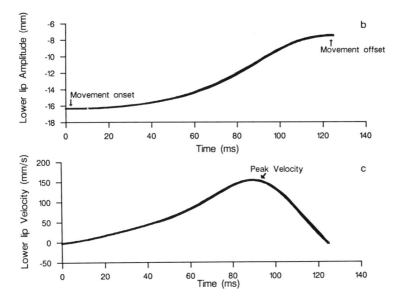

Figure 5. Graphic representations of lower lip closing from /aɪ/ in /baɪ/ to /b/ in /babi/ for one normal speaker. Average phase plane trajectory (a) relating lower lip movement amplitude on the abscissa to movement velocity on the ordinate is plotted. Movement onset, offset, and peak velocity are marked to compare with amplitude and velocity time histories presented in graphs (b) and (c), respectively.

figures. The lines encircling the average trajectories represent one standard deviation from the mean.

The amplitude-velocity relation for this opening gesture was represented by a relatively smooth, unimodal curve for all groups. Disordered speakers showed greater variability from the average trajectories than normal speakers for this opening gesture (Figure 8).

The relationship between movement amplitude and velocity in the closing gesture varied more with subject group than the trajectories for

Table 1. Median ranking of pathological subjects on the basis of perceived magnitude of apraxia of speech

1. A4	6. D3
2. A1	7. A2
3. A3,D4	8. C4
4. D1	9. N1,N3
5. D2	10. N2,N4

A = apraxic, C = conduction aphasic, D = ataxic dysarthric, N = normal.

the opening gesture. This is shown in Figure 12 through Figure 15, with the closing gesture starting in the lower left of each graph. As with the opening gesture, all normal speakers showed a smooth, unimodal relation between movement amplitude and velocity throughout the closing gesture. The relation between movement amplitude and velocity was not unimodal for the majority of apraxic speakers as seen in Figure 13. Subjects A1 and A4 had distinctly bimodal relations between amplitude and

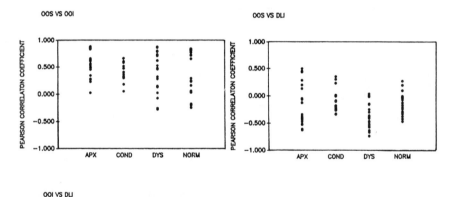

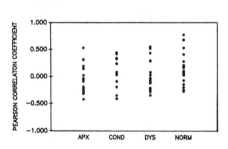

Figure 6. Correlation coefficients for agonist (OOS-OOI) and antagonist (OOI-DLI) muscles for each group. Correlations greater than +.15 suggest co-contraction; less than −.15, reciprocal contraction; between +.15 and −.15, not classified as either. (APX = apraxic; COND = conduction aphasic; DYS = ataxic dysarthric; NORM = normal.)

Table 2. Summary of activation patterns indexed by correlation coefficients for antagonist muscle pairs for each group

	Coefficient		
Group	< −.15	−.15 to +.15	> +.15
Apraxic	9	6	5
Aphasic	3	4	7
Dysarthric	6	7	7
Normal	4	6	10

Correlation coefficients greater than +.15 indicate co-contraction; less than −.15, reciprocal contraction; between +.15 and −.15 coefficients are ambiguous.

velocity, and this shape was also apparent in the curve for subject A3. This bimodal curve for the closing gesture was evident in 1 ataxic dysarthric speaker (D4) and, to a slight extent, in 1 conduction aphasic speaker (C2). Phase planes for the simpler gestures (e.g., /a/ to /b/ in /babi/) were qualitatively similar to those displayed in Figures 12–15 for the more complex gestures. Consistent with the data for the more complex gesture, the amplitude-velocity relation for the simpler gestures varied more for the disordered speakers than the normal speakers.

Careful inspection of Figure 8 through Figure 15 revealed differences among groups in opening and closing peak velocities. For normal speakers (Figure 8 and Figure 12), peak velocity was greater for the closing gesture (closing/opening peak velocity = 1.3 average), as would be predictable from previous research (Kuehn & Moll, 1976). By contrast, three apraxic speakers (A1, A2, and A3) had peak velocities higher for the opening gesture than for the closing gesture in /baɪ b/. The ratio of peak closing

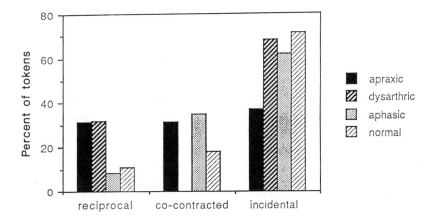

Figure 7. Percent of DLI and OOI patterns that were reciprocal, antagonist co-contraction, or incidental co-contraction by group.

Lower lip opening /baI/

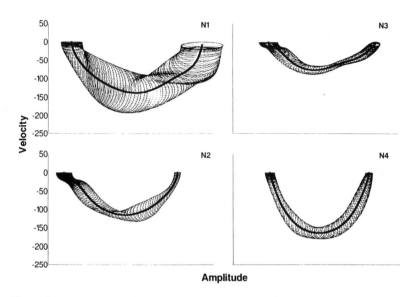

Figure 8. Average phase plane trajectory (solid line) of lower lip movement in the opening gesture from /b/ to /aI/ in "Buy" for each normal speaker. (Onset is displayed in the upper right of each graph, and encircling lines represent 1 standard deviation from the mean relating movement amplitude [*x* dimension] to movement velocity [*y* dimension].)

and opening velocity was .94 for the apraxic group in this sequence. In other speaker groups, only subjects D4 and C2 demonstrated greater peak velocity for the opening, compared to closing, gesture. Phase plane trajectories indicated and the perceptual rating of D4 confirmed that these speakers had apraxic speech qualities. It should be noted, however, that this relation for closing and opening velocities was found only in the sequence /baI b/. For less complex sequences in this sentence, closing velocity was higher than opening velocity.

Figure 16 presents the relation between voicing and movement termination for /aI/ to /b/ in "Buy Bobby" for one normal speaker who was representative of all normal, dysarthric, and conduction aphasic speakers. Voicing terminated around the time of peak closing velocity, approximately 50 ms prior to the end of the gesture. In Figure 17, the relationship between voicing and closing movement termination is displayed for one apraxic speaker. It should be noted that the time scale on this figure is twice as long as the scale on the previous display. For this speaker, voicing terminated approximately 300 ms prior to the end of the closing gesture. This speaker, who was perceived to be the most apraxic speaker in the group, was unique in showing this long latency between voicing and movement termination.

Lower lip opening /baI/

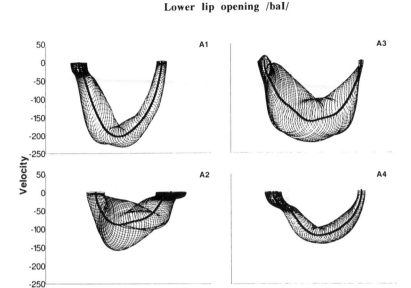

Figure 9. Average phase plane trajectory (solid line) of lower lip movement in the opening gesture from /b/ to /aɪ/ in "Buy" for each apraxic speaker. (Onset is displayed in the upper right of each graph, and encircling lines represent 1 standard deviation from the mean relating movement amplitude [x dimension] to movement velocity [y dimension].)

CONCLUSIONS

Although there is reason to believe that AOS is manifested by motor impairments (Adams, McNeil, & Weismer, 1989; Kent & Rosenbek, 1983; McNeil & Adams, 1990), it does not appear that the existence of antagonistic co-contraction is a hallmark of this disorder as suggested by Fromm et al. (1982) and Keller (1987). Based on the work of Fromm et al. (1982), antagonistic co-contraction should correspond to perceived magnitude of apraxia, a prediction not substantiated by the present data. In fact, there appeared to be no relation between patterns of muscle activity and perceived magnitude of apraxia of speech. General issues of EMG analysis should be considered in interpreting these findings because EMG activity patterns differ across speakers, with repeated insertions within the same speaker, and with different placements within the same muscle. To a large extent, these factors cannot be controlled, so interpretation of between-subject or between-group comparisons must be approached with caution.

Present results are consistent with data on jaw muscle activity reported by Moore, Smith, and Ringel (1988) in showing co-contraction in

Lower lip opening /baI/

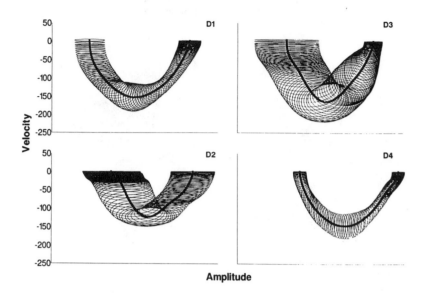

Figure 10. Average phase plane trajectory (solid line) of lower lip movement in the opening gesture from /b/ to /aɪ/ in "Buy" for each ataxic dysarthric speaker. (Onset is displayed in the upper right of each graph, and encircling lines represent 1 standard deviation from the mean relating movement amplitude [x dimension] to movement velocity [y dimension].)

Lower lip opening /baI/

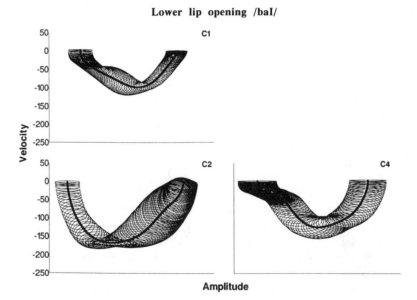

Figure 11. Average phase plane trajectory (solid line) of lower lip movement in the opening gesture from /b/ to /aɪ/ in "Buy" for each conduction aphasic speaker. (Onset is displayed in the upper right of each graph, and encircling lines represent 1 standard deviation from the mean relating movement amplitude [x dimension] to movement velocity [y dimension].)

Lower lip closing /aI b/

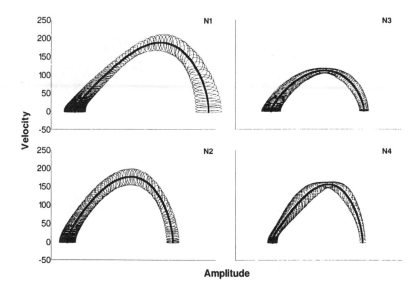

Figure 12. Average phase plane trajectory (solid line) of lower lip movement in the closing gesture from /aɪ/ in "Buy" to the first /b/ in "Bobby" for each normal speaker. (Onset is displayed in the lower left of each graph, and encircling lines represent one standard deviation from the mean relating amplitude [x dimension] to movement velocity [y dimension].)

Lower lip closing /aI b/

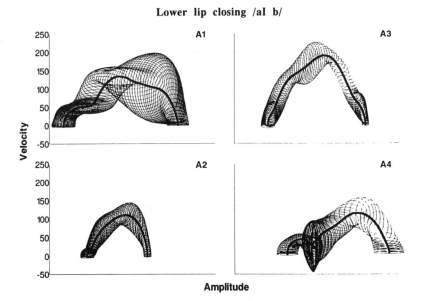

Figure 13. Average phase plane trajectory (solid line) of lower lip movement in the closing gesture from /aɪ/ in "Buy" to the first /b/ in "Bobby" for each apraxic speaker. (Onset is displayed in the lower left of each graph, and encircling lines represent one standard deviation from the mean relating amplitude [x dimension] to movement velocity [y dimension].)

Lower lip closing /aɪ b/

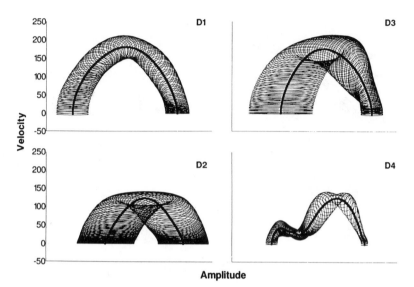

Figure 14. Average phase plane trajectory (solid line) relating lower lip movement in the closing gesture from /aɪ/in "Buy" to the first /b/ in "Bobby" for each ataxic dysarthric speaker. (Onset is displayed in the lower left of each graph, and encircling lines represent one standard deviation from the mean relating amplitude [x dimension] to movement velocity [y dimension].)

Lower lip closing /aɪ b/

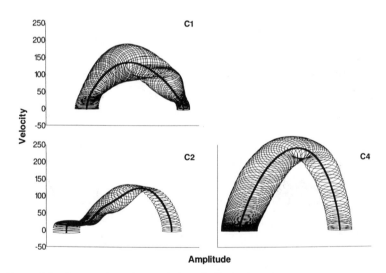

Figure 15. Average phase plane trajectory (solid line) for lower lip movement in the closing gesture from /aɪ/ in "Buy" to /b/ in "Bobby" for each conduction aphasic subject. (Onset is displayed in the lower left of each graph, and encircling lines represent one standard deviation from the mean relating amplitude [x dimension] to movement velocity [y dimension].)

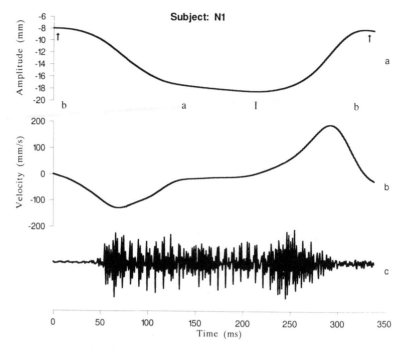

Figure 16. Relation between lower lip amplitude (a), velocity (b), and voicing (c) in /baɪ b/ by normal speaker. (Arrows in graph mark movement onset and offset.)

normal movement. The conclusion to be drawn from these and other studies (e.g., Darling, Cooke, & Brown, 1989; Smith, 1981) is that co-contraction may be a desirable feature of normal motor control rather than a sign of a disordered system. As Smith (1981) asserts, "The general idea that antagonist muscles cease to function when agonists contract . . . is clearly a gross oversimplification of muscular activity in voluntary movements" (p. 733). In fact, co-contraction in normal individuals has been shown to increase muscular force (Walmsley, Hodgson, & Burke, 1978; Zomlefer, Zajac, & Levine, 1977), movement velocity (Bouisset & Lestienne, 1974), and displacement (Patton & Mortensen, 1971), which are inconsistent with descriptions of AOS.

Continuous, undifferentiated EMG in AOS subjects (Fromm et al., 1982) has also been suggested as a distinguishing feature of apraxic speakers. Although this feature was judged qualitatively in the present study and in the work of Fromm et al., differences between groups in the frequency of occurrence did not appear (Figure 7). Rather than a feature of neurologic impairment, continuous, undifferentiated EMG probably characterizes muscle activity in general, in older adults suggested by Darling et al. (1989) and Kamen and DeLuca (1989).

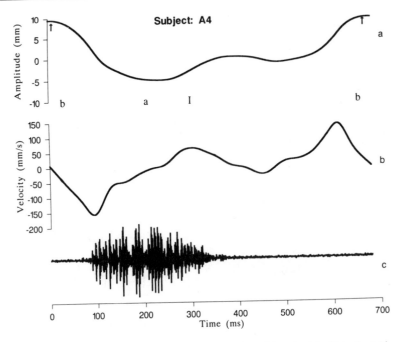

Figure 17. Relation between lower lip amplitude (a), velocity (b), and voicing (c) in /baɪ b/ by an apraxic speaker. (Arrows in graph mark movement onset and offset.)

It is difficult to conceptualize any group characteristics concerning AOS on the basis of the EMG data because each speaker displayed individual patterns of muscle activity. By contrast, kinematic analyses revealed some consistency across speakers as well as striking similarities between AOS in these speakers and previous reports of limb apraxia (Poizner et al., 1990). For example, phase plane trajectories for closing gestures produced by apraxic speakers indicated decoupling of the spatial-temporal relations that are prominent in normal movement control. Apraxic trajectories for lip movement were characterized by inconsistent relations between movement amplitude and velocity (Figure 13) contrasted with the tight coupling of these parameters associated with normal movement (Figure 12). Decoupling of spatial-temporal indices have been noted in complex arm movements in individuals with limb apraxia (Poizner et al., 1990) and related to disturbance in the planning of those trajectories. Furthermore, this spatial-temporal decoupling may represent a less efficient organization of the motor control system than is found in neurologically normal adults (Poizner et al., 1990; Viviani & Terzuolo, 1982).

Decomposition of multiarticulate movements is evidenced in complex arm trajectories produced by apraxic subjects (Poizner et al., 1990) and was present in speech articulation in this study. In arm trajectories, apraxic individuals perform the gesture with rotation of the proximal joint and little if any movement at more distal joints. When movement occurred simultaneously at two or more joints, there was marked discoordination. Rather than discoordination between the joints, apraxic speakers may lack coordination between phonatory and articulatory control. For example, one apraxic speaker terminated voicing approximately 300 ms before the articulatory gesture was completed (Figure 17) whereas normal speakers terminated voicing approximately 50 msec before the end of lower lip movement. Perhaps this represents a decomposition of speech into its subcomponents whereby vocal fold adduction cannot occur with the articulatory gesture of vocal tract closure. In acoustic terms, this lack of coordination between voicing and movement may represent syllable segregation as described by Kent and Rosenbek (1983) in which syllables were separated by predominantly silent intervals. This study reveals that syllable segregation may be a combination of transition lengthening and uncoordinated glottal and supraglottal activity, features of AOS noted by Kent and Rosenbek (1983).

Correspondence between median perceptual ratings and phase plane trajectories suggests that the disruption of the amplitude-velocity relation during the closing gesture either may have perceptual consequences or relate to other kinematic events associated with AOS qualities. This assertion is supported by the rating of speaker D4, who had phase plane trajectories resembling apraxic speakers. Listeners perceived D4 to be more apraxic than other dysarthric or aphasic speakers and, more interesting, D4 was perceived to be more apraxic than A2, whose phase planes resembled those of normal speakers.

It is possible that the abnormal amplitude-velocity relation found in apraxic speakers reflects speaking rate reductions in this group (see McNeil & Adams, 1990). Research has shown that slow speech rate, even in normal speakers, results in alterations in velocity profiles (Adams, 1990). Specifically, slow speaking rate in normal speakers is manifested in multimodal velocity profiles, compared with unimodal velocity profiles that characterize conversational speech. Additional investigation of the influence of speaking rate on the phase plane trajectories of normal and disordered speakers is in progress.

Finally, the observation that apraxic speakers have more difficulty with complex sequences was substantiated by comparing opening and closing velocities. In the sequence /baɪ b/, apraxic speakers had lower closing than opening velocities, counter to what is found in normal speakers. In simpler sequences (e.g., /a/ to /b/ in /babi/), apraxic speakers showed the expected relation between opening and closing velocities.

This investigation found that patterns of contraction between agonist and antagonist muscle pairs may not be a good indicator of the neurological state of a speaker, as researchers previously suggested (Fromm et al., 1982; Keller, 1987). Both qualitative and quantitative analyses reveal no differences in these muscle activity patterns for neurogenically impaired versus normal speakers or for different groups of impaired speakers.

Observations of the dynamic aspects of lower lip movement measured by phase plane trajectories suggest differences between the normal and apraxic speakers, particularly in the production of complex closing gestures. These findings are consistent with observations of limb apraxia and suggest some features common to these two forms of apraxia. The suggestion can also be made that other neurologically impaired speakers exhibit apraxic-like characteristics, a suggestion that is bolstered by the perceptual judgments that found a correspondence between apraxic-like phase planes and an apraxic quality to speech. These types of analyses need to be conducted with more speakers, more repetitions per speaker, other articulators, and other movement dimensions (e.g., anterior-posterior) to verify this observation.

It appears that no simple neuromotor explanation for speech apraxia can be invoked. This investigation points to the need for more research in this area with larger groups of well-defined subjects. There is the suggestion, however, that investigation of the dynamic elements of articulation, in parallel with perceptual judgments of the produced speech may be fruitful in the understanding of neurologically impaired speakers.

REFERENCES

Abbs, J.H., Hunker, C.J., & Barlow, S.M. (1983). Differential speech motor subsystem impairments with suprabulbar lesions: Neurophysiological framework and supporting data. In W.R. Berry (Ed.), *Clinicial dysarthria* (pp. 21–56). San Diego: College-Hill Press.

Adams, S.G. (1990). *Rate and clarity of speech: An x-ray microbeam study.* Unpublished doctoral dissertation, University of Wisconsin-Madison.

Adams, S.G., McNeil, M.R., & Weismer, G. (1989, November). *Speech movement velocity in neurogenic speech disorders.* Paper presented at the American Speech-Language-Hearing Association Convention, St. Louis, MO.

Barlow, S.M., Cole, K., & Abbs, J.H. (1983). A new headmounted lip-jaw movement transduction system for the study of motor speech disorders. *Journal of Speech and Hearing Research, 26*, 283–288.

Blair, C., & Smith, A. (1986). EMG recording in human lip muscles: Can single muscles be isolated? *Journal of Speech and Hearing Research, 29*, 256–266.

Blumstein, S., & Baum, S. (1987). Consonant production deficits in aphasia. In J. Ryalls (Ed.), *Phonetic approaches to speech production in aphasia and related disorders.* (pp. 137–162). San Diego: College-Hill Press.

Blumstein, S., Cooper, W., Goodglass, H., Statlender, S., & Gottlieb, J. (1980). Production deficits in aphasia: A voice-onset time analysis. *Brain and Language, 9*, 153–170.

Blumstein, S., Cooper, W., Zurif, E., & Caramazza, A. (1977). The perception and production of voice onset time in aphasia. *Neuropsychologia, 15*, 371–383.

Borkowski, J.G., Benton, A.L., & Spreen, O. (1967). Word fluency and brain damage. *Neuropsychologia, 5,* 135–140.

Bouisset, S., & Lestienne, F. (1974). The organization of a simple voluntary movement analysed from its kinematic properties. *Brain Research, 71,* 451–458.

Dabul, B. (1979). *Apraxia battery for adults.* Tigard, OR: C.C. Publications, Inc.

Darley, F.L. (1982). *Aphasia.* Philadelphia: W.B. Saunders.

Darley, F.L., Aronson, A.E., & Brown, J.R. (1975). *Motor speech disorders.* Philadelphia: W.B. Saunders.

Darling, W.G., Cooke, J.D., & Brown, S.H. (1989). Control of simple arm movements in elderly human subjects. *Neurobiology of Aging, 10,* 149–157.

Duffy, J., & Gawle, C. (1984). Apraxic speakers' vowel duration in consonant-vowel-consonant syllables. In J.C. Rosenbek, M.R. McNeil, & A.E. Aronson (Eds.), *Apraxia of speech: Physiology, acoustics, linguistics, management* (pp. 1–72). San Diego: College-Hill Press.

Fromm, D., Abbs, J.H., McNeil, M.R., & Rosenbek, J.C. (1982). Simultaneous perceptual-physiological method for studying apraxia of speech. In R.H. Brookshire (Ed.), *Clinical aphasiology* (pp. 155–171). Minneapolis: BRK Publishers.

Goodglass, H., & Kaplan, E. (1972). *The assessment of aphasia and related disorders.* Philadelphia: Lea & Febiger.

Itoh, M., Sasanuma, S., Hirose, H., Yoshioka, H., & Ushijima, T. (1980). Abnormal articulatory dynamics in a patient with apraxia of speech: X-ray microbeam observation. *Brain and Language, 11,* 66–75.

Itoh, M., & Sasanuma, S. (1987). Articulatory velocities of aphasia patients. In J. Ryalls (Ed.), *Phonetic approaches to speech production in aphasia and related disorders* (pp. 137–162). San Diego: College-Hill Press.

Itoh, M., Sasanuma, S., Tatsumi, I.F., Murakami, S., Fukusako, Y., & Suzuki, T. (1982). Voice onset time characteristics in apraxia of speech. *Brain and Language, 17,* 193–210.

Itoh, M., Sasanuma, S., & Ushijima, T. (1979). Velar movements during speech in a patient with apraxia of speech. *Brain and Language, 7,* 227–239.

Johns, D., & Darley, F. (1970). Phonemic variability in apraxia of speech. *Journal of Speech and Hearing Research, 13,* 556–583.

Kamen, G., & DeLuca, C.J. (1989). Unusual motor unit firing behavior in older adults. *Brain Research, 482,* 136–140.

Keller, E. (1987). The cortical representation of motor processes of speech. In E. Keller & M. Gopnik (Eds.), *Motor and sensory processes of language* (pp. 125–162). Hillsdale, NJ: Lawrence Erlbaum Associates.

Kent, R.D., & Rosenbek, J.C. (1983). Acoustic patterns of apraxia of speech. *Journal of Speech and Hearing Research, 26,* 231–249.

Kennedy, J.G., & Abbs, J.H. (1979). Anatomic studies of the perioral motor system: Foundations for studies in speech physiology. In N.E. Lass (Ed.), *Speech and language: Advances in basic research and practice 1* (pp. 211–270). New York: Academic Press.

Kuehn, D.P., & Moll, K. L. (1976). A cineradiographic study of VC and CV articulatory velocities. *Journal of Phonetics, 4,* 303–320.

LaPointe, L.L., & Johns, D.F. (1975). Some phonemic characteristics of apraxia of speech. *Journal of Communication Disorders, 8,* 259–269.

Loeb, G.E., Pratt, C.A., Chanaud, C.M., & Richmond, F.J.R. (1986). Cross-correlation of EMG reveals widespread synchronization of motor units during some slow movements in intact cats. *Journal of Neuroscience Methods, 17,* 207–208.

Martin, A.D. (1974). Some objections to the term apraxia of speech. *Journal of Speech and Hearing Disorders*, *39*, 53–64.

McClean, M., Goldsmith, H., & Cerf, A. (1984). Lower-lip EMG and displacement during bilabial disfluencies in adult stutterers. *Journal of Speech and Hearing Research*, *27*, 342–349.

McNeil, M.R., & Adams, S. (1990). A comparison of speech kinematics among apraxic, conduction aphasic, ataxic dysarthric and normal geriatric speakers. In T.E. Prescott (Ed.), *Clinical aphasiology* (pp. 279–294). Austin: PRO-ED.

McNeil, M.R., Weismer, G., Adams, S., & Mulligan, M. (1990). Oral structure nonspeech motor control in normal, dysarthric, aphasic, and apraxic speakers: Isometric force and static position control. *Journal of Speech and Hearing Research*, *33*, 255–268.

McNeil, M.R., Caligiuri, M.A., & Rosenbek, J.C. (1989). A comparison of labiomandibular kinematic durations, displacements, velocities and dysmetrias in apraxic and normal adults. In T.E. Prescott (Ed.), *Clinical aphasiology* (pp. 173–193). San Diego: College-Hill Press.

McNeil, M.R., & Prescott, T.E. (1978). *Revised Token Test*. Baltimore: University Park Press.

Moore, C.A., & Scudder, R.R. (1989). Coordination of jaw muscle activity in parkinsonian movement: Description and response to traditional treatment. In K. Yorkston & D. Beukelman (Eds.), *Clinical dysarthria* (pp. 147–163). San Diego: College-Hill Press.

Moore, C.A., Smith, A., & Ringel, R.L. (1988). Task-specific organization of activity in human jaw muscles. *Journal of Speech and Hearing Research*, *31*, 670–680.

Munhall, K.G. (1989). Articulatory variability. In P. Square-Storer (Ed.), *Acquired apraxia of speech in aphasic adults* (pp. 64–84). London: Taylor and Francis.

Odell, K., McNeil, M.R., Hunter, L., & Rosenbek, J.C. (1990). Perceptual characteristics of consonant production by apraxic speakers. *Journal of Speech and Hearing Disorders*, *55*, 345–359.

Patton, N.J., & Mortensen, O.A. (1971). An electromyographic study of reciprocal activity of muscles. *Anatomy Review*, *170*, 255–268.

Poizner, H., Mack, L., Verfaellie, M., Rothi, L.J., & Heilman, K.M. (1990). Three-dimensional computergraphic analysis of apraxia. *Brain*, *113*, 85–101.

Porch, B.E. (1967). *Porch Index of Communicative Ability: Vol. II. Administration and scoring*. Palo Alto, CA: Consulting Psychologist Press.

Raven, J.C. (1962). *Coloured Progressive Matrices*. London: H.K. Lewis.

Robin, D.A., Bean, C., & Folkins, J.W. (1989). Lip movement in apraxia of speech. *Journal of Speech and Hearing Research*, *32*, 512–523.

Rosenbek, J.C., Kent, R.D., & LaPointe, L.L. (1984). Apraxia of speech: An overview and some perspectives. In J.C. Rosenbek, M.R. McNeil, & A.E. Aronson (Eds.), *Apraxia of speech: Physiology, acoustics, linguistics, management* (pp. 1–72). San Diego: College-Hill Press.

Shewan, C.M. (1980). Verbal dyspraxia and its treatment. *Human Communication*, *5*, 3–12.

Smith, A.M. (1981). The coactivation of antagonist muscles. *Canadian Journal of Physiology and Pharmacology*, *59*, 733–747.

Viviani, P., & Terzuolo, C. (1982). Trajectory determines movement dynamics. *Neuroscience*, *7*, 431–437.

Walmsley, B., Hodgson, J.A., & Burke, R.E. (1978). Forces produced by medial gastrocnemius and soleous muscles during locomotion in freely moving cats. *Journal of Neurophysiology, 41*, 1203–1216.

Zomlefer, M.R., Zajac, F.E., & Levine, W.S. (1977). Kinematics and muscular activity of cats during maximum height jumps. *Brain Research, 126,* 563–566.

Dysarthria and Apraxia of Speech:
Perspectives on Management
edited by Christopher A. Moore, Ph.D., Kathryn M. Yorkston, Ph.D.,
and David R. Beukelman, Ph.D.
copyright © 1991   Paul H. Brookes Publishing Co., Inc.
Baltimore · London · Toronto · Sydney

Measurement of Tongue Strength and Endurance in Normal and Articulation Disordered Subjects

Donald A. Robin,
Lori B. Somodi, and Erich S. Luschei

SPEECH-LANGUAGE PATHOLOGISTS routinely ask questions about the structure and function of the oral mechanism during speech and in nonspeech activities. A host of measures are collected during an oral examination, including estimates of maximal and submaximal performance of the articulators. While the empirical data are limited, these measures are often deemed useful in diagnosing problems of the speech production system and, more generally, of the nervous system (e.g., Darley, Aronson, & Brown, 1975). For instance, it is not unusual for a speech clinician to refer a patient for neurological assessment based on findings from an oral mechanism examination, because symptoms of neuropathology may appear first in speech or the speech mechanism. As well, a neurologist might refer a patient to a speech-language pathologist to confirm a neurological diagnosis. Information about structure and function of the oral mechanism is useful in understanding factors that contribute to speech impairment.

We wish to thank Melinda Mohr and Nancy Rogers for their assistance in data collection. We also thank Colleen Gardner for her secretarial support.

Although caution is warranted in interpreting maximal performance tests in speech-language pathology (see Kent, Kent, & Rosenbek, 1987), one clinical measure frequently obtained is strength of the articulatory muscles, particularly the tongue. However, two problems limit the utility of these measures. First, there is limited data on the relation of tongue strength to the performance of skilled movements, such as those in speech. Second, most strength measurements are made subjectively by the clinician. For example, the patient is asked to press as hard as possible against a tongue blade, and this action can be performed in an anterior direction, at midline, or laterally. From this, judgments are made about the absolute strength of the tongue, as well as about its symmetry, but subtle weakness or assymetry may not be detected by such subjective means. Moreover, decreases or increases in strength related to disease progression or therapy are subjective and difficult to document. Finally, subjective impressions of tongue strength do not allow for study of the relation between maximal strength and speech production, particularly articulatory precision.

MEASURES

A small number of studies point to the potential of tongue strength measures in diagnosing and understanding speech disorders. One of the first attempts to examine tongue strength (Palmer & Osborn, 1940) had subjects press as hard as possible with their tongues against a hard rubber bulb. The pressure acted on a mercury-filled manometer, and the height of the mercury was used as an index of maximal tongue strength. Both normally speaking individuals and those with speech problems were tested, and results showed that subjects with speech problems had reduced tongue strength.

Dworkin (1978, 1980a), using a force transduction system in which subjects pressed their tongues against a metal lever, found that children with lisps had reduced tongue strength compared to normal children. Dworkin and Culatta (1985), however, found no differences in tongue strength between normally speaking children and those diagnosed with functional articulation problems. Dworkin's procedure required subjects to hold a force for 5 seconds, on three separate trials. The peak of each trial was considered as the maximal force, and peak forces were averaged across three trials. Averaging across trials would not have yielded a maximum performance measure which, by definition should have been the highest force achieved.

Data for dysarthric speakers are likewise limited. Dworkin and Aronson (1986) integrated the force curve generated by having normal and dysarthric speakers sustain a maximal tongue force for 5 seconds. While dysarthric speakers had less area under the curve than normal speakers, no relation between the integral of tongue strength and speech intelligibility, or alternate motion rates was established. Dworkin, Aronson, and Mulder (1980) found reduced maximal tongue strength in dysarthric speakers with amyotrophic lateral sclerosis. Using a force transducer system, Barlow and Abbs (1983) reported that two speakers with dysarthria had poorer tongue force control (greater variability around a target force) than normal speakers.

Because of limited data, speech-language pathologists have not developed a standard of tongue strength (see Luschei, chap. 1, this volume). Development of such a standard should consider the variables of gender (examined by Dworkin [1978, 1980a] with conflicting results), height, weight, hand size, and occupation (e.g., professional trumpet player). The relation between tongue and limb strength should also be examined to assist in understanding the relation between general muscular conditioning and condition of the oral musculature.

Muscle endurance or fatigue may also be a critical factor in diagnosing neuromotor speech problems. We refer to the length of time that a certain force level is sustained as endurance because there are numerous factors that may affect an individual's performance, of which muscle fatigue is just one. Such factors include motivation and central recruitment of motor units. Kent et al. (1987, p. 377) have noted, "Few, if any, data have been published on these or similar measures of endurance or fatigue although it could be important clinically to make these determinations, especially for clients with neurological disorders." Subjective or objective measures of endurance are not part of a routine speech mechanism examination. Extent of individual fatigue, time frame, and recovery could contribute to assessing the function of articulatory muscles. Very rapid fatigue might lead to an inability to achieve or maintain accurate articulatory postures during speech. Changes in fatigue noted in periodic reassessments might aid in determining the course of a disease or the results of treatment.

In this preliminary report, we focus on strength and endurance of the anterior tongue, and compare this measure to an index of general muscle strength and endurance by measuring hand performance in the same individuals. We have developed an inexpensive, portable, and easy to use device to measure oral performance. Our approach is to measure the pressure an individual produces by compressing a small rubber bulb with oral structures or hands. Using a pliable bulb to measure pressure eliminates the potential shearing of sensitive tissue against a hard edge, which can cause discomfort and limit the ability to produce a maximal effort.

As a first step toward the development of a standard, this study was undertaken with the following goals:

1. To estimate intra-subject and inter-subject variability of: 1) maximal tongue pressure (P_{max-t}) and maximal hand pressure (P_{max-h}), and 2) endurance of the tongue and hand in sustaining a pressure equal to 50% of P_{max}

2. To determine the relation between the dependent measures (P_{max} or endurance) and certain subject variables, such as weight

3. To determine if young children can understand the instructions and perform the tasks in a reliable manner

Because a long-term goal is to evaluate the clinical utility of these measures, we also sought to determine if measures of strength and endurance distinguish individuals with known articulation problems from normal speakers.

METHODS

Subjects

Thirty-eight individuals were studied. The group included 26 normally speaking adults ages 20–49 (5 males and 21 females), 6 normally speaking children ages 6–12 (4 males and 2 females), 5 children with articulation disorders (identified as developmental apraxia of speech [DAS] by University of Iowa clinical faculty members) ages 8–10 (4 males and 1 female), and 1 neurologically impaired female, age 26, with a mild mixed spastic-flaccid dysarthria resulting from traumatic brain injury sustained in a car accident.

Apparatus

The instrument for measuring tongue and hand strength and endurance was an air-filled soft rubber bulb connected to a pressure transducer. Pressure was transduced and displayed digitally as pascals (Pa). Since the physical characteristics of the bulb are standard for all measurements, pressure measures are meaningful force measures. In addition to the advantage of squeezing a soft material, using modern pressure transducers, compared to force transducers, greatly lowers the cost of the device. Moreover, using pressure allowed measurement of oral strength and limb strength with the same system.

Pressure bulbs for tongue measures were made from 1 mL latex rubber pipette bulbs. A 0.040 cm-diameter silastic rubber tube was sealed in the bulb, and then the unit was gas sterilized. The bulb was sheathed in a clean polyethylene sleeve that was heat sealed.

Hand bulbs were made by placing the 1 mL bulb inside a 10 mL rubber syringe bulb. The bulbs were filled with a silicone fluid and sealed.

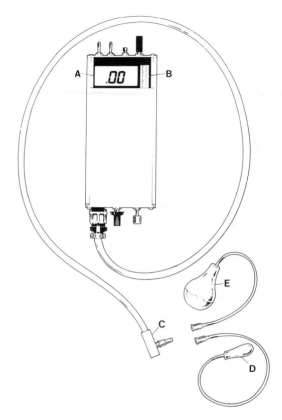

Figure 1. Portable pressure transduction system (7.5 cm × 16.5 cm). (A = liquid crystal display, B = light-emitting diodes that display pressure generated, C = pressure transducer, D = 1 mL tongue bulb, E = 10 mL hand bulb.)

Although individuals were tested using three sizes of bulbs, there were no differences, so data from the 10 mL bulb only are reported.

Amplifiers for the pressure transducer and display were enclosed in a small metal case (Figure 1), and powered by two 9 V batteries. Thus, the entire system was portable.

Procedure

Information about gender, age, weight, height, hand span, and medical history was recorded prior to testing. To measure maximal tongue strength, subjects were instructed to "use the front of your tongue to squeeze the bulb against the roof of your mouth as hard as you can." A peak-holding circuit in the device displayed maximal pressure (P_{max-t}), which the experimenter recorded on a standard form. After a 1-minute rest, this procedure was repeated. The greater of the two values was taken as P_{max-t}. To measure tongue endurance, subjects were asked to look at the device and apply enough pressure to maintain light-emitting diodes at 50% P_{max-t}, represented by a white line at the 5th light. Subjects were then asked to sustain the 50% P_{max-t} for as long as possible and were timed with a stopwatch. Timing began when individuals reached 50% and ended when they terminated trials or when there was a persistent drop greater than 10% (more than two lights).

Hand strength was measured in a similar manner. An individual used the preferred hand (typically the right) and produced two maximal trials by compressing the bulb. Hand endurance was measured by having the subjects hold 50% P_{max-h} for as long as possible. If individuals sustained 50% P_{max-h} for more than 1 minute, the trial was stopped. This period was felt to be indicative of normal performance, and allowing subjects to continue would only increase the length of the procedure without yielding clinically useful data. The order of testing was randomized.

All individuals, except for the adult with dysarthria, were tested several times over 3–5 days. This established an estimate of intra-subject variability.

RESULTS

Normal Speakers

Figure 2 shows data for maximal tongue strength for normal children and adults. The ordinate represents P_{max} in kPa, and the abscissa, subject weight in kg. There are two striking features. Recall that each data point represents three to five trials for a single speaker. The standard deviation was quite small for each individual.

It is also striking that the correlation is quite low ($r = .38$). Thus, the P_{max-t} of a child who weighs 25 kg was not radically different from that of an 80 kg adult. The spread of data points around the regression line is relatively small, thus inter-subject variability is also quite low.

Data on maximal hand strength in these individuals are shown in Figure 3. Similar to data for P_{max-t}, the intra-subject variability for maximal hand strength is quite low, indicated by the standard deviation bars for individual subjects. Inter-subject variability was also relatively low, with most data points falling close to the regression line. The remarkable difference between the two graphs is found in the correlation of strength and weight. Tongue strength by weight yielded a relatively low correlation, but as weight increased, maximal hand strength also increased, so the correlation was quite high ($r = .76$) and twice that of tongue strength.

Children sustained 50% P_{max-t} for an average of 24.03 s ($SD = 4.13$ s) while adults averaged 36.31 s ($SD = 10.13$ s). These differences, statis-

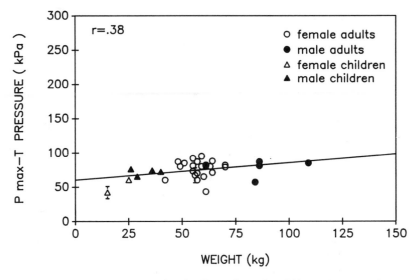

Figure 2. Maximal tongue pressures (kPa) for all normally speaking children and adults as a function of weight (kg). Each symbol represents each individual's average maximal tongue pressure across 3–5 trials.

tically analyzed using a *t*-test, were significant ($p < .05$). There were no statistically significant differences related to gender or weight within these groups.

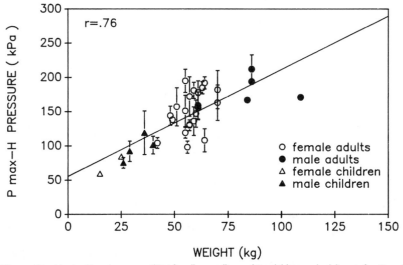

Figure 3. Maximal hand pressures (kPa) for all normally speaking children and adults as a function of weight (kg). Each symbol represents each individual's average maximal hand pressure across 3–5 trials.

By contrast, endurance times for hand strength were significantly longer than for tongue strength ($p < .05$). Children maintained 50% P_{max-h} for an average of 48 s ($SD = 10.14$ s) while adults averaged of 56.49 s ($SD = 13.70$ s). Differences were not statistically significant between children and adults for the hand endurance measure.

Children with DAS

Data for the 4 children with DAS and the 6 normally speaking children are shown in Figure 4. P_{max-t} is plotted as a function of age. Mean tongue strength of the DAS children was 46 kPa and for normally speaking children, 65 kPa. This difference was not statistically significant. Two apraxic speakers had P_{max-t} three times lower than that of the children with normal speech and two times lower than other DAS children (mean approximately 25 kPa).

Results for P_{max-h} are shown in Figure 5. There were no statistically significant differences between the two groups, and the 2 DAS children with low tongue strength did not have low hand strength. Inter-subject and intra-subject variability were quite low.

As a group, the DAS children were able to sustain a 50% maximal effort for 9.1 s ($SD = 4.84$) compared with 24.03 s ($SD = 4.13$) for the group of normally speaking children. A t-test revealed that this difference

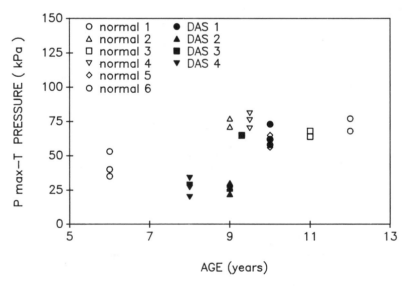

Figure 4. Maximal tongue pressures for all normally speaking and DAS children as a function of age. Each symbol represents a single trial for one individual.

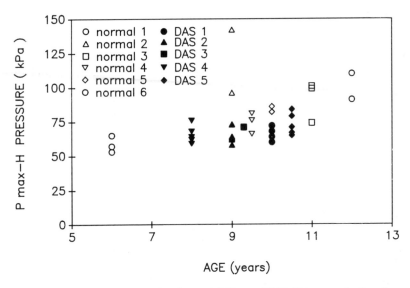

Figure 5. Maximal hand pressures for all normal children and DAS children as a function of age. Each symbol represents a single trial for one individual.

was significant ($p < .05$). Even the 2 DAS children who could produce a maximal effort similar to normal speakers could not sustain 50% for very long. The DAS children also had difficulty sustaining 50% maximal pressure with their hands (DAS mean = 11.57 s, SD = 6.96 s; normal speaker mean = 48 s, SD = 10.14 s), although they had maximal pressures within the range of the normally speaking group. These differences were statistically significant ($p < .05$).

Dysarthric Speaker

A woman with a mild dysarthria following traumatic brain injury was tested once. Her primary speech articulation problem was in production of tongue tip sounds. Her sentence intelligibility as measured by the Assesment of Intelligibility of Dysarthric Speech (Yorkston & Beukelman, 1981) was 83%. Her speaking rate was 137.5 words per minute. Her data were compared with a control speaker matched in age, weight, height, and sex. The dysarthric speaker was not able to generate as much pressure with her tongue as the control speaker, although hand strength was similar. Her P_{max-t} was 44 kPa (normal speaker, 71 kPa) and her P_{max-h} was 132 kPa (normal speaker, 110 kPa). Nevertheless, her ability to sustain 50% P_{max-t} (25 s) and P_{max-h} (56 s) was comparable to that of normal speakers.

CONCLUSIONS

We explored maximal anterior tongue strength and endurance in normal speakers, focusing on variability, age, subject size, hand size, and differences between tongue strength and hand strength. We are encouraged by the initial results suggesting that standardization of measures is possible because: 1) intra-subject and inter-subject variability was quite low; and 2) the device was simple to use, and all individuals could follow instructions and perform the task. Data from disordered speakers suggest clinical usefulness for measures of strength and endurance.

Hand size does not appear to be a critical variable associated with measures of hand strength or endurance in normal speakers. Weight did have to be considered in comparing tongue with hand strength, and, interestingly, tongue strength was not related to weight while hand strength was. Thus, a child of 25 kg was able to exert as much pressure with the tongue, but not with the hand, as an adult of 80 kg. It may be that the growth rate differs for the two structures, and the tongue reaches full growth earlier than the hand, or the tongue may actually receive more exercise than the hand, and thus weight differences are not critical. It is also of interest that individuals sustained 50% efforts with their tongues approximately half as long as with their hands. Tongue muscles may fatigue more rapidly than hand muscles, but other factors are associated with submaximal pressure, including motivation and activation of motor units. Differences in muscle fiber composition might contribute to these results as well.

Because there are no standards for tongue strength or endurance, comparisons of disordered speakers to normal speakers must be guarded. Previous studies (e.g., Dworkin, 1978, 1980a & b; Dworkin & Aronson, 1986; Palmer & Osborn, 1940) found, as we did, that speakers with known speech disorders had lower tongue strength, tongue endurance, or both, compared with normal speakers. These studies also should be conservatively interpreted.

Data from children with DAS bear special comment. These children are presumed to have faulty motor control systems, resulting in poor volitional control of the speech musculature (e.g., Rosenbek & Wertz, 1972). They are not thought to be dysarthric. Yet, 2 DAS children had lower tongue strengths than normally speaking children, though a measure of general body strength (maximal hand pressure) was normal. It may be possible to describe these 2 children as dysarthric, not apraxic, although more data are needed to arrive at this conclusion. It is interesting that examinations of their tongue strengths during 3 years of routine, clinical oral mechanism examinations did not suggest weaknesses.

It is also interesting to note that all the DAS children maintained 50% pressure with their tongues and hands for significantly less time than did normal speakers. This suggests that a DAS speaker may have a muscle system that fatigues more than a normal system, and this affects not just the speech system but musculature in general. It is also possible that DAS children do not have the volitional control to sustain the pressures, and cannot accurately program the articulators to achieve maximal pressure. EMG studies of the tongue, examining the growth of EMG activity as a function of time, could directly test the hypothesis that these children are more fatigable. If the muscle fatigued EMG activity would be increased. If EMG activity did not increase, then a hypothesis would be needed that a mechanism other than fatigue caused submaximal efforts.

To propose a relation between measures of strength and endurance and speech disorders requires more data than has been presented here. Our preliminary results do suggest, however, that study of these factors may be fruitful. The use of a standardized instrument that can provide objective measures may eventually make these procedures clinically useful and cost-effective. In addition, the ease of data collection and interpretation enables use of a large sample and questions about the relation of oral muscle strength to skilled performance can be answered using these instruments.

REFERENCES

Barlow, S.M., & Abbs, J.H. (1983). Force transducers for the evaluation of labial, lingual, and mandibular motor impairments. *Journal of Speech and Hearing Research, 26*, 616–621.

Darley, F., Aronson, A.E., & Brown, J. (1975). *Motor speech disorders*. Philadelphia: W.B. Saunders.

Dworkin, J.P. (1978). Protrusive lingual force and lingual diadochokinetic rates: A comparative analysis between normal and lisping speakers. *Language, Speech, and Hearing Services in Schools, 9*, 8–16.

Dworkin, J.P. (1980a). Characteristics of frontal lispers clustered according to severity. *Journal of Speech and Hearing Disorders, 45*, 37–44.

Dworkin, J.P. (1980b). Tongue strength measurement in patients with amyotrophic lateral sclerosis: Qualitative vs quantitative procedures. *Archives of Physical Medicine and Rehabilitation, 61*, 422–444.

Dworkin, J.P., & Aronson, A. (1986). Tongue strength and alternate motion rates in normal and dysarthric subjects. *Journal of Communication Disorders, 19*, 115–132.

Dworkin, J.P., Aronson, A., & Mulder, D.W. (1980). Tongue strength in normal subjects and dysarthric patients with amyotrophic lateral sclerosis. *Journal of Speech and Hearing Research, 23*, 828–837.

Dworkin, J.P., & Culatta, R.A. (1985). Oral structural and neuromuscular characteristics in children with normal and disordered articulation. *Journal of Speech and Hearing Disorders, 50*, 150–156.

Kent, R.D., Kent, J.F., & Rosenbek, J.C. (1987). Maximum performance tests of speech production. *Journal of Speech and Hearing Disorders, 52,* 367–387.

Palmer, M.F., & Osborn, C.D. (1940). A study of tongue pressures of speech defective and normal speaking individuals. *Journal of Speech Disorders, 5,* 133–140.

Rosenbek, J.C., & Wertz, R.T. (1972). A review of 50 cases of developmental apraxia of speech. *Language, Speech, and Hearing Services in Schools, 3,* 23.

Yorkston, K.M., & Beukelman, D.R. (1981). *Assessment of intelligibility of dysarthric speech.* Austin, TX: PRO-ED.

Dysarthria and Apraxia of Speech:
Perspectives on Management
edited by Christopher A. Moore, Ph.D., Kathryn M. Yorkston, Ph.D.,
and David R. Beukelman, Ph.D.
copyright © 1991   Paul H. Brookes Publishing Co., Inc.
Baltimore · London · Toronto · Sydney

Chapter 14 _____

Aerodynamic and Temporal Measures of Continuous Speech in Dysarthric Speakers

James A. Till and Linda A. Alp

The activation of the speech neural mechanisms with *meaningful speech* may be the only valid test of function for the speech motor system. (Netsell, 1983, p. 10)

DYSARTHRIA IS A neurogenic disorder of speech resulting from abnormal movements in the pulmonary, laryngeal, velopharyngeal, or orofacial articulatory systems during speech production. The locus and nature of defective speech muscular control (Hardy, 1967) and compensatory activity by the dysarthric speaker (Netsell, 1983; 1986) partially determine the specific pattern of speech deviance. The complexity of the speech and required interactions of the speech motor systems also affect the speech pattern. This chapter provides a rationale for using continuous speech in the diagnostic evaluation of dysarthria and presents data describing continuous speech disruption in dysarthric speakers when compared with normal speakers.

The purposes of diagnostic evaluation of communication disorders, as stated by various authors, include: 1) determining presence of a communication problem and describing its nature, 2) determining cause(s) if possible, and 3) stating a prognosis and recommendations for management (e.g., Darley & Spriestersbach, 1978; Emerick & Hatten, 1974;

This work was supported in part by the Rehabilitation Research & Development Service, Project C468-R, Department of Veterans Affairs, Washington, D.C.

Johnson, Darley, & Spriestersbach, 1952, 1963; Nation & Aram, 1977, 1984). Diagnostic evaluation of dysarthria should satisfy these same purposes. Determining the presence of dysarthria may be accomplished simply by listening to a speaker known to have neurological damage (Yorkston, Beukelman, & Bell, 1988). In most clinical settings, the neurologic damage or disease accompanying the dysarthria already has been identified by medical professionals through neurologic examinations and imaging. Identifying neurologic etiology is not usually the primary task of the clinician charged with dysarthria evaluation and management. A major task for the speech-language pathologist is to describe the nature of the communication problem. This requires a detailed description of the existing speech signs and symptoms that led to the complaint and likely will be the focus of treatment.

Initial focus on speech function rather than disordered movement is advantageous during diagnostic evaluation of dysarthria for a variety of reasons. Careful speech assessment acknowledges the patient's concern and motivation in seeking professional services. Typically, the dysarthric speaker — or someone else — has noticed decrements in speech intelligibility, speech naturalness, or both. In addition, the effort required to speak may cause concern. Speaking difficulties in daily verbal interaction are the source of most patients' concern. For all but the most severely dysarthric speakers, day-to-day speech is characterized by one or more breath groups of connected syllables during dyadic exchange. Our patients do not complain about sudden loss of ability to produce /pʌtəkə/ with adequate speed, range, and symmetry of motion; they do not complain of inadequacy in producing pitch range glissandos; and they do not express concern about weakness of tongue lateralization pressure against a tongue blade. Identification of neuromuscular abnormalities in various motor subsystems may be a reasonable goal in dysarthria evaluation (Rosenbek & LaPointe, 1978), and some nonspeech tasks may be useful for this purpose. An initial assessment of speech deviance in connected speech, however, provides guidance and justification for additional procedures that test neuromuscular integrity. Speech patterns may implicate malfunction in the pulmonary, laryngeal, velopharyngeal, or orofacial articulatory systems. By assessing speech function first, unnecessary diagnostic procedures can be avoided.

There are no universal standards for assessing speech function in dysarthria. Unlike audiologists, speech-language pathologists do not have a standard, calibrated diagnostic instrument, or American National Standards Institute standards for speech assessment (e.g., ANSI, 1970). In dysarthria evaluation, speaking tasks, methods of measurement, and foci of measurement vary from clinical setting to setting. Speaking tasks that replicate daily speech have particular appeal for diagnostic evaluation of dysarthria because of high face validity. Monologue requires cognitive, pragmatic, semantic, syntactic, prosodic, and motor organization and execution. These requirements make continuous speaking difficult to control and likely to reflect breakdowns in conversation (Baken, 1987). Although reading more precisely controls content, oral reading can result in speech characteristics different from those of continuous speech (Horii & Cooke, 1978; Till & Goff, 1986). We collected continuous monologue data for trials lasting at least 1 minute. Individual breath groups in monologue appear to have speech characteristics similar to those in conversational interchange (Till & Alp, 1990). Improvements in computer capabilities have improved cost-effectiveness of acquiring, storing, and analyzing lengthy samples of speech and speech-related signals. As software is developed that allows rapid analysis of continuous speech, objective physical measurements may replace less reliable subjective judgments of certain speech attributes (Bradford, Brooks, & Shelton, 1964; Davis, 1979; Kreiman, Gerratt, & Precoda, 1990; Wolfe & Ratusnik, 1988).

Aerodynamic and temporal measures of monologue speech are presented for a group of dysarthric speakers who exhibit laryngeal hypovalving. These data are contrasted with data from normal speakers. The data are not meant to characterize patterns specific to dysarthric speakers with a common neuropathology. Instead, the data reflect effects of poor laryngeal breath stream management in dysarthric speakers who have a variety of neurologic etiologies.

METHODS

Subjects

Twelve male dysarthric speakers were studied. Each had been identified as having a breathy voice by a certified speech-language pathologist. None had a history of speech deficit prior to neurological damage. Five had frank unilateral vocal fold paralyses that had been verified by an otolaryngologist. Four had been diagnosed for cerebral vascular accident by a neurologist. One had suffered traumatic head injury, and one was in the early stages of amyotrophic lateral sclerosis. None of the dysarthric speakers had clinically significant language deficits reported by the examining clinician. None was reported to have severe vocal tract valving problems at locations other than laryngeal. Specifically, 2 speakers were reported to have mild inconsistent hypernasality with mild articulatory distortions, and 3 other speakers were reported to have mild articulatory distortions. The mean speech airflow for these 5 speakers (323.3 mL/s) was essentially equal to that of the other speakers with laryngeal involvement only (323.9 mL/s). Therefore, these speakers were not analyzed as a separate group. The age of the dysarthric speakers ranged from 22 to 72 years.

Data are also reported for 19 normal speakers, 8 males and 11 females. These data are presented to provide a general indication of expected values for the measures from the dysarthric group. These were native speakers of American English with no history of speech, hearing, pulmonary, cognitive, or neuromotor disorder. They ranged in age from 22 to 39 years. It is recognized that both age and gender could affect certain measures obtained from the monologue. We have insufficient data for older, normally speaking men to allow age-matched comparisons with dysarthric speakers. Our pilot data suggest there would be mild increases in airflow during speech epochs and in the inspiration rate for older speakers. Neither of these mild effects would alter the statistically significant group differences reported below.

Procedures

Each individual was seated in a sound booth and asked to speak conversationally on a topic of his choice for 1 minute. An experimenter was present as a "live listener" to ensure conversational effort levels. Data presented are based on at least three 1-minute trials for all except 1 speaker, for whom only a single monologue trial was available. There was at least a 3-minute interval between trials.

Speakers wore a single-chamber pneumotachographic mask connected to a differential pressure transducer and electronics, which gave voltage linearly proportional to airflow over the measured range. This system was calibrated using a mannequin and cylinder-driven respirator modified to deliver 1,000 mL (+/− 10 mL) of cyclic inspiratory and expiratory volume at a variety of flow rates. Between each 1-minute trial the mask was removed and air-dried. A microphone was mounted on a cantilever that extended from the mask approximately 75 mm in front of the speaker's mouth. Figure 1 shows the mask assembly mounted on the calibration mannequin.

Measurement

Airflow and acoustic signals were simultaneously digitized at 100 Hz. Figures 2 and 3 show speech and airflow signals for representative normally speaking and dysarthric individuals. The airflow signal associated with monologue has a general cyclical pattern of inspiration, followed by valved expiration during speech. Software was developed to determine measures for each breath group unit, which included the period of inspiratory airflow and of valved expiration, with either speech or a pause. Figure 4 shows a complete breath group for a normal speaker with the pause period marked. Inspiration was defined as a negative airflow event exceeding 300 ms in duration with integrated volume greater than 50 mL. Previous experiments (Till & Goff, 1986) had suggested that short dura-

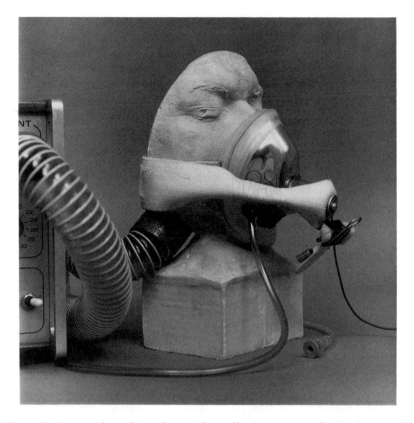

Figure 1. Pneumotachographic mask mounted on calibration mannequin showing placement of microphone on cantilever.

tion negative flow events with < 50 mL volume were produced by buccal and lingual movement and were not pulmonary in nature. Pauses were defined as periods in the acoustic signal between successive inspirations that exceeded 200 ms (Canter, 1965) and remained less than ⅓ of the *rms* voltage for ambient noise in the experimental environment. Speech expiration partition of a breath group was the data remaining above the noise floor not classified as either inspiration or pause.

Table 1 shows 17 measures extracted from the monologue trials organized by the breath group placement of inspiration, speech, or pause. Means and standard deviations were obtained by pooling measures across all analyzed breath group monologue samples. Volumes for inspiration, expiration, and pause periods were obtained by integrating the airflow signal for those events. The measures expressed in minutes (MINVOL, CPM, PPM, and PSEMINVOL) were based on observed rates and volumes extrapolated to a full minute of speaking.

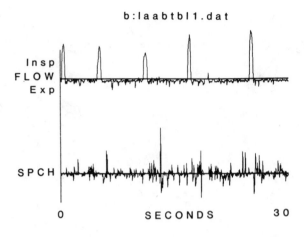

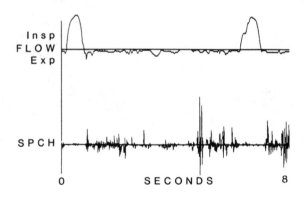

Figure 2. Thirty-second and expanded eight-second epoch of acoustic and airflow data for a normal speaker.

RESULTS

Significant differences between groups were inferred from independent, one-way analyses of variance for each measure. The between-group F ratios are shown in Tables 2–4. Because of the large number of analyses, the critical F value associated with an alpha level of 0.001 ($F = 13.39$, df 1,29) was used to infer significant group difference. As indicated in the tables, 5 of the 17 measures resulted in significant group differences using this conservative procedure.

Inspiratory Results

Table 2 shows inspiratory means and standard deviations for each group. Minute volume (MINVOL) was significantly higher for the dysarthric

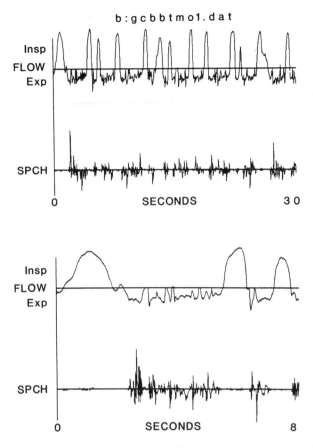

Figure 3. Thirty-second and expanded eight-second epoch of acoustic and airflow data for a dysarthric speaker, hypovalvular at the laryngeal level only. Airflow cessation in the 8-second plot corresponds to articulatory valving.

group, which inspired more than twice the volume of the normal group. This occurred presumably because of increased expiratory airflow during speech, as discussed below. Figure 5 shows the bivariate plot of SPCHFLO and MINVOL for both groups. Correlations between SPCHFLO and MINVOL were high for both the normal ($r = 0.94$) and the dysarthric ($r = 0.94$) speakers.

Inspiratory minute volume can be increased by increasing inspiration rate (CPM), increasing average volume per inspiration (INSPVOL), or increasing both CPM and INSPVOL. Table 2 shows that groups differed significantly for inspiration rate ($F = 49.55$), but did not differ significantly at the $p = .001$ level for mean inspiratory volume ($F = 3.05$). The bivariate relationship of MINVOL and CPM (Figure 6) was analyzed to examine

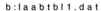

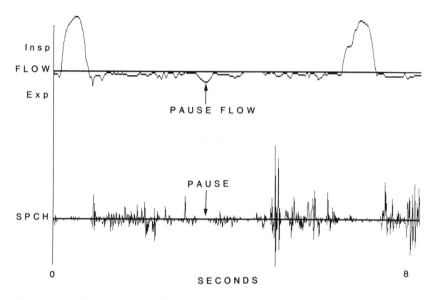

Figure 4. Eight-second display of a single breath group for a normal speaker showing the three analysis partitions: inspiration, valved expiration during speech, and pause.

Table 1. Breath group measures for inspiration, speech, and pause periods

Breath group partition	Measure
Inspiration	Minute volume (MINVOL)
	Mean inspiratory volume (INSPVOL)
	Mean inspiratory airflow (INSPFLO)
	Breath groups (cycles) per minute (CPM)
	Mean inspiratory duration (INSPDUR)
	Mean inspiratory percent (PCNTINSP)
Speech	Mean speech volume (SPCHVOL)
	Mean speech airflow (SPCHFLO)
	Mean duration per breath group (SPCHDUR)
	Speech percent (PCNTSPCH)
	Mean dB-SPL for speech epochs (INTENSITY)
Pause	Mean expiratory volume during pause (PSEVOL)
	Mean expiratory airflow during pause (PSEFLO)
	Pause minute volume (PSEMINVOL)
	Mean pause per minute (PPM)
	Mean pause duration (PSEDUR)
	Mean pause percent (PCNTPSE)

Table 2. Means, standard deviations, and F ratios for inspiratory measures

			Measure			
Group	MINVOL (L)	INSPVOL (mL)	INSPFLO (mL/s)	CPM	INSPDUR (ms)	PCNTINSP (%)
Normal						
M	7.4	619	1038	12.2	604	11.9
SD	1.6	135	221	2.6	110	2.4
Dysarthric						
M	15.0	719	1146	21.3	653	22.5
SD	3.8	186	322	4.7	140	4.4
F ratio	56.22[a]	3.05	1.23	49.55[a]	1.21	76.45[a]

[a]Significant at $P < 0.001$.

Table 3. Means, standard deviations, and F ratios for speech measures

			Measure		
Group	SPCHVOL (L)	SPCHFLO (mL/s)	SPCHDUR (ms)	PCNTSPCH (%)	INTENSITY (dB)
Normal					
M	617	143	4,030	77.6	79.6
SD	146	33	1,000	7.1	3.7
Dysarthric					
M	761	351	2,073	69.7	78.8
SD	214	91	582	8.8	5.4
F ratio	4.95	83.03[a]	37.61[a]	7.49	0.27

[a]Significant at $P < 0.001$.

Table 4. Means, standard deviations, and *F* ratios for pause measures

Group	PSEMINVOL (L)	PSEVOL (mL)	PSEFLO (mL/s)	PSEDUR (ms)	PCNTPSE (%)	PPM (n)
			Measure			
Normal						
M	13.2	71	170	394	10.5	15.1
SD	1.6	57	114	79	6.1	7.1
Dysarthric						
M	14.8	122	376	349	7.7	12.9
SD	1.0	63	214	78	5.7	9.1
F ratio	0.09	5.38	12.25ª	2.35	1.55	0.54

ªSignificant at P < 0.01.

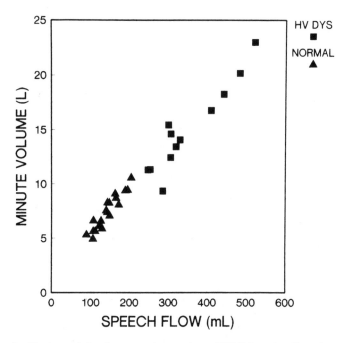

Figure 5. Bivariate relation between minute volume (MINVOL) and airflow during speech (SPCHFLO) for the normal and dysarthric speakers.

individual data. Both groups had relatively low positive correlations between these two variables ($r = 0.47$ and $r = 0.39$, respectively). This suggests that despite the insignificant group difference for INSPVOL, increased INSPVOL contributed to increased MINVOL for some speakers. To investigate this, the relation between MINVOL and INSPVOL (Figure 7) was examined. The correlations of 0.58 for the dysarthric speakers and 0.55 for the normal speakers suggest that increased INSPVOL contributed to increased MINVOL for some speakers. Finally, the contributions of INSPFLO and INSPDUR to increased INSPVOL were examined. Results suggest that when INSPVOL was increased, INSPFLO was more likely to increase ($r = 0.61$) than was INSPDUR ($r = 0.28$). This may relate to a study (Simpson, Till, & Goff, 1988) in which a dysarthric patient modified inspiratory airflow more successfully than inspiratory duration.

Table 2 also shows a significant group difference in time spent inspiring (PCNTINSP). The above analyses suggest that this was related to increased breathing rate (CPM). Increased inspiratory duration (INSPDUR) would also increase this measure, but, as shown, there was not a significant difference in INSPDUR.

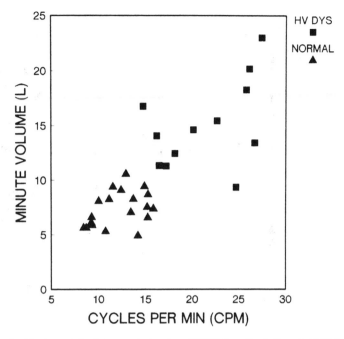

Figure 6. Bivariate relation between minute volume (MINVOL) and inspiration rate (CPM) for normal and dysarthric speakers.

Speech Results

The main purpose of this study was to investigate effects of laryngeal hypovalving on continuous speech, so the measure of speech airflow was of special interest. The dysarthric speakers were selected on the basis of a clinical perception of breathy voice, without other severe vocal tract valving problems. Because we assumed the clinical judgment generally to be accurate, we expected the significant group difference for speech airflow (Table 3). The mean speech airflow (SPCHFLO) for the dysarthric group was approximately 2.5 times the mean airflow for the normal group. Individual data (Figure 5) showed no overlap between groups.

Logically, increased SPCHFLO would result in reduced speech duration (SPCHDUR) in a breath group, unless inspiratory volume was increased to compensate. Data in Table 3 show a reduction of approximately 50% in mean speech duration for the dysarthric group relative to the normal group. The dysarthric group demonstrated mean speech airflow 2.45 times that of the normal group. This increased airflow predicts an approximate 60% reduction in speech duration, rather than the 50% observed. The dysarthric group, however, had a mean inspiratory volume

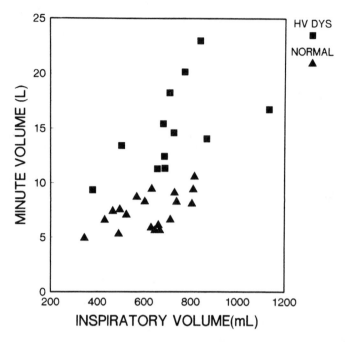

Figure 7. Bivariate relation between minute volume (MINVOL) and inspiratory volume (INSPVOL) for normal and dysarthric speakers.

approximately 100 mL greater than that of the normal group. This approximately 16% increase in INSPVOL probably helped yield a 50% reduction in speech duration, rather than the 60% reduction predicted by increased airflow alone. The remaining extra inspiratory volume for the dysarthric speakers probably was expired during pauses.

The relation between speech airflow and intensity is complicated (cf., Isshiki, 1964) by factors such as subglottal pressure, fundamental frequency, and laryngeal mechanics. These factors were not measured in this present study, but several findings regarding intensity deserve comment. We had expected diminished speech intensity for the hypovalvular group relative to the normal group, but no such difference was observed (Table 3). The dysarthric speakers maintained speech intensities within normal limits, despite impaired laryngeal function. We also examined the relation between speech airflow and speech intensity for the hypovalvular group. We hypothesized that the subjects with higher airflow rates would have lower speech intensities. There was a moderate correlation between INTENSITY and SPCHFLO ($r = -0.59$).

Intensity data for the normal speakers are more difficult to interpret. The normal group showed negative correlations between INTENSITY and SPCHFLO ($r = -0.44$). This finding may relate to other reports that increased subglottal pressure and increased glottal resistance result in greater sound pressure (Isshiki, 1964), but not necessarily greater airflow (Baken, 1987; Isshiki, 1964). Although our data do not directly address the issue, it is possible that the normal speakers with the most efficient (van den Berg, 1956) voices produced greater intensity with less airflow.

Finally, both groups exhibited a negative correlation between IN-TENSITY and SPCHDUR ($r = -0.58$ and $-.035$, respectively). One reason for shortened speech duration in more intense speech might be assumed to be increased airflow. As discussed, this probably did not occur in either group. An explanation related to subglottal pressure requirements is more likely. Weismer (1985), based on data from Hixon, Goldman, and Mead (1973, 1976), has suggested that speakers generally strive for economy of muscular effort when combining the pulmonary relaxation pressures and muscular pressures that produce conversational speech. More specifically, Weismer (1985) suggested that loud conversation might be initiated and terminated at higher lung volume levels than those used for less intense conversation. It is possible that the more intense normal and dysarthric speakers in this study used a higher, but truncated, lung volume range when producing speech. Using a restricted high lung volume could perhaps increase subglottal driving pressure with less muscular effort. One logical ramification of this strategy would be increased breaths per minute (CPM). We observed positive correlations between INTENSITY and CPM both for the normal group ($r = 0.64$) and for the dysarthric group ($r = 0.24$).

Pause Results

The pause measures did not result in significant statistical group differences using the .001 alpha level (Table 4). Means and F ratio data, however, show trends toward increased expiratory airflow (PSEFLO, $F = 12.25$) and air volume (PSEVOL, $F = 5.38$) during pauses for the dysarthric group. Because the dysarthric speakers showed only a slightly lower mean pause rate (PPM) and mean pause duration (PSEDUR) compared to normal speakers, the minute volume expired during pause (PSEMINVOL) was very similar for the two groups. We do not have data that directly explain these trends. Our conjectures are: 1) dysarthric speakers with vocal tract hypovalving may have more difficulty retaining pulmonary volume during pauses than do normal speakers, and 2) dysarthric speakers with vocal tract hypovalving may produce fewer pauses than do normal speakers because they may lose pulmonary air, or pauses might encroach on already reduced speaking time. Mild support for this latter possibility comes from negative correlations observed in dysarthric speakers between pauses per minute (PPM) and factors associated with increased hypovalving, MINVOL ($r = -0.62$), SPCHFLO ($r = -0.44$), and INSPFLO ($r = -0.76$). This is especially interesting considering much weaker correlations in the normal group for these same variables (MINVOL, $r = -0.17$; SPCHFLO, $r = -0.01$; INSPFLO, $r = -0.39$). For both groups the between-subject variability for pause measures was larger than that observed for inspiration or speech measures. This has been true in previous studies also and may suggest greater individual variation in pause behavior than for speech inspiration and valved expiration.

CONCLUSIONS

The data describe differences in monologue speech of a group of normal speakers and a group of dysarthric speakers. The dysarthric speakers had disparate neurologic etiologies, yet were very similar in terms of speech signs and symptoms. Some studies of dysarthric patients with common neuropathologies (e.g., Kent, Netsell, & Abbs, 1979) failed to find sufficient similarity to justify group statistical description. In contrast, between-subject variability for many measures in this dysarthric group approached that of the normal group. For certain purposes, perhaps even for treatment, it may be advantageous to group patients on the basis of speech signs and symptoms, rather than on the basis of neurologic etiology.

All disordered speakers studied had higher than expected (Horii & Cooke, 1978) mean airflow values during continuous speech. Because of difficulty in managing the expiratory speech airstream, these speakers had other abnormal temporal and aerodynamic characteristics of continuous speech. They inspired approximately twice the mean volume of air per minute of normal speakers. Increased air exchange requires extra work and extra time. This effort explains to some extent the relatively common complaint of these speakers that talking is difficult. Increased minute volume was accomplished largely by increased breaths per minute. Additional breathing time reduces available time for production of meaningful content, and mean speech duration per breath group was approximately one-half that of the normal group. There were less obvious indications that inspiratory volume was increased to compensate for laryngeal hypovalving. When inspiratory volume increased, inspiratory airflow increased more often than did inspiratory duration. Trends in the data suggest that the dysarthric group had abnormal pause characteristics. They expired more air during pauses than did the normal group. Perhaps related to this, the dysarthric group showed trends of reduced pause frequency and duration. Possibly, pause frequency is diminished because hypovalvular speakers have difficulty avoiding expulsion of pulmonary air during a pause. Additionally, pauses may be avoided to use the available, but diminished, time for speech.

Although some of the reported measures could be useful to quantify responses to surgical or behavioral management, others might more directly quantify disrupted cyclicity in continuous speech. In a general sense, coefficients of variation for temporal and aerodynamic aspects of breath groups quantify certain aspects of regularity. We are investigating additional statistics that directly reflect adjacent cycle-to-cycle variation in speech and airflow signals, as well as "meta" periodicities related to multiple-breath group patterns. Some measures would be similar to jitter and shimmer statistics derived from the acoustic voice signal. Faster sampling rates and improved analysis algorithms will lead to finer measures of acoustic signals to describe continuous speech. It is possible to measure fundamental frequency and identify syllables at faster sampling rates. Estimates of syllabic rate, variations in syllable intensity and fundamental frequency, and measures related to phrase declination in fundamental frequency should increase the ability to describe continuous speech and acknowledge its rhythmic nature. Speech production theorists view speech as a rhythmic or cyclic behavior (cf. Fowler, 1985; Kelso, Tuller, & Harris, 1983). Yet, surprisingly little clinical attention has been given to describing cyclic, coordinated behaviors in the speech of disordered speakers. Disruptions in normal cyclicity undoubtedly underlie some of the perceived speech deviance in dysarthria. Partial or complete restoration of normal speech cyclicity may be a reasonable therapeutic goal in dysarthria.

REFERENCES

American National Standards Institute. (1970). *Specifications for audiometers* (ANSI S3.6–1969,R–1970). New York: Author.

Baken, R.J. (1987). *Clinical measurement of speech and voice*. San Diego: College-Hill Press.

Bradford, L., Brooks, A., & Shelton, R. (1964). Clinical judgement of hypernasality in cleft palate children. *Cleft Palate Journal, 1*, 329–335.

Canter, G.J. (1965). Speech characteristics of patients with Parkinson's disease, II. Physiological support for speech. *Journal of Speech and Hearing Disorders, 30*, 44–49.

Darley, F.L., & Spriestersbach, C. (1978). *Diagnostic methods in speech pathology* (2nd ed.). New York: Harper & Row.

Davis, S. (1979). Acoustic characteristics of normal and pathological voices. In N. Lass (Ed.), *Speech and language: Advances in basic research and practice, Vol. 1* (pp. 271–335). New York: Academic Press.

Emerick, L.L., & Hatten, J.T. (1974). *Diagnosis and evaluation in speech pathology*. Englewood Cliffs, NJ: Prentice Hall.

Fowler, C.A. (1985). Current perspectives on language and speech production: A critical review. In R.G. Daniloff (Ed.), *Speech science: Recent advances* (pp. 193–278). San Diego: College-Hill Press.

Hardy, J. (1967). Suggestions for physiologic research in dysarthria. *Cortex, 3*, 128–156.

Hixon, T., Goldman, M., & Mead, J. (1973). Kinematics of the chest wall during speech production: Volume displacements of the rib cage, abdomen, and lung. *Journal of Speech and Hearing Research, 16,* 78–115.

Hixon, T., Mead, J., & Goldman, M. (1976). Dynamics of the chest wall during speech production: Function of the thorax, rib cage, diaphragm and abdomen. *Journal of Speech and Hearing Research, 19,* 297–356.

Horii, Y., & Cooke, P.A. (1978). Some airflow, volume, and duration characteristics of oral reading. *Journal of Speech and Hearing Research, 21,* 470–481.

Isshiki, N. (1964). Respiratory mechanism of voice intensity variation. *Journal of Speech and Hearing Research, 7,* 17–29.

Johnson, W., Darley, F., & Spriestersbach, D. (1952). *Diagnostic manual in speech correction.* New York: Harper & Brothers.

Johnson, W., Darley, F., & Spriestersbach, D. (1963). *Diagnostic methods in speech pathology.* New York: Harper & Row.

Kelso, J.A.S., Tuller, B., & Harris, K. (1983). A "dynamic pattern" perspective on the control and coordination of movement. In P. MacNeilage (Ed.), *The production of speech* (pp. 137–166). New York: Springer-Verlag.

Kent, R., Netsell, R., & Abbs, J. (1979). Acoustic characteristics of dysarthria associated with cerebellar disease. *Journal of Speech and Hearing Disorders, 22,* 627–648.

Kreiman, J., Gerratt, G., & Precoda, K. (1990). Listener experience and perception of voice quality. *Journal of Speech and Hearing Research, 33,* 103–115.

Nation, J.E., & Aram, D.M. (1977). *Diagnosis of speech and language disorders.* Saint Louis: C.V. Mosby.

Nation, J.E., & Aram, D.M. (1984). *Diagnosis of speech and language disorders* (2nd ed.). San Diego: College-Hill Press.

Netsell, R.K. (1983). Speech motor control: Theoretical issues with clinical impact. In W.R. Berry (Ed.), *Clinical dysarthria* (pp. 1–19). San Diego: College-Hill Press.

Netsell, R.K. (1986). *A neurobiologic view of speech production and the dysarthrias.* San Diego: College-Hill Press.

Rosenbek, J., & LaPointe, L. (1978). The dysarthrias: Description, diagnosis, and treatment. In D. Johns (Ed.), *Clinical management of neurogenic communicative disorders* (pp. 251–310). Boston: Little, Brown.

Simpson, M.A., Till, J.A., & Goff, A.M. (1988). Long-term treatment of severe dysarthria: A case study. *Journal of Speech and Hearing Disorders, 53,* 433–440.

Till, J.A., & Alp, L.A. (1990, November). *Aerodynamic and temporal measures of monologue and dyadic speech.* Paper presented at the annual meeting of the American Speech-Language-Hearing Association, Seattle.

Till, J.A., & Goff, A.M. (1986, November). *Variables affecting temporal structure and respiratory patterns in speech.* Paper presented at the annual meeting of the American Speech-Language-Hearing Association, Detroit.

van den Berg, J.W. (1956). Direct and indirect determination of the mean subglottic pressure. *Folia Phoniatrica, 8,* 1–14.

Weismer, G. (1985). Speech breathing: Contemporary views and findings. In R.D. Daniloff (Ed.), *Speech science: Recent advances* (pp. 47–72). San Diego: College-Hill Press.

Wolfe, V., & Ratusnik, D. (1988). Acoustic and perceptual measurements of roughness influencing judgments of pitch. *Journal of Speech and Hearing Disorders*, *53*, 15–22.

Yorkston, K., Beukelman, D., & Bell, K. (1988). *Clinical management of dysarthric speakers*. Boston: College-Hill Press.

Dysarthria and Apraxia of Speech:
Perspectives on Management
edited by Christopher A. Moore, Ph.D., Kathryn M. Yorkston, Ph.D.,
and David R. Beukelman, Ph.D.
copyright © 1991   Paul H. Brookes Publishing Co., Inc.
Baltimore · London · Toronto · Sydney

Chapter 15 _____

Oral-Facial
Sensorimotor Function
in Spasmodic Dysphonia

Michael P. Cannito,
George V. Kondraske, and Donnell F. Johns

_____

SPASMODIC DYSPHONIA (SD) is an uncommon, poorly understood
disorder of laryngeal speech motor control that is characterized by
strained, intermittent voice stoppages with laryngealized and aspirate
phonatory perturbation (Cannito & Johnson, 1981). In contrast, nonspeech vocalizations (e.g., laughing or sighing) as well as whispering and
phonation at high pitch levels remain relatively unimpaired (Aronson,
1985). SD does not respond to conventional voice therapy or psycho-
therapy and has remained a subject of heated controversy in clinical literature for over 100 years (see Schaefer, 1983). Although traditionally regarded as psychogenic (Bloch, 1965; Boone, 1977; Brodnitz, 1976;
Heaver, 1959), researchers have turned their attention toward finding a
neuromotor basis for SD (Aminoff, Dedo, & Izdebsky, 1978; Aronson,
Brown, Litin, & Pearson, 1968; Aronson & Hartman, 1981; Blitzer, Lovelace, Brin, Fahn, & Fink, 1985; Cannito, 1989; Cannito & Kondraske,
1990; Feldman, Nixon, Finitzo-Hieber, & Freeman, 1984; Finitzo &
Freeman, 1989; Ludlow & Connor, 1987; Reich & Till, 1983; Robe,
Brumlik, & Moore, 1960; Rosenfield, 1988), perhaps hoping to provide a
rational framework for medical interventions involving neurosurgery or
neuropharmacology.

_____

    This research was supported by NIH Grant NS 18276. The authors acknowledge
principal investigators, Dr. Frances J. Freeman and Dr. Terese Finitzo, for their encourage-
ment and assistance with this work. Additional support was provided by a Biomedical Science
Research Grant from the University Research Institute of the University of Texas at Austin.

In this pursuit of neuromotor correlates of spasmodic dysphonia, two broad lines of research have evolved. First, laryngeal behaviors have been studied to determine if the violent laryngospasms of SD are comparable to those of known (though poorly understood) neurologic diseases such as dystonia or essential tremor. Laryngeal behavior has been studied indirectly using acoustic analyses of the phonatory signal, and directly, using technologies such as electromyography, cinefluorography, fiberoptic endoscopy, and electroglottography (Aronson & Hartman, 1981; Blitzer et al., 1985; Freeman, Cannito, & Finitzo-Hieber, 1985; Ludlow & Connor, 1987; McCall, Skolnik, & Brewer, 1971; Shipp, Izdebsky, Reed, & Morrissey, 1985). A problem with this line of research is that it remains difficult to determine unequivocally whether abnormal laryngeal behavior is functional or neuropathophysiologic. A second line of research seeks evidence of neuromotor abnormalities *external* to the larynx in patients with SD. As Cannito and Kondraske (1990) observed:

> The implicit rationale for such investigations is that if the uncontrollable laryngospasms of SD result from central neuromotor system pathology, it is unlikely that dysfunction would be confined to a single end organ in the majority of cases. Whereas absence of extralaryngeal involvement in SD cannot preclude the possibility of focal organic involvement, it has been recognized that documentation of more generalized motor findings across multiple samples of SD subjects would strengthen arguments in favor of a neuromotor interpretation of the disorder. (p. 123)

Studies of extralaryngeal motor function in SD patients have typically involved clinical observations of neurologic signs and symptoms by a single examiner, usually a neurologist. As early as 1985, Schnitzler reported two SD patients who also exhibited synkinesis of the facial muscles and abnormal movements of the arms and legs (Schaefer et al., 1985). Since then, investigators have reported a high incidence of abnormal neuromotor symptoms external to the larynx in SD. Table 1 reviews the frequency of occurrence reported in these studies. Abnormalities are most frequently interpreted to be of extrapyramidal origin within the CNS (e.g., dystonia and essential tremor), and to a lesser extent of pyramidal origin (e.g., hyperreflexia, bilateral asymmetry, and weakness). Peripheral nerve, bulbar, and cerebellar signs are rarely reported.

To validate clinical observations of extralaryngeal motor abnormalities in SD, researchers employed quantitative objective measurement techniques for statistical comparison of SD patients to matched groups of normal controls. Feldman et al. (1984) reported statistically significant differences between SD and normal speakers in visceral motor functions, including cardiac vagal reflex and gastric acid secretion. Reich and Till (1983) examined manual reaction times in SD and normal speakers but found no difference for a simple finger lift response. Similarly, Cannito

Table 1. Incidence of extrapyramidal/pyramidal neuromotor signs external to the larynx in clinical studies of patients with SD

Study	N	Incidence (%)
Chritchley, 1939[a]	3	100
Robe, Brumlik, & Moore, 1960[a]	10	100
Aronson, Brown, Litin, & Pearson, 1968[b]	27	74
Aminoff, Dedo, & Izdebsky, 1978[b]	12	50
Aronson & Hartman, 1981[a]	22	50
Hartman & Aronson, 1981[c]	17	59
Rosenfield, 1988[b]	41	59
Total	132	58

[a]Adductor SD cases only.
[b]Both adductor and abductor SD cases.
[c]Abductor SD cases only.

and Kondraske (1990) found no difference between groups for simple finger lift reaction time, but did find significant differences for more complex activities involving rates of finger tapping and peg placement (i.e., Purdue Pegboard Test). Cannito and Kondraske's (1990) data were part of a broader study of extralaryngeal motor functions in SD (Cannito, 1986). This chapter presents additional data from that study, focusing on quantitative measures of oral-facial motor performance and the relation of those measures to more conventional clinical observational assessments of oral-facial sensorimotor function. Oral-facial structures are closely related to laryngeal structures because of their integral role in speech production and proximity of their neural representations within the CNS.

EXTRALARYNGEAL MOTOR PERFORMANCE IN SD

Cannito (1986) administered a battery of psychomotor tests to a group of 18 female SD speakers and matched normal speakers to quantify a range of extralaryngeal motor functions in the SD sample. These measures included simple reaction time, rapid sequential movement, postural steadiness, visual pursuit ramp tracking, and step tracking. Analogous activities of the upper extremities and oral-facial region were selected to test a hypothesized *disassociation of functions* predicated on an extrapyramidal (i.e., cortical-basal gangliar-thalamic) model of SD. (For discussion, see Cannito [in press].)

This model suggests that small, variable lesions that disrupt pathways of premotor programming of speech and other complex motor behaviors may account for many signs and symptoms associated with SD. On this basis, it was predicted that SD patients would perform more poorly than the control group for tasks involving complex coordination, but would perform simple, isolated motor gestures as well as the control group. The specific tasks and predictive hypotheses are provided in Table 2. It should be noted that of 19 motor tasks, 11 were predicted to be impaired in SD and 8 were predicted to be normal. To evaluate overall statistical significance of the multivariate distribution with respect to the model-generated predictions, two Hotelling's T^2 statistics (the multivariate analog of the t-test) were computed. Results indicate a significant between-group effect in measures for which differences were predicted ($T^2 = 36.51$; $df = 8,27$; $p = 0.045$; two-tailed), but no difference in measures for which similar group performance was predicted ($T^2 = 12.13$, $df = 8.27$, $p = 0.441$). A stepwise discriminant function analysis revealed that a linear combination of four motor measures could differentiate speaker groups with 86% accuracy ($F = 7.22$; $df = 8,27$; $p < 0.001$). These striking results, however, did not entirely support the model of SD. Univariate repeated measures ANOVAs ($p < 0.05$) indicate that differences were limited to rapid sequential movements of the upper extremities (Cannito & Kondraske, 1990) and vocal tract, and to vocal tract steadiness (Cannito, 1989). Slow visual pursuit ramp tracking and sustained upper extremity steadiness remained unimpaired, as did the simple isolated movement tasks. The relation among predictions, actual outcomes, and associated motor variables are given in Figure 1. Expanded binomial probability (Guilford, 1954) is a means of determining the joint probability of n out of N significant directional

Table 2. Experimental hypotheses from Cannito (1986)

Hypothesis number	Predictions[a]	Experimental tasks[b]
1	SD speakers will exhibit: 1) unimpaired finger reaction times, but 2) impaired finger tapping speed.	RTD, RTN, FTD, FTN
2	SD speakers will exhibit impaired complex movement sequencing of the: 1) upper extremities, and 2) vocal tract.	PBD, PBN, WTS
3	SD speakers will exhibit impaired slow graded movements of the: 1) upper extremities, and 2) vocal tract.	SRTD, SRTN, SRTJ
4	SD speakers will exhibit impaired maintenance of sustained position of the: 1) upper extremities, and 2) vocal tract.	UESD, UESN, FFS
5	SD speakers will exhibit no impairment of isolated ballistic movement of the: 1) upper extremities or 2) vocal tract.	SID, SIN, SIJ SMD, SMN, SMJ

[a]In comparison to matched normal controls at alpha level 0.05, two-tailed.

[b]RT = reaction time, FT = fingertapping, PB = pegboard, WT = whispered trisyllables, SRT = slow ramp tracking, UES = upper extremity sustension, FFS = formant frequency steadiness, SI = step track initiation, SM = step movement completion, D = dominant upper extremity, N = nondominant upper extremity, J = jaw.

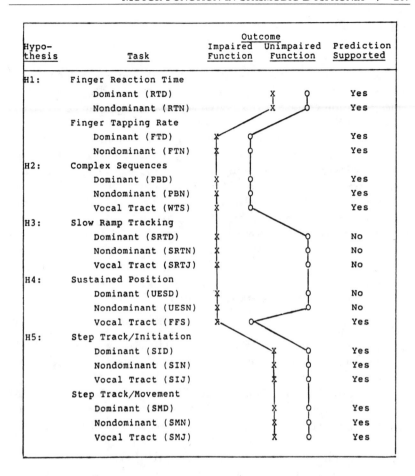

Hypo-thesis	Task	Outcome Impaired Function	Unimpaired Function	Prediction Supported
H1:	Finger Reaction Time			
	Dominant (RTD)			Yes
	Nondominant (RTN)			Yes
	Finger Tapping Rate			
	Dominant (FTD)			Yes
	Nondominant (FTN)			Yes
H2:	Complex Sequences			
	Dominant (PBD)			Yes
	Nondominant (PBN)			Yes
	Vocal Tract (WTS)			Yes
H3:	Slow Ramp Tracking			
	Dominant (SRTD)			No
	Nondominant (SRTN)			No
	Vocal Tract (SRTJ)			No
H4:	Sustained Position			
	Dominant (UESD)			No
	Nondominant (UESN)			No
	Vocal Tract (FFS)			Yes
H5:	Step Track/Initiation			
	Dominant (SID)			Yes
	Nondominant (SIN)			Yes
	Vocal Tract (SIJ)			Yes
	Step Track/Movement			
	Dominant (SMD)			Yes
	Nondominant (SMN)			Yes
	Vocal Tract (SMJ)			Yes

Figure 1. Pattern of predicted and obtained outcomes (Cannito, 1986). (X = predicted, O = obtained.)

predictions, using the alpha levels of the original comparisons. For the pattern of extralaryngeal motor findings reported in Cannito (1986), the expanded binomial probability was less than 0.001. In addition, the abnormal motor performance observed in SD could not be attributed to aging, or to affective involvement, as standardized test scores for anxiety and depression were uncorrelated with the motor variables deficient in SD.

This chapter will discuss five quantitative measures of oral-facial function, the results of conventional clinical assessments of oral-facial sensorimotor integrity, and the relation of these two measurements to each other, and to type, severity, age at onset, and duration of SD.

METHOD

Subjects

Eighteen female English-speaking adults with diagnosis of SD, confirmed by speech-language pathologists and an otolaryngologist, were studied. Voice inclusion characteristics as well as type, severity, age at onset, and duration of SD symptoms have been detailed in Cannito and Kondraske (1990). These individuals had no history of psychiatric and communicative disorders (other than SD), or symptomatic neurologic diseases (e.g., Parkinson's disease or spastic paralysis). Histories suggestive of hereditary familial tremor were ruled out. Eighteen nondysphonic females closely matched to the SD individuals on the bases of age and handedness, constituted the control group. The mean age of each group was 48.5 years (range = 25–65 years). SD subjects were additionally classified into subgroups by type of laryngospasm (adductor, $n = 6$; abductor, $n = 4$; mixed, $n = 8$) and presence ($n = 10$) or absence ($n = 8$) of audible voice tremor. The average age at onset of SD symptoms was 38.3 years ($SD = 14.24$), while the average time post-onset was 10.8 years ($SD = 9.72$).

Procedures

Two subjective clinical examinations of oral-facial sensimotor function were conducted and four quantitative assessments of oral-facial sensorimotor performance were employed.

Whispered Diadochokinetic Rate Subjects repeated whispering the trisyllable sequence /tukipa/ as rapidly as possible without sequencing errors. Whispering was employed because SD speakers have little difficulty with this voicing mode. Speech was recorded in a sound-isolated booth using a head-mounted Countryman EM101 electret condenser microphone with an Otari 5050 audio tape recorder. Acoustic signals were digitized (10,000 samples/sec) using a DEC PDP-11/73 laboratory computer. Timing measurements, from release of /t/ in the first trisyllable to the termination of /a/ in the fifth trisyllable, were made with the Interactive Laboratory System (Signal Technology, 1985) and were accurate to ± 10 msec. Four trials were obtained from each speaker. Figure 2 shows five repetitions of the whispered trisyllable sequence.

Second Formant Steadiness Subjects sustained the vowel /a/ for 8 seconds using an artificial voice source (Cooper Rand Intraoral Electrolarynx). The artificial voice source minimized the influence of laryngospasms on vowel articulation. The electrolarynx was supported by a free-standing boom so that the intraoral tube was positioned in the corner of the speaker's mouth, with her head supported by a headrest. These precautions reduced potential movement artifact. Acoustic signals were recorded and digitized as described. The time course of the second

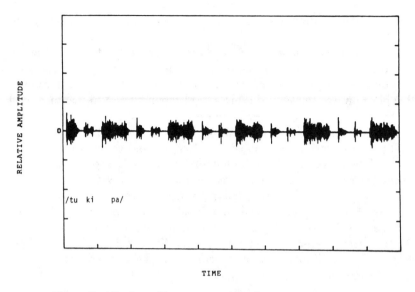

Figure 2. Waveform of five repetitions of the whispered sequence /tukipa/.

formant frequency was obtained using linear predictive coding algorithms, and the root mean squared variability was statistically derived. (See Figure 3.) Four trials were obtained from each speaker. Details of

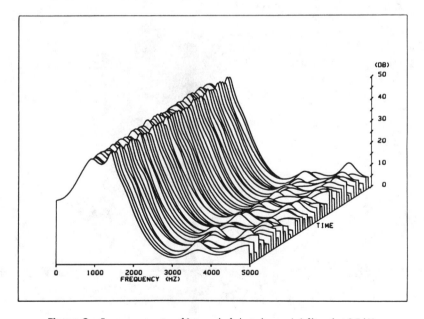

Figure 3. Frequency spectra of 1 second of electrolarynx /a/, filtered at 2.5 kHz.

instrumentation and analysis for this experiment were reported in Cannito (1989).

Mandibular Visual Ramp Tracking   The speaker followed a target cursor that moved vertically across a CRT in a slow, quasi-random manner by controlling a tracking cursor derived from jaw movement. Mandible position was transduced using a head-mounted system that measured rotation about the temporo-mandibular joint with a fixture clamped to the teeth and chin. This structure was coupled to a potentiometer with cable and pulley (a spring maintained cable tension and compensated for the mass of the moveable clamp and frame). Figure 4 illustrates the jaw movement transduction apparatus. The output signal provided a transducer sensitivity of 5.2 V/degree, linear throughout the total displacement range of 1 to 11 degrees. The output signal was digitized and provided on-line control of the tracking cursor. The dependent measure was the integrated average error between cursors. Four 20-second tracking trials were obtained. Additional system specifications have been provided in Kondraske, Potvin, Tourlette, and Syndulko (1984).

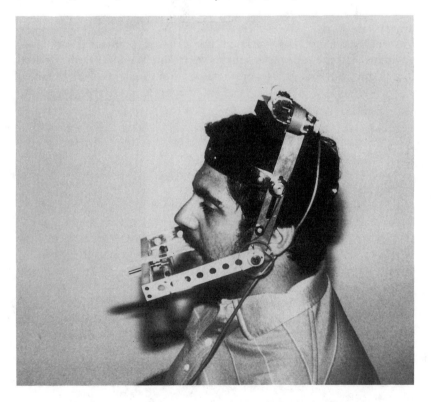

Figure 4.   Jaw movement transducer used in mandibular visual tracking tasks.

Mandibular Visual Step Tracking The same jaw movement transducer was used by the speaker to pursue a stimulus cursor that jumped vertically across the CRT screen at random intervals of 4–7 seconds. Movement initiation and movement completion times were measured. Movement initiation time was defined as elapsed msec between the onset of movement of the target cursor and onset of movement of the tracking cursor. Movement completion time was defined as elapsed msec between the onset and offset of tracking cursor movements. The fastest 8 of 10 step tracking measurements were averaged to constitute one trial and four such trials were obtained. Additional system specifications can be found in Kondraske et al. (1984).

Each speaker had a motor speech evaluation using the Dworkin-Culatta Oral Mechanism Examination (Dworkin & Culatta, 1980). Items relating to musculoskeletal structure were unremarkable for either group, so that only items associated with neuromotor function of the facies, lips, mandible, and velopharynx were tabulated for further analysis. The examination was supplemented with an assessment of oral-facial reflexes, nonspeech sequencing ability, and neck muscle function (see Appendix A). Each item was rated on a 4-point scale (Darley, Aronson, & Brown, 1975) and a cumulative rating of dysfunction computed for each speaker. Rating was considered useful for two reasons: 1) it included severity information lacking in a simple incidence count; 2) since deviations were infrequent in either group, the increased variation provided by the rating made correlation and regression procedures more feasible.

The clinical somatosensory evaluation comprised three tasks: 1) oral form identification by stereognostic-to-visual matching (Rosenbek, Wertz, & Darley, 1973; Weinberg, Lyons, & Liss, 1967); 2) labial and lingual two-point discrimination (Ringel, 1967) using a hand-held aesthesiometer, and 3) bucco-facial graphesthesia, adapted from Rey's procedure for testing manual graphesthesia (Lezak, 1976). A composite oral-facial somatosensory score was obtained by the sum of stereognostic errors, two-point thresholds for lip and tongue, and graphesthetic errors from both sides of the face.

Reliability

Test-retest reliability of the quantitative motor measures was estimated from inter-trial correlations for each variable using the Spearman-Brown formula (Guilford, 1954). Coefficients were as follows: whispered trisyllable speed, $r = .96$; second formant frequency steadiness, $r = .85$; mandibular ramp tracking, $r = .96$; step track initiation time, $r = .93$; and step track movement time, $r = .92$. All values were significant beyond alpha $=$ 0.01. Reliability measures were not obtained for the clinical examinations, but, a high level of clinical agreement for the oral mechanism examination had been established between the first and third authors prior to this research. In addition, the oral mechanism examination has been shown to be a reliable instrument (Dworkin & Culatta, 1985).

RESULTS

Overall means and standard deviations for quantitative performance measures and clinical examinations are provided for each subject group (Table 3). Each of the quantitative variables was subjected to a three-way repeated measures ANOVA (group x age x trials). Aging was included as a treatment within the statistical design because motor performance is known to decline with age (Potvin, Syndulko, Tourlette, Lemmon, & Potvin, 1980), and it is particularly interesting to explore interactions of SD and aging (Cannito & Kondraske, 1990). Significant between-group differences were obtained for second formant steadiness ($F = 5.50$; $df = 1,32$; $p = 0.026$) and for whispered diadochokinetic rates ($F = 4.53$; $df = 1,32$; $p = 0.041$). No significant differences were noted for the mandibular visual pursuit tracking measures ($p > 0.10$). Age significantly affected the whispered trisyllable rate, mandibular ramp tracking accuracy, and mandibular movement initiation time, but did not produce a between-group difference.

Table 3. Summary statistics for qualitative and quantitative measures of oral-facial sensorimotor functions in spasmodic dysphonic and normal females

Measurement	Units	Group	Mean	SD	Range
Motor speech examination	Severity rating sum	CN[a]	3.83	2.38	1.0–9.0
		SD[b]	8.94	5.72	3.0–27.0
Orofacial somasthesia	Error score composite	CN	8.11	2.17	4.0–11.0
		SD	9.58	3.07	4.0–14.5
Whispered diadochokinesis	Sec per five trisyllables	CN	3.09	0.31	2.69–3.79
		SD	3.35	0.47	2.74–4.14
Formant steadiness[c]	rms F2 in Hz	CN	9.00	5.40	2.44–19.98
		SD	13.48	8.24	2.09–37.53
Slow ramp tracking	Integrated avg error[d]	CN	1.44	0.55	0.65–2.78
		SD	1.27	0.44	0.83–2.35
Step track initiation	Time in msec	CN	330.2	37.9	268–400
		SD	347.2	68.1	276–551
Step track completion	Time in msec	CN	102.1	51.5	33.0–242.0
		SD	98.1	47.2	35.0–213.0

[a]CN = control normal (n = 18).
[b]SD = spasmodic dysphonic (n = 18).
[c]Originally reported in Cannito (1989).
[d]In degrees.

Means and standard deviations were computed for the raw numbers of oral motor deviations and for weighted ratings. To assess the possibility of an examiner's bias, ratios of unweighted to weighted cumulative oral motor scores were computed for each group. The SD group exhibited a ratio of 97 : 161, or 0.602. The control group exhibited a ratio of 43 : 67, or 0.642. These proportions did not differ significantly, but there was a slight bias toward weighting severity scores more for the control group. In addition, a correlation computed between raw and weighted oral motor scores indicated that they were monotonic ($r = .97$). These probes suggest that systematic error was not introduced into oral motor data by the severity rating. Means and standard deviations were also computed for somatosensory composite scores for each group (Table 4). Fisher's t-tests for independent samples were computed between groups for the clinical motor and somatosensory examinations. A significant difference was obtained between groups for the oral motor ratings ($t = 3.50$, $df = 34$, $p = 0.0013$), but not for the somatosensory examination ($p > 0.10$).

Analysis was undertaken to determine whether the distributional pattern of deviant oral motor findings by peripheral structure differed between the two groups (Table 5). Comparison of mean severity ratings by structure for each group is presented in Figure 5. Severity ratings greater than two were regarded as clinically significant. Statistically significant differences between groups (Mann-Whitney U tests) were observed for the velar and labiofacial loci only ($p < 0.01$). For other structures, motor deviations were distributed similarly for both groups. Abnormal oral-facial motor findings in SD are listed in Table 6. These were identified either

Table 4. Somatosensory examination subtest results

Task	Group	Mean	SD	Range
Two-point discrimination[a]				
labial	CN[d]	3.11	0.83	2–5
	SD[e]	3.67	1.14	2–6
lingual	CN	2.39	0.70	1–4
	SD	2.89	1.37	1–5
Buccal graphesthesia[b]				
right	CN	0.28	0.46	0–1
	SD	0.56	0.86	0–3
left	CN	0.78	1.26	0–2
	SD	0.61	0.70	0–2
Oral stereognosis[c]				
	CN	1.83	10.1	0–3.5
	SD	1.86	1.41	0–5

[a] In millimeters.
[b] Number incorrect.
[c] Number incorrect to visual matching. Half points reflect correct shape but incorrect size identification.
[d] CN = control normal ($n = 18$).
[e] SD = spasmodic dysphonic ($n = 18$).

Table 5. Mean raw scores[a], weighted scores[b], and incidence distributions[c] of motor speech deviations (%) across structures

Structures	Group		
	Spasmodic dysphonics	Normal controls	Combined groups
Labio-facial			
Raw number	27	6	17
Weighted score	50	9	30
%	28	14	24
Mandibular			
Raw number	9	5	7
Weighted score	9	5	7
%	9	12	10
Lingual			
Raw number	24	17	20
Weighted score	38	29	34
%	25	39	29
Velar			
Raw number	29	11	20
Weighted score	51	19	35
%	30	26	28
Cervico-brachial			
Raw number	8	4	6
Weighted score	13	5	9
%	8	9	9

[a] Raw number of deviant findings.
[b] Weighted deviation score based on severity ratings.
[c] Percent distribution by structure.

because they did not occur in the control speakers, or because they received a clinically significant severity rating. Two or more clinically significant motor deviations were exhibited by 72% of the SD group, but by only 33% of the control group. Cumulative motor ratings of seven SD speakers exceeded two standard deviations above the control group mean ($p < 0.05$). No single abnormality or pattern of abnormalities typified the SD group. The abnormal findings, however, were most compatible with a surpranuclear localization rather than lower motor neuron involvement. No evidence of flaccidity, atrophy, or fasiculation of the cranial musculature was observed in any speakers studied.

Pearson product-moment correlations indicate that the oral motor examination was significantly correlated (r-crit = 0.418, $df = 35$, $p < 0.01$) with second formant steadiness ($r = .451$), mandibular step movement initiation time ($r = 0.446$), and mandibular step movement completion time ($r = .521$). Multiple regression analysis yielded a combination of step movement completion and second formant steadiness ($F = 8.67$; $df = 2,34$; $p < 0.001$) that accounted for approximately 35% of

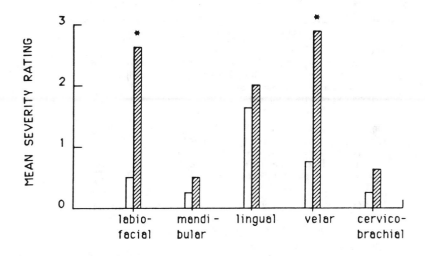

PERIPHERAL STRUCTURE

Figure 5. Mean severity of motor speech deviations across structures (starred contrasts are statistically significant. White = control normal, cross-hatched = spasmodic dysphonia.)

the variance in oral motor examinations (20% of variance was attributable to $F2$ steadiness alone). Aging was correlated with ramp tracking ($r = .626$) and step movement initiation ($r = .460$). No other correlations achieved statistical significance, nor did any variables differ among SD subcategories on the basis of laryngospasm type or voice tremor.

CONCLUSIONS

SD speakers in this study differed from matched normal speakers on clinical ratings of oral-facial motor dysfunction, but not on the somatosensory examination. Motor dysfunction was most affected in the tongue and labiofacial and velar structures, but only the latter two differentiated speaker groups. In addition, SD speakers differed on two quantitative measures of speech motor performance: whispered diadochokinetic rate for trisyllables, and sustained vowel formant steadiness using an electrolarynx. No differences were noted for nonspeech measures of mandibular visual pursuit tracking. Finally, the subjective clinical ratings were significantly correlated with three quantitative performance measures.

These findings are compatible with previous studies (see Table 1) that report a high incidence of extralaryngeal motor abnormalities in patients with SD. While these studies did not focus specifically on oral-facial

Table 6. Oral-facial abnormalities exhibited by SD speakers uncharacteristic of control speakers

Labial findings
  labial assymetry (reduced unilateral retraction with lip corner droop)
  slow and irregular diadochokinesis for /b/ (whispered)
  labial weakness (for smacking and resistance to force)
  flattening of nasolabial fold
  labial tremor on protrusion

Lingual findings
  reduced tongue strength and range of motion
  lingual tremor on protrusion
  lingual writhing movements and tics at rest
  slow and irregular diadochokinesis for /k/ (whispered)

Velar findings
  velar assymetry (low unilaterally with uvular deviation to opposite side)
  hyperactive gag reflex[a]
  velar tremor on sustained phonation

Facial and mandibular findings
  bilateral facial ptosis
  occulomotor spasms
  reduced jaw strength (to resistance on opening and closing)
  nocturnal bruxism (reported)

Cervical findings
  reduced platysmal function (on contraction)
  reduced sternocleidomastoid function (head turning against resistance)
  tics and tremors of the head

Complex sequential findings
  alternating motion rate (pucker and smile) impaired
  errors on three part oral facial commands
  difficulty repeating complex word (whispered)

[a]Hypoactive gag reflexes were common to both groups.

function, most include oral-facial signs and symptoms within their inventories. As in previous studies, this study also reports a predominance of extrapyramidal and pyramidal motor signs (compared with relatively few peripheral nerve, bulbar, or cerebellar signs), implicating a supranuclear locus of dysfunction in SD. Lack of somatosensory involvement fails to support a somatosensory model of SD (cf. Izdebsky & Shipp, 1985) or claims of parietal lobe involvement in SD (Finitzo & Freeman, 1989; Robe et al., 1960).

Quantitative measures were able to account for variation in clinical examinations, which suggests the validity of using both assessment techniques, but correlated variance was small and partly related to factors other than SD. Furthermore, no oral-facial motor measure bore any statistical relation to actual voice symptoms of SD. At most, it may be inferred that phonatory symptoms and associated extralaryngeal abnormalities could arise on the basis of size and location of some, as yet unspecified, neurologic lesion(s). More direct evidence of underlying brain pathology in SD is accumulating (Cannito, Finitzo, Freeman, & Pool, 1985; Chapman et al., 1989; Feldman et al., 1985; Finitzo & Freeman, 1989; Schaefer et al., 1985) but remains difficult to interpret. Multifocal and variable lesion explanations have been advanced to accommodate the diverse neurologic signs and symptoms that are associated with SD (Cannito, in press; Finitzo & Freeman, 1989; Schaefer, 1983).

Prevalence of adventitious movements in SD patients (Rosenfield, 1988) has led authors to speculate that SD may be a dystonia (Aronson et al., 1968; Blitzer et al., 1985; Chritchley, 1939; Freeman et al. 1985; McCall, 1974; Ludlow & Connor, 1987; Marsden & Sheehy, 1982; Rosenfield, 1988), with the implication that it is a basal ganglia disorder. If SD is a dystonia, however, it is a *focal* and *function specific* dystonia. The violent laryngospasms that define the syndrome are specific to phonated speech.

SD shares characteristics of focal dystonias (with which it often occurs), including association with essential tremor (Baxter & Lal, 1979; Couch, 1976), emergence of dystonia elsewhere in the body (Marsden, 1976b), in addition to idiopathic adult onset. Many authors regard SD as an isolated manifestation of oral-facial-cervical dystonia or Meige syndrome (Jankovic & Ford, 1982; Marsden & Sheehy, 1982; Rosenfield, 1988). However, focality alone is insufficient to describe SD. Most SD patients do not have laryngospasms when swallowing or breathing, or in nonspeech vocalizations such as laughing or crying. Therefore, SD has been compared to "action induced" dystonias (Blitzer et al., 1985) such as dystonic writer's cramp or dystonia for walking forward but not backward (Rothwell, Obeso, Day, & Marsden, 1983). As Rothwell et al. (1983) observe: "The abnormality producing dystonic spasms in these patients cannot lie in the motor outflow pathway since some categories of movement are unaffected. A fault must also lie in the production of the motor command as well" (p. 862). Similarly, Sheehy and Marsden (1982) suggested the breakdown of a brain mechanism for generating an "engram of our script independent of which muscles are required, and of sensory feedback" (p. 478) as a basis for dystonic writer's cramp.

In this regard, it is important that in this study, the impaired oral-facial performances were limited to speech-like tasks. Within the broader study (Cannito, 1986), upper extremity findings parallelled those for speech — only complex, rapid sequential movements were impaired (Cannito & Kondraske, 1990). Analogous findings have also been reported for laryngeal movements in SD. Reich and Till (1983) found no significant difference in phonatory reaction time for the vowel /ʌ/ but significantly prolonged latencies for the more complex word /ʌpɚ/ in SD speakers compared with normal speakers. Similarly, Ludlow and Connor (1987) found that simple laryngeal movement initiation was not delayed in SD, but attainment of "correct production of laryngeal position and force for phonation, after initiating a response" (p. 204) was. Collectively, quantitative motor findings argue that SD is neither a peripheral nerve disorder (cf. Dedo, Townsend, & Izdebsky, 1978), nor a brainstem disorder (cf. Izdebsky & Shipp, 1985; Schaefer, Finitzo-Hieber, Gerling, & Freeman, 1983), but a supranuclear disorder disrupting the voluntary pathways for phonation and, sometimes articulation and manual control. A selective impairment of complex motor functions of this type, in the presence of intact isolated ballistic and slow ramp gestures, appears to implicate very high levels of motor information processing within the CNS. The underlying neuropathophysiology of such impairments in SD, however, continues to remain obscure.

The etiologic basis of other focal, function-specific dystonias is equally uncertain. Like SD, they are not characteristically hereditary (in contrast to generalized torsion dystonia), nor has their pathophysiologic basis been identified (Hallett & Ravits, 1986; Marsden, 1976a). Penney and Young (1983) proposed a model of basal ganglia function that accounts for hyperkinesias of extrapyramidal disease by disruption of premotor cortical-striatal-pallidal-thalamic-cortical circuits for voluntary movement control. Interestingly, the same circuits are thought to be involved in the premotor organization of complex voluntary sequential movements (Evarts, 1980; Palliard, 1960). The idea of a disruption in the cortical-subcortical loop that produces vocal manifestations of SD and a variety of sensory and motor symptoms (depending on the location of disruption), is compelling because it accounts for both the heterogeneous and homogeneous characteristics of the disorder. The proximity of extrapyramidal and pyramidal structures and pathways within the CNS might explain the frequent occurrence of these symptoms in SD patients. Such an interpretation is consistent with the selective deficits reported for complex laryngeal, articulatory, and manual coordination in SD. It may also explain some of the diversity and apparent inconsistency of brain imaging findings in the literature. Finally, it should be acknowledged that: 1) truly "spastic" dysphonias (i.e., pyramidal dysarthria in which the laryngeal component dominates), as well as some psychogenic dysphonias, sometimes are diagnosed as SD; and 2) that these are difficult, if not impossible, to differentiate from extrapyramidal dysphonias on the basis of vocal output alone. Continued heuristic experimentation should elucidate these complex diagnostic and theoretic issues toward a comprehensive model of the spasmodic dysphonias.

REFERENCES

Aminoff, M.J., Dedo, H.H., & Izdebsky, K. (1978). Clinical aspects of spasmodic dysphonia. *Journal of Neurosurgery and Psychiatry*, *41*, 361–365.

Aronson, A.E. (1985). *Clinical voice disorders: An interdisciplinary approach* (2nd ed.). New York: Thieme, Inc.

Aronson, A.E., Brown, J.R., Litin, M.E., & Pearson, J.S. (1968). Spastic dysphonia: I. Voice, neurologic, and psychiatric aspects. *Journal of Speech and Hearing Disorders, 33,* 203–218.

Aronson, A.E., & Hartman, C. (1981). Adductor spastic dysphonia as a sign of essential (voice) tremor. *Journal of Speech and Hearing Disorders, 46,* 52–58.

Baxter, D.W., & Lal, S. (1979). Essential tremor and dystonic syndromes. In L.H. Poirier, T.L. Sourkes, & P.J. Bedard (Eds.), *Advances in neurology* (Vol. 24, pp. 373–377). New York: Raven Press.

Blitzer, A., Lovelace, R., Brin, M., Fahn, S., & Fink, M. (1985). Electromyographic findings in focal laryngeal dystonia (spastic dysphonia). *Annals of Otology, Rhinology and Laryngology, 94,* 591–594.

Bloch, P. (1965). Neuro-psychiatric aspects of spastic dysphonia. *Folia Phoniatrica, 17,* 301–364.

Boone, D.R. (1977). *The voice and voice therapy.* Englewood Cliffs, NJ: Prentice Hall.

Brodnitz, F.S. (1976). Spastic dysphonia. *Annals of Otorhinolaryngology, 85,* 210–214.

Cannito, M.P. (1986). *Extralaryngeal functions in spasmodic dysphonia: Vocal tract and manual control.* Unpublished doctoral dissertation, University of Texas at Dallas.

Cannito, M.P. (1989). Vocal tract steadiness in spasmodic dysphonia. In K. Yorkston & D. Beukelman (Eds.), *Recent advances in clinical dysarthria* (pp. 243–262). Boston: Little, Brown.

Cannito, M.P. (in press). Neurobiological interpretations of spasmodic dysphonia. In D. Vogel & M.P. Cannito (Eds.), *Treating disordered speech motor control: For clinicians by clinicians.* Austin, TX: PRO-ED.

Cannito, M.P., Finitzo, T., Freeman, F., & Pool, K. (1985). Brain electrical activity mapping in adductor spasmodic dysphonia. *Journal of the Acoustical Society of America, 77* (Suppl. 1: S87) 4:37.

Cannito, M.P., & Johnson, J.P. (1981). Spastic dysphonia: A continuum disorder. *Journal of Communication Disorders, 14,* 215–223.

Cannito, M.P., & Kondraske, G.V. (1990). Rapid manual abilities in spasmodic dysphonic and normal female subjects. *Journal of Speech and Hearing Research, 33,* 123–133.

Chapman, S.D., Watson, B.C., Pool, K., Devous, M.D., Freeman, F., Schaefer, S.D., Konraske, G.V., Mendelsohn, D.B., Close, L.G., & Finitzo, T. (1989). Multifocal cortical dysfunction in spasmodic dysphonia. In K. Yorkston & D. Beukelman (Eds.), *Recent advances in clinical dysarthria.* Boston: College-Hill Press.

Chritchley, M. (1939). Spastic dysphonia ("inspiratory speech"). *Brain: A Journal of Neurology, 62,* 96–103.

Couch, J.R. (1976). Dystonia and tremor in spasmodic torticollis. In R. Eldridge & S. Fahn (Eds.), *Advances in neurology* (Vol. 14). NY: Raven Press.

Darley, F.L., Aronson, A.E., & Brown, J.R. (1975). *Motor speech disorders.* Philadelphia, W.B. Saunders.

Dedo, H.H., Townsend, J.J., & Izdebsky, K. (1978). Current evidence for the organic etiology of spastic dysphonia. *Otolaryngology, 86* (6) 875–880.

Dworkin, J.P., & Culatta, R.A. (1980). *Dworkin-Culatta Oral Mechanism Examination.* Nicholasville, KY: Edgewood Press.

Dworkin, J.P, & Culatta, R.A. (1985). Oral structural and neuromuscular characteristics in children with normal and disordered articulation. *Journal of Speech and Hearing Disorders, 50,* 150–156.

Evarts, E.V. (1980). Brain mechanisms in voluntary movement. In D. McFadden (Ed.), *Neural mechanisms in behavior* (pp. 232–252). New York: Springer-Verlag.

Feldman, M., Nixon, J.V., Finitzo-Hieber, T., & Freeman, F.J. (1984). Abnormal parasympathetic vagal function in patients with spasmodic dysphonia. *Annals of Internal Medicine, 100,* 401–495.

Finitzo, T., & Freeman, F.J. (1989). Spasmodic dysphonia, whether and where: Results of seven years of research. *Journal of Speech and Hearing Research, 32,* 541–555.

Freeman, F.J., Cannito, M.P., & Finitzo-Hieber, T. (1985). Classification of spasmodic dysphonia by perceptual-acoustic-visual means. In G.A. Gates (Ed.), *Spasmodic dysphonia: The state of the art, 1984* (pp. 5–18). New York: The Voice Foundation.

Guilford, J.P. (1954). *Psychometric methods.* New York: McGraw-Hill.

Hallett, M., & Ravits, J.H. (1986). Involuntary movements. In A.K. Asbury, G.M. McKhann, & W.I. McDonald (Eds.), *Diseases of the nervous system: Clinical neurobiology* (pp. 452–460). Philadelphia: W.B. Saunders.

Heaver, L. (1959). Spastic dysphonia: II. Psychiatric considerations. *Logos, 2,* 15–24.

Izdebsky, K., & Shipp, T. (1985). Model of spastic dysphonia. In G.A. Gates (Ed.), *Spastic dysphonia: The state of the art, 1984.* New York: The Voice Foundation.

Jankovic, J., & Ford, J. (1982). Blepharospasm and orofacial-cervical dystonia: Clinical and pharmacological findings in 100 patients. *Annals of Neurology, 13,* 402–411.

Kondraske, G.V., Potvin, A.R., Tourlette, W.W., & Syndulko, K.A. (1984). A computer based system for automated quantification of neurologic function. *IEEE Transactions in Biomedical Engineering, 31,* 401–414.

Lezak, M.D. (1976). *Neuropsychological assessment.* New York: Oxford University Press.

Ludlow, C., & Connor, N. (1987). Dynamic aspects of phonatory control in spasmodic dysphonia. *Journal of Speech and Hearing Research, 30,* 197–206.

Marsden, C.D. (1976a). Dystonia: The spectrum of the disease. In M.D. Yahr (Ed.), *The basal ganglia* (pp. 351–367). New York: Raven Press.

Marsden, C.D. (1976b). The problem of adult-onset ideopathic torsion dystonia and other isolated dyskinesias in adult life (including blepharospasm oromandibular dystonia, dystonic writer's cramp, and torticollis or axial dystonia.) In R. Eldridge & S. Fahn (Eds.), *Advances in neurology* (Vol. 14). New York: Raven Press.

Marsden, C.D., & Sheehy, M.P. (1982). Spastic dysphonia, Meige disease and torsion dystonia. (Letter to the editor). *Neurology, 32,* 1202.

McCall, G.N. (1974). Spasmodic dysphonia and the stuttering block: Commonalities or possible connections. In L.M. Webster & L.C. Furst (Eds.), *Vocal tract dynamics and dysfluency* (pp. 124–151). New York: Speech & Hearing Institute.

McCall, G., Skolnik, L., & Brewer, D. (1971). A preliminary report of some atypical movement patterns in the tongue, palate, hypopharynx and larynx of patients with spasmodic dysphonia. *Journal of Speech and Hearing Disorders, 36,* 466–470.

Palliard, J. (1960). The patterning of skilled movements. In J. Field, H. Magoun, & V. Hall (Eds.), *Handbook of physiology,* (Vol. 3, pp. 1679–1708). Washington, DC: American Physiological Society.

Penney, J.G., & Young, A.B. (1983). Speculations on the functional anatomy of basal ganglia disorders. *Annual Review of Neuroscience, 6*, 73–94.

Potvin, A.R., Syndulko, K., Tourlette, W.W., Lemmon, J.A., & Potvin, J.H. (1980). Human neurologic function and the aging process. *American Geriatrics Society, 28*, 1–9.

Reich, A., & Till, J. (1983). Phonatory and manual reaction times of women with ideopathic spasmodic dysphonia. *Journal of Speech and Hearing Research, 26*, 10–18.

Ringel, R.L. (1967). Oral region two-point descrimination in normal and myopathic subjects. In J.F. Bosma (Ed.), *Second symposium on oral sensation and perception.* Springfield, IL: Charles C Thomas.

Robe, E., Brumlik, J., & Moore, P. (1960). A study of spastic dysphonia: Neurologic and electroencephalographic abnormalities. *Laryngoscope, LXX*, 219–245.

Rosenbek, J.C., Wertz, R.T., & Darley, F.L. (1973). Oral sensation and perception in apraxia of speech and aphasia. *Journal of Speech and Hearing Research, 16*, 22–36.

Rosenfield, D.B. (1988). Spasmodic dysphonia. In J. Jankovic & E. Tolosa (Eds.), *Advances in Neurology: Vol. 49. Facial dyskinesias* (pp. 323–327). New York: Raven Press.

Rothwell, J.C., Obeso, J.A., Day, B.L., & Marsden, C.D. (1983). Pathophysiology of dystonias. In J.E. Desmedt (Ed.), *Motor control mechanisms in health and disease* (pp. 851–863). New York: Raven Press.

Schaefer, S.D. (1983). Neuropathology of spasmodic dysphonia. *Laryngoscope, 93*, 1183–1204.

Schaefer, S.D., Finitzo-Hieber, T., Gerling, I.J., & Freeman, F.J. (1983). Brainstem conduction abnormalities in spasmodic dysphonia. *Annals of Otology, Rhinology, and Laryngology, 92*, 59–63.

Schaefer, S., Freeman, F., Finitzo, T., Close, L., Cannito, M., Ross, E., Reisch, J., & Miravella, K. (1985). Magnetic resonance imaging findings and correlations in spasmodic dysphonia patients. *Annals of Otology, Rhinology and Laryngology, 94*, 595–601.

Sheehy, M.P., & Marsden, C.D. (1982). Writers' cramp — A focal dystonia, *Brain, 105*, 461–480.

Shipp, T., Izdebsky, K., Reed, C., & Morrissey, P. (1985). Intrinsic laryngeal muscle activity in a spastic dysphonia patient. *Journal of Speech and Hearing Disorders, 50* (1-) 54–59.

Signal Technology. (1985). *Interactive Laboratory System Version 5* [Computer program].

Weinberg, B., Lyons, M.J., & Liss, G.M. (1967). Studies of oral, manual, and visual form identification in children and adults. In J.F. Bosma (Ed.), *Second symposium on oral sensation and perception* (pp. 340–349). Springfield, IL: Charles C Thomas.

Dysarthria and Apraxia of Speech:
Perspectives on Management
edited by Christopher A. Moore, Ph.D., Kathryn M. Yorkston, Ph.D.,
and David R. Beukelman, Ph.D.
copyright © 1991   Paul H. Brookes Publishing Co., Inc.
Baltimore · London · Toronto · Sydney

Appendix A

Neuro-speech Supplement for Spasmodic Dysphonia

I. Pathologic Oral Reflexes
Jaw Jerk Reflex
The jaw jerk reflex is a stretch reflex of the muscles of mastication (Masseter/temporalis) in which contractions result from sudden stretching of muscle. The patient is instructed to let the jaw relax in a half open position. The examiner's finger, placed on the chin and pressing downward, is struck sharply with a rubber mallet. The jaw reflex is difficult to obtain. Consequently, if it is visible, it is probably increased. Exaggeration of this reflex is evidence of corticobulbar disease.
Absent _____ Present _____

Snout Reflex
The snout reflex is a pathologic reflex that emerges in bilateral upper motor neuron disease. Have the patient relax his lips and breathe gently through his mouth. Tapping with a rubber mallet or briskly stroking the upper lip (from corner of mouth to center with a tongue blade) will result in puckering of the lips in a quick transient bilateral contraction of the obicularis oris.
Absent _____ Present _____

Meyerson's Reflex
In spasticity and sometimes in rigidity (parkinsonism), tapping about the forehead and especially the glabella will result in exaggerated muscle response.
Absent _____ Present _____

II. Oral-Facial Sequences*
1. Open your mouth/then puff your cheeks/then blow.
   _____   _____   _____

2. Wiggle your tongue/then close your eyes/then bare your teeth.
   _____   _____   _____

3. Lick your lips/then wink/then clear your throat.
   Number of Sequenced Errors: Command: _____   Imitation: _____

III. Strength and Symmetry*
1. Jaw resistance
   To opening   _____
   To closing   _____

2. Eyelid resistance to opening
   Right   _____
   Lef.   _____
3. Platysma
   Right   _____
   Left   _____
4. Trapezius   _____
5. Sterno-cleido-mastoid
   Right   _____
   Left   _____
6. Lingual range of motion
   Circumoral   _____
   Retroflexion   _____

---

note: *to be scored as + = normal, − = abnormal.

Chapter 16 _____

Botulinum Treatment for Orolingual-Mandibular Dystonia
Speech Effects

Geralyn M. Schulz and Christy L. Ludlow

PATIENTS WITH OROLINGUAL-mandibular dystonia (OLMD) have abnormal movements of the vocal tract, including sustained tongue movements, clenched jaw, and/or forced jaw opening (Jankovic, 1988b; Tolosa & Marti, 1988). These abnormal movements are characterized by sustained, repetitive muscle spasms (Marsden, 1976) and the heightened activity of particular muscles (Thompson, Obeso, Delgado, Gallego, & Marsden, 1986). OLMD has its onset in adulthood, usually between the ages of 40 and 60, and has a 3:1 female occurrence (Fahn, 1988). OLMD often occurs with blepharospasm (Jankovic, 1988b) but may occur as an isolated focal dystonia (Lagueny, Deliac, Julien, Demotes-Mainard, & Ferrer, 1989). The complex, including both oromandibular symptoms and blepharospasm, has been variously referred to as Meige syndrome, cranial-cervical dystonia, Brueghel's syndrome, and Wood's syndrome (Jankovic, 1988b).

Similar to other focal dystonias such as writer's cramp (Sheehy, Rothwell, & Marsden, 1988) and spasmodic dysphonia (Cohen, Ludlow, et al., 1989), patients with OLMD have abnormal blink reflexes that indicate hyperexcitability of brainstem interneurons (Berardelli, Rothwell, Day, & Marsden, 1988).

Mandibular dyskinesias and dystonias have been associated with dental problems and temporomandibular joint syndrome (Koller, 1983). In-

This chapter is in the public domain.

stances of blepharospasm and cranial dystonias have been reported subsequent to lesions involving the brainstem and/or basal ganglia (Jankovic & Patel, 1983; Keane & Young, 1985), while other cases are reported to be familial (Jankovic & Nutt, 1988). Idiopathic OLMD is often spontaneous, however, with no evident etiology, and can be distinguished from hemifacial spasms (Gottleib & May, 1984; Jankovic, 1988c), drug-induced orofacial movement disorders such as tardive dyskinesia (Marsden & Fahn, 1987), other secondary dystonias (Calne & Lang, 1988), facial chorea (Kurlan & Shoulson, 1988), and psychogenic dystonia (Fahn & Williams, 1988). Abnormal movements in OLMD may interfere with, or be precipitated by, voluntary actions such as speaking and chewing, and patients may be free of abnormal movements at rest in early stages of the disorder (Marsden, 1976).

In their review of the dysarthrias of movement disorders, Hartman and Abbs (1988) identified only two studies that measured perceived speech difficulties in OLMD patients (Darley, Aronson, & Brown, 1975; Golper, Nutt, Rau, & Coleman, 1983). Darley et al. (1975) found that phonation, articulation, and prosody were significantly disturbed in dystonia. Golper et al. (1983) in perceptual evaluations of 10 patients with OLMD and/or Meige syndrome found that 6 had abnormal speech symptoms, including slow speech rate, inappropriate silences and pauses, abnormal stress, and imprecise consonants, and 5 had reduced speech intelligibility.

Drug therapies for treatment of OLMD have had mixed benefits (Gimenez-Roldan, Mateo, Orbe, Munoz-Blanco, & Hipola, 1988; Klawans & Tanner, 1988; Tanner, Wilson, Goetz, & Shannon, 1988; Tolosa & Kulisevsky, 1988), and surgical approaches have had similarly mixed results (Fahn & Marsden, 1987; Waltz, 1982). The treatment of choice for many forms of focal dystonia is botulinum toxin injected into the affected muscles. Botulinum toxin reduces muscle activity by temporarily blocking the release of acetylcholine at the neuromuscular junction (Bandyopadhyay, Clark, DasGupta, & Sathyamoorthy, 1987; Wright, 1955). Muscle activity returns usually within 3–4 months with the sprouting of new terminals. Botulinum toxin has been used to treat blepharospasm (Scott, 1980), writer's cramp (Cohen, Hallett, Geller, & Hochberg, 1989), spasmodic dysphonia (Ludlow, Naunton, Sedory, Schulz, & Hallett, 1988), hemifacial spasm (Brin et al., 1987; Tolosa, Marti, & Kulisevsky, 1988), spasmodic torticollis (Tsui et al., 1985), Meige syndrome (Mauriello, 1985), and OLMD (Blitzer, Greene, Brin, & Fahn, 1989; Jankovic, 1988a; Tsui & Calne, 1988). No studies have evaluated the effect of botulinum toxin in OLMD patients, and Jankovic (1989) noted the difficulty of demonstrating objective improvement in this population.

This study proposed to determine if botulinum toxin injected into hypertonic muscles would objectively change the speech of patients with OLMD. More specifically, based on reports of speech difficulties in OLMD, we investigated the acoustic durations of syllables, words, and sentences prior to treatment, and at 2 week and 3 month intervals following treatment. To determine clinical effectiveness of botulinum toxin treatment, we also examined the severity ratings of perceptual dimensions at the same intervals.

METHODS

Subjects

Three subjects had focal dystonia affecting the orofacial or mandibular musculature only, and two had OLMD and blepharospasm (Table 1). Patient 1 was a former auctioneer and thus had a history of overuse of the speech production mechanism. Movement abnormalities occurred only during speech and his nonspeech oral movements were normal. He demonstrated increased posterior tongue elevation and jaw depression that worsened with continued speaking, resulting in a fixed oral posture. Patients 2 and 3 had undergone extensive dental work and had cases of edentulous orofacial dyskinesia (Koller, 1983). Although both had movement abnormalities at rest and during speech, patient 2 had continuous jaw clenching while patient 3 maintained a constantly depressed jaw position. Patient 4 had Meige syndrome with blepharospasm, facial grimacing, tongue elevation, and jaw depression that was exacerbated by speaking. Patient 5 also had Meige syndrome and presented similar clinical movement abnormalities, without tongue elevation. All five patients complained of difficulty in speaking prior to treatment. Five normal control subjects, matched in age and sex and without histories of neurologic or speech problems, were also studied.

Procedures

Each speaker repeated the individual syllables /pɑ/ /tɑ/ /kɑ/; the words "potato," "tomato," and "baggage"; and the sentences "I have the baggage," and "I thought about my sister," for 7 seconds. These tasks were employed to produce speech of varying length and containing problematic phonemes. Bilabial consonants (/p/, /b/, /m/) would be difficult to produce by patients with abnormal lip and jaw opening or closing; and lingual consonants (/t/, /k/, /g/, /θ/, /s/) would be difficult for patients with abnormal tongue movement. Subjects were instructed to repeat these stimuli at their regular speaking rate and volume. The acoustic signal was

Table 1. Subject characteristics

	Orolingual-mandibular dystonia					Normal
Sex/age	Clinical description	Diagnosis	Years post-onset	Injected muscle(s)	Dosage	Sex/age
1. M/46	Excessive tongue elevation	OLMD	4	Genioglossus, styloglossus	40U 20U	1. M/51
2. F/75	Excessive jaw closing	OLMD	2	Medial pterygoid, masseter	20U 20U	2. F/70
3. F/59	Excessive jaw opening	OLMD	4	Ant. belly digastric, masseter	40U	3. F/48
4. F/69	Excessive tongue elevation, Lip pulling	Meige	15	Genioglossus Risorius	30U 10U	4. F/61
5. F/59	Excessive jaw closing	Meige	2	Medial pterygoid, masseter	15U 30U	5. F/30

recorded on FM tape and digitized at 10K samples/second with a 4.5 kHz anti-aliasing filter. Commercial hardware and software systems (Mac-Speech Lab, GW Instruments) were used for analysis.

Botulinum toxin injections were administered in two or three sessions to produce a clinical muscle weakness. The units injected per muscle and patient are listed in Table 1. Injection procedures were similar to those for laryngeal injections described by Ludlow ét al. (1988). Non-speech verification gestures were used for all.

The OLMD patients' speech was recorded at three intervals: prior to injection, 2 weeks after injection, and 3 months after injection. To assess speech impairment, we compared the baseline measures of OLMD to normal controls. To assess injection effects, we compared baseline measures with those made 2 weeks post-injection. To assess effects of treatment withdrawal, we compared baseline measures to those made 3 months after injection.

Acoustic Measures

For each 7-second syllable, word, or sentence repetition task, the duration between voicing onset (first glottal pulse) and offset (last glottal pulse) was measured from oscillographic tracings of acoustic waveforms. Figure 1 illustrates the duration measurement of one repetition of "potato" by a normal speaker and an OLMD patient. This did not include the plosive burst for the initial stop consonant, but did include pauses that occurred between syllables within the word and sentence repetitions.

Perceptual Measures

For perceptual measurement, a listening tape was made using "potato" and the sentence, "I have the baggage." This tape contained all uniden-

NORMAL PRODUCTION "POTATO"

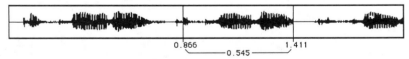

ORO-LINGUAL-MANDIBULAR PRODUCTION "POTATO"

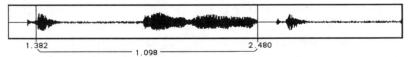

Figure 1. Measurement illustration for production of the word "potato" by a control subject and a patient with orolingual-mandibular dystonia. (2 sec total duration.)

tified randomly ordered, 7-second samples from normal speakers and from pre-injection, post-injection, and follow-up patients. The total samples (five patients × two speech items × three recording intervals, plus five controls × 2 speech items) was 37, not 40, because one patient did not repeat the sentence at baseline, and one patient was unable to return at the 3-month interval. Intensity of the tape was monitored with the VU meter on the recorder between −3 and +2 V for all samples. Listening playback was set at a loudness level comfortable for the judges that was maintained throughout the listening session. The three judges listened to the tape through speakers and were allowed to listen again to samples if they felt they could not make accurate ratings after the first listening. This was necessary for the initial three samples only.

Four perceptual rating dimensions were selected, based on the cluster analysis results of Darley et al. (1975) for patients with dystonia. They found two clusters important for classifying the speech of dystonia patients. From the first cluster, articulatory inaccuracies, we selected the dimension most severely impaired, imprecise consonants. From the second cluster, prosodic excess, we selected prolonged phonemes, inappropriate silences, and overall speech rate. These dimensions were chosen because they were unrelated as well as severely impaired in their patients. The perceptual study by Golper et al. (1983) also identified these perceptual dimensions as impaired in OLMD.

Three experienced speech pathologists rated each of the 37 speech samples on the four dimensions using a 7-point interval scale. A rating of 1 represented normal speech, and 7, severe impairment. Raters were not familiar with any of the subjects. Percent agreement was calculated as the number of times that a listener gave identical ratings or ratings differing by 1 point. The mean percentage agreement for the three raters across conditions for word repetitions was 77%, and for the sentence repetitions, 80%, giving an overall agreement for the three raters of 79%.

RESULTS

Durations

OLMD patients' pre-injection measures were compared with those of the normal controls to determine differences on each speech task. Two-way ANOVAs were used to examine group and task effects. An asterisk beside the duration measure in the first column of Table 2 indicates a significant difference ($p \leq 0.001$) between normal and patients' pre-injection measures. Group differences varied across tasks, and patients' pre-injection durations were longer than those of normal speakers on word and sentence repetition but not on the syllable repetition.

Table 2. Group means and standard deviations for acoustic duration in milliseconds

		Control	OLMD		
		Normal	Pre-	Post-	Follow-up
Syllable	X̄	284	231	267*	216*
	SD	84	128	93	88
Word	X̄	520*	597	485*	460*
	SD	76	269	117	80
Sentence	X̄	1,278*	1,925	1,413*	1,328*
	SD	216	744	425	266

*$p \leq 0.001$ compared to patient pre-injection measures.

To determine if measures changed with botulinum toxin treatment, responses to treatment were examined using a three-way ANOVA to test for patient, treatment, and task effects. Significant patient differences were found ($F = 182$, $df = 4$, $p = 0.001$), so a repeated analysis of variance was performed with blocking on patients to examine treatment effects within each task. Post-injection syllable durations were significantly longer (toward normal) than pre-injection durations, while word and sentence durations were significantly shorter and also closer to normal (column 3, Table 2). Group mean data also indicated that at 3 months, syllable, word, and sentence durations were significantly shorter than pre-injection (column 4, Table 2), and also closer to normal.

Since there were significant differences between subjects on all three analyses, individual mean durations for each subject were plotted before and after treatment. The stippled area in Figures 2, 3, and 4 represent the

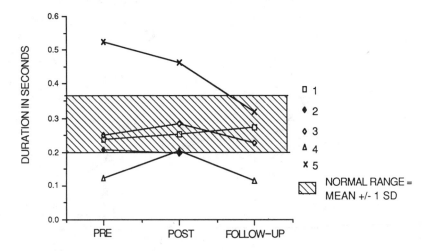

Figure 2. Mean syllable durations for patients before and after botulinum toxin treatment. The stippled area represents normal control mean syllable duration plus and minus 1 standard deviation.

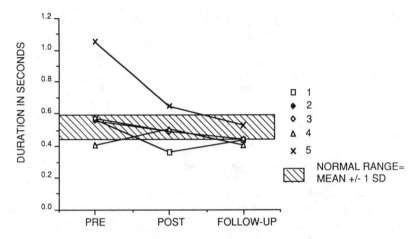

Figure 3. Mean word durations for patients before and after botulinum toxin treatment. The stippled area represents normal control mean word duration plus and minus 1 standard deviation.

range of 1 standard deviation above and below the normal mean duration for syllables, words, and sentences. Before botulinum toxin treatment, one patient had longer than normal durations for both syllables and words. Following injection, four patients' mean syllable durations, and three patients' mean word durations, were within or next to the normal range (Figures 2 and 3). On follow-up, all except one were within normal range. (Patient 2 did not return for personal reasons.)

Unlike syllable and word durations, four of five patients' pre-injection sentence durations were longer than normal by at least one *SD* above

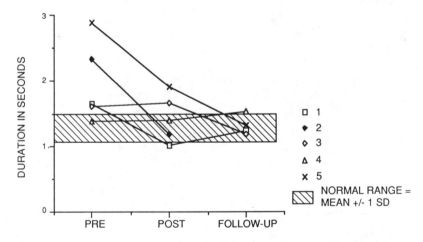

Figure 4. Mean sentence durations for patients before and after botulinum toxin treatment. The stippled area represents the normal control mean sentence duration plus and minus 1 standard deviation.

the mean (Figure 4). After injection, two were outside normal range. At follow-up, three of the four remaining patients were within the normal range.

Perceptual Ratings

Figure 5 displays means and standard deviations of the listener ratings of imprecise consonants for words and sentences before and after treatment. Because of the nature of the rating scale, the Mann-Whitney U test was used to compare the mean pre-injection ratings of OLMD subjects to the mean ratings of normal controls. The Wilcoxon signed ranks test was used to compare patients' pre-injection, post-injection, and follow-up mean ratings for each dimension.

Since each group comparison was made for four perceptual dimensions, a significance level of 0.02 was chosen. Prior to treatment, patients were judged to have less precise consonant production (Figure 5) and more prolonged phonemes (Figure 6) in both words and sentences than control subjects. The ratings did not change from pre-injection levels on these dimensions at post-injection or follow-up.

Listeners rated the patients' pre-injection inappropriate silences and speech rate as significantly different from normal (Figures 7 and 8). Two

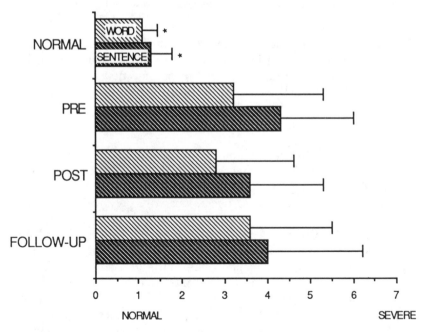

Figure 5. Listener ratings for imprecision of consonant production in "potato" and "I have the baggage." (*$p \leq 0.02$ compared to pre-injection.)

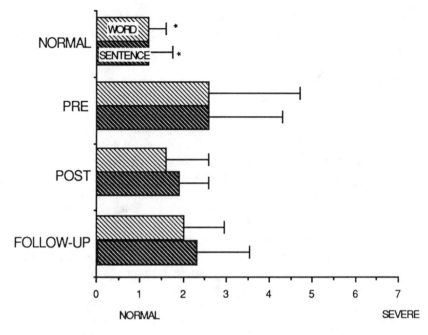

Figure 6. Listener ratings for prolongation of phonemes in "potato" and "I have the baggage." (*p ≤ 0.02 compared to pre-injection.)

weeks following botulinum treatment, patients were rated significantly less severe on both dimensions. At follow-up, patients tended to be less severe on these dimensions compared to pre-injection ratings, but the most severely impaired patient did not return for follow-up.

CONCLUSIONS

The effects of botulinum toxin on the speech of OLMD patients can be objectively assessed. In this study two acoustic and two perceptual measures reflected changes in the speech of OLMD patients following botulinum toxin treatment. These dimensions were polysyllabic word and sentence durations and inappropriate silences and speech rate. Prior to treatment, OLMD patients produced longer polysyllabic words and sentences than normal subjects and differed in the precision of consonant articulation, prolongation of phonemes, intrusion of inappropriate silences, and overall speech rate. These results agree with those of Darley et al. (1975) and Golper et al. (1983), who reported similar perceptual problems in patients with OLMD (e.g., inappropriate silences were noted in the two patients who had the highest bizarreness rating). With botulinum toxin treatment, patients in our study had shorter multisyllabic utterances

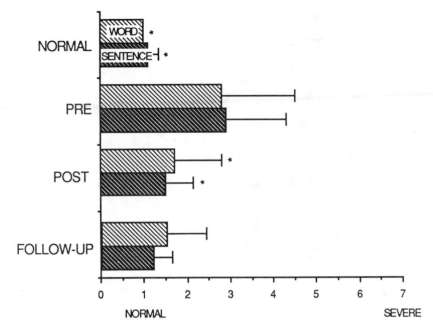

Figure 7. Listener ratings for inappropriate silences in "potato" and "I have the baggage." (*$p \leq 0.02$ compared to pre-injection.)

and were rated perceptually as less severe for inappropriate silences and overall speech rate. The efficacy of botulinum toxin treatment for these patients was substantiated and quantified in a relatively easy and effective manner.

Our results demonstrate that OLMD patients before treatment had less difficulty with single syllable utterances than with polysyllabic words and sentences. Before treatment, the patients' syllable durations did not differ significantly from normal, while polysyllabic word and sentence durations were significantly increased. This discrepancy suggests that patients may have paused longer than normal between syllables in the multisyllabic utterances. Such pausing may be due to difficulty with initiating movements or to increased plosive durations.

We computed Pearson product-moment correlations between polysyllabic word and sentence mean durations and each perceptual mean rating (Table 3). Correlations between mean word durations and prolonged phonemes and inappropriate silences ratings were similar. The correlation between mean sentence duration and inappropriate silences was greater than that between mean sentence duration and prolonged phonemes. For both types of utterance, high correlations (greater than 0.60) were obtained for mean durations and overall speech rate, and very

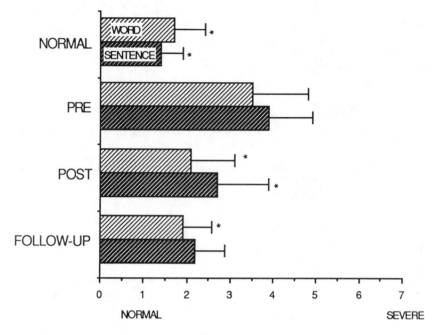

Figure 8. Listener ratings for speaking rate of "potato" and "I have the baggage." (*p ≤ 0.02 compared to pre-injection.)

low correlations were obtained for these durations and imprecise consonants. These correlations suggest that pauses between words in the sentence may have contributed to the increased sentence durations, although pauses between syllables may not have contributed to increased word durations. Future research should investigate physiologic events during inappropriate silences to determine whether abnormal muscle activity and/or static postures interfere with speech production in OLMD patients.

Our results did not demonstrate a return to baseline following treatment withdrawl on the 3-month follow-up. Three or more months after treatment, patients maintained shorter durations for polysyllabic utter-

Table 3. Person product-moment correlations for the mean durations of polysyllabic utterances "potato" and "I have the baggage" with the mean rating of the four perceptual measures

Perceptual measure	Potato	I have the baggage
Imprecise consonants	−0.183	−0.084
Prolonged phonemes	0.398	0.539
Inappropriate silences	0.360	0.851
Overall speech rate	0.656	0.794

ances and tended to maintain reduced severity ratings for inappropriate silences and overall speech rate. This finding contrasts with the results of Jankovic (1988a) who noted improvement lasting for only 5 weeks, but agrees with results of Brin et al. (1987) who noted 4 months of improvement in one patient. Although a double-blind study of botulinum toxin effects in OLMD has been performed (Jankovic, 1988a), a double-blind crossover study in this patient group would be necessary to demonstrate fully the effects of the toxin, because measurements made at 3 months did not return to baseline.

REFERENCES

Bandyopadhyay, S., Clark, A.W., DasGupta, B.R., & Sathyamoorthy, V. (1987). Role of heavy and light chains of botulinum neurotoxin in neuromuscular paralysis. *Journal of Biological Chemistry, 262,* 2660–2663.

Berardelli, A., Rothwell, J.C., Day, B.L., & Marsden, C.D. (1988). The pathophysiology of cranial dystonia. In S. Fahn (Ed.), *Advances in neurology: Vol. 50. Dystonia 2* (pp. 525–535). New York: Raven Press.

Blitzer, A., Greene, P.E., Brin, M.F., & Fahn, S. (1989). Botulinum toxin injection for the treatment of oromandibular dystonia. *Annals of Otology, Rhinology and Laryngology, 98,* 93–97.

Brin, M.F., Fahn, S., Moskowitz, C., Friedman, A., Shale, H.M., Greene, P.E., Blitzer, A., List, T., Lange, D., Lovelace, R.E., & McMahon, D. (1987). Localized injections of botulinum toxin for the treatment of focal dystonia and hemifacial spasm. *Movement Disorders, 2,* 237–254.

Calne, D.B., & Lang, A.E. (1988). Secondary dystonia. In S. Fahn (Ed.), *Advances in neurology: Vol. 50. Dystonia 2* (pp. 9–33). New York: Raven Press.

Cohen, L.G., Hallett, M., Geller, B.D., & Hochberg, F. (1989). Treatment of focal dystonias of the hand with botulinum toxin injections. *Journal of Neurology, Neurosurgery and Psychiatry, 52,* 355–363.

Cohen, L.G., Ludlow, C.L., Warden, M., Estequi, M., Agostino, R., Sedory, S.E., Holloway, E., Dambrosio, J.A., & Hallett, M. (1989). Blink reflex curves in patients with spasmodic dysphonia. *Neurology, 39,* 572–577.

Darley, F.L., Aronson, A.E., & Brown, J.R. (1975). *Motor speech disorders.* Philadelphia: W.B. Saunders.

Fahn, S. (1988). Concept and classification of dystonia. In S. Fahn (Ed.), *Advances in neurology: Vol. 50. Dystonia 2* (pp. 1–8). New York: Raven Press.

Fahn, S., & Marsden, C.D. (1987). The treatment of dystonia. In C.D. Marsden & S. Fahn (Eds.), *Movement disorders 2* (pp. 359–382). London: Butterworths.

Fahn, S., & Williams, D.T. (1988). Psychogenic dystonia. In S. Fahn (Ed.), *Advances in neurology: Vol. 50. Dystonia 2* (pp. 431–455). New York: Raven Press.

Gimenez-Roldan, S., Mateo, D., Orbe, M., Munoz-Blanco, J.L., & Hipola, D. (1988). Acute pharmacologic tests in cranial dystonia. In J. Jankovic & E. Tolosa (Eds.), *Advances in neurology: Vol. 49. Facial dyskinesias* (pp. 451–465). New York: Raven Press.

Golper, L.A.C., Nutt, J.G., Rau, M.T., & Coleman, R.O. (1983). Focal cranial dystonia. *Journal of Speech and Hearing Disorders, 48,* 128–134.

Gottlieb, J.S., & May, M. (1984). Blepharospasm-oromandibular dystonia (Meige's syndrome) misdiagnosed as secondary hemifacial spasm. *American Journal of Otology, 5,* 206–655.

Hartman, D.E., & Abbs, J.H. (1988). Dysarthrias of movement disorders. In J. Jankovic & E. Tolosa (Eds.), *Advances in neurology: Vol. 49. Facial dyskinesias* (pp. 289–306). New York: Raven Press.

Jankovic, J. (1988a). Botulinum A toxin in the treatment of blepharospasm. In J. Jankovic & E. Tolosa (Eds.), *Advances in neurology: Vol. 49. Facial dyskinesias* (pp. 467–472). New York: Raven Press.

Jankovic, J. (1988b). Cranial-cervical dyskinesias: An overview. In J. Jankovic & E. Tolosa (Eds.), *Advances in neurology: Vol. 49. Facial dyskinesias* (pp. 1–13). New York: Raven Press.

Jankovic, J. (1988c). Etiology and differential diagnosis of blepharospasm and oromandibular dystonia. In J. Jankovic & E. Tolosa (Eds.), *Advances in neurology: Vol. 49. Facial dyskinesias* (pp. 103–117). New York: Raven Press.

Jankovic, J. (1989). Blepharospasm and oromandibular-laryngeal-cervical dystonia: A controlled trial of botulinum A toxin therapy. In S. Fahn (Ed.), *Advances in neurology: Vol. 50. Dystonia 2* (pp. 583–591). New York: Raven Press.

Jankovic, J., & Nutt, J.G. (1988). Blepharospasm and cranial-cervical dystonia (Meige's syndrome): Familial occurrence. In J. Jankovic & E. Tolosa (Eds.), *Advances in neurology: Vol. 49. Facial dyskinesias* (pp. 117–123). New York: Raven Press.

Jankovic, J., & Patel, S.C. (1983). Blepharospasm associated with brain stem lesions. *Neurology, 33,* 1237–1240.

Keane, J.R., & Young, A.B. (1985). Blepharospasm with bilateral basal ganglia infarction. *Archives of Neurology, 42,* 1206–1208.

Klawans, H.L., & Tanner, C.M. (1988). Cholinergic pharmacology of blepharospasm with oromandibular dystonia (Meige's syndrome). In J. Jankovic & E. Tolosa (Eds.), *Advances in neurology: Vol. 49. Facial dyskinesias* (pp. 443–450). New York: Raven Press.

Koller, W.C. (1983). Endentulous oro-dyskinesia. *Annals of Neurology, 13,* 97–100.

Kurlan, R., & Shoulson, I. (1988). Differential diagnosis of facial chorea. In J. Jankovic & E. Tolosa (Eds.), *Advances in neurology: Vol. 49. Facial dyskinesias* (pp. 225–237). New York: Raven Press.

Lagueny, A., Deliac, M.M., Julien, J., Demotes-Mainard, J., & Ferrer, X. (1989). Jaw closing spasms — a form of focal dystonia? An electrophysiological study. *Journal of Neurology, Neurosurgery and Psychiatry, 52,* 652–655.

Ludlow, C.L., Naunton, R.F., Sedory, S.E., Schulz, G.M., & Hallett, M. (1988). Effects of botulinum toxin injections on speech in adductor spasmodic dysphonia. *Neurology, 38,* 1220–1225.

Marsden, C.D. (1976). The problem of adult-onset idiopathic torsion dystonia and other isolated dyskinesias in adult life (including blepharospasm, oromandibular dystonia, dystonic writer's cramp, and torticollis, or axial dystonia). In R. Eldridge & S. Fahn (Eds.), *Advances in neurology: Vol. 14* (pp. 259–276). New York: Raven Press.

Marsden, C.D., & Fahn, S. (1987). Problems in the dyskinesias. In C.D. Marsden & S. Fahn (Eds.), *Movement disorders 2* (pp. 305–312). London: Butterworths.

Mauriello, J.A. (1985). Blepharospasm, Meige syndrome, and hemifacial spasm: Treatment with botulinum toxin. *Neurology, 35,* 1499–1500.

Scott, A.B. (1980). Botulinum toxin injection into extraocular muscles as an alternative to strabismus surgery. *Ophthalmology, 87,* 1044–1047.

Sheehy, M.P., Rothwell, J.C., & Marsden, C.D. (1988). Writer's cramp. In S. Fahn

(Ed.), *Advances in neurology: Vol. 50. Dystonia 2* (pp. 457–472). New York: Raven Press.

Tanner, C.M., Wilson, R.S., Goetz, C.G., & Shannon, K.M. (1988). The predictive value of acute antimuscarinic drugs in adults with focal dystonia. In S. Fahn (Ed.), *Advances in neurology: Vol. 50. Dystonia 2* (pp. 557–560). New York: Raven Press.

Thompson, P.D., Obeso, J.A., Delgado, G., Gallego, J., & Marsden, C.D. (1986). Focal dystonia of the jaw and the differential diagnosis of unilateral jaw and masticatory spasm. *Journal of Neurology, Neurosurgery and Psychiatry, 49*, 651–656.

Tolosa, E., & Kulisevsky, J. (1988). Dopaminergic mechanisms in cranial dystonia. In J. Jankovic & E. Tolosa (Eds.), *Advances in neurology: Vol. 49. Facial dyskinesias* (pp. 433–441). New York: Raven Press.

Tolosa, E., & Marti, M.J. (1988). Blepharospasm-oromandibular dystonia syndrome (Meige's syndrome): Clinical aspects. In J. Jankovic & E. Tolosa (Eds.), *Advances in neurology: Vol. 49. Facial dyskinesias* (pp. 225–237). New York: Raven Press.

Tolosa, E., Marti, M.J., & Kulisevsky, J. (1988). Botulinum toxin injection therapy for hemifacial spasm. In J. Jankovic & E. Tolosa (Eds.), *Advances in neurology: Vol. 49. Facial dyskinesias* (pp. 479–491). New York: Raven Press.

Tsui, J.K., & Calne, D.B. (1988). Botulinum toxin in cervical dystonia. In J. Jankovic & E. Tolosa (Eds.), *Advances in neurology: Vol. 49. Facial dyskinesias* (pp. 473–468). New York: Raven Press.

Tsui, J.K., Eisen, E., Mak, J., Scott, A., & Calne, D.B. (1985). A pilot study on the use of botulinum toxin in spasmodic torticollis. *Canadian Journal of Neurological Sciences, 12*, 314–316.

Waltz, J.M. (1982). Surgical approach to dystonia. In C.D. Marsden & S. Fahn (Eds.), *Movement disorders* (pp. 300–307). London: Butterworths.

Wright, G.P. (1955). The neurotoxins of *Clostridium botulinum* and *Clostridium tetani*. *Pharmacology Review, 7*, 413.

Dysarthria and Apraxia of Speech:
Perspectives on Management
edited by Christopher A. Moore, Ph.D., Kathryn M. Yorkston, Ph.D.,
and David R. Beukelman, Ph.D.
Paul H. Brookes Publishing Co., Inc.
Baltimore · London · Toronto · Sydney

APRAXIA OF SPEECH

RESEARCHERS AND CLINICIANS involved with apraxic speakers continue to grapple with diagnostic and taxonomic distinctions. Experimentally, many researchers continue to classify patients according to site of lesion (with medical imaging), acoustic analyses, perceptual analyses, and standardized testing. Square-Storer and Apeldoorn present such a study in Chapter 18. Alternatively, some clinical researchers, dissatisfied with conventional diagnostic distinctions, suggest adjustments, even elimination, of the contemporary taxonomy in disorders of speech motor control. With the wide variation in severity and symptomatology, and the routine occurrence of several speech and language deficits (i.e., dysarthria, dementia, and aphasia), there is considerable motivation for such a reevaluation. In Chapter 19 Rosenbek and McNeil provide this reappraisal. Weismer and Liss, applying the principles of qualitative patient description set forth in Chapter 2, demonstrate how research might proceed if released from the constraints of a priori classification and diagnostic taxonomies. These chapters evidence the persistent struggles in research in apraxia and, perhaps, foreshadow the resolution of these problems.

Chapter 17

Acoustic/Perceptual Taxonomies of Speech Production Deficits in Motor Speech Disorders

Gary Weismer and Julie M. Liss

ONE GOAL OF speech motor control research is to acquire an understanding of normal and disordered speech production behaviors so that informed predictions and productive hypotheses can be proposed. This goal necessitates developing methodologies for identification and measurement of important aspects of speech production, those phenomena that have to be explained by a theory. Although technological capabilities allow measurements at different levels of speech production (physiologic, aerodynamic, kinematic, and acoustic), the important aspects have eluded our grasp. This may stem, in part, from restrictions inherent in quantitative analyses.

One example of restriction was evident in the investigation reported by Liss and Weismer (1989). We sought to document the effects on speech production of contrastive stress drills, a therapy technique wherein speakers with motor speech disorders are taught to selectively emphasize words to enhance intelligibility and convey important information by quantifying selected acoustic events. The acoustic analysis included measurements of total utterance durations, segment durations, and transition extents. These measurements were chosen because they are easy to obtain and have been used to describe the acoustic signal and articulatory performance of various normal and disordered speaker groups (Weismer, 1984;

This work was supported by NIH Grant NS 18797. We would like to thank Shirley Hunsaker for her technical assistance.

Weismer, Kent, Hodge, & Martin, 1988). When we tried to make sense of the segment duration and formant patterns across four apraxic speakers and four normal speakers, however, the major effect seemed to be that every speaker did something different. The lack of systematic effects across speakers was typical of all utterances examined. In other words, inter-subject variability, even among normal speakers, dominated the data. Examination of repetition variability within subjects also suggested great intra-subject variability in performance, and while this was true for the normal speakers (compared to data reported for younger adults [Weismer & Ingrisano, 1979]), it was an outstanding feature of the apraxic speakers.

We concluded in Liss and Weismer (1989) that this approach to understanding articulatory behavior in persons with motor speech disorders was, at one level, seriously misguided. By "this approach," we mean quantification of speech production phenomena for cases in which idiosyncratic statistical effects and within-subject variability are the rule, rather than the exception. Moreover, almost all quantitative analyses of motor speech disorder phenomena must be restricted to error-free (or fluent) utterances. As Sussman, Marquardt, MacNeilage, and Hutchinson (1988) suggested, much important information about the nature of motor speech disorders is lost under such restrictions. This problem is not exclusive to acoustic analysis, because our experience with physiologic measures (e.g., McNeil, Weismer, Adams, & Mulligan, 1990) indicates a similar problem. Speech production phenomena in persons with neurologic disease tend to be extremely variable when indexed parametrically, thus making the experimental psychology model of research difficult to justify for the kinds of information we seek to obtain.

Having reached this conclusion, we considered other analyses that might provide information about the nature and cause of speech production deficits in motor speech disorders. This chapter presents an approach that we feel has more theoretical power than the classical parametric analysis. The greater theoretical power derives, in our opinion, both from a coarser grain of analysis than is typically used in parametric work, and from the more direct comparison of the acoustic analysis with perceptual data. The coarser grain of analysis should reveal immediately accessible characteristics of apraxic speech production and point to quantitative analyses that might refine understanding of these phenomena. This approach is documented with utterances from 4 normal speakers and 4 speakers with apraxia of speech, under the same "contrastive stress" condition studied quantitatively by Liss and Weismer (1989). It should be noted here that a similar qualitative approach to the analysis of apraxic speech disturbances was undertaken several years ago by Kent and Rosenbek (1983). A major difference between their work and ours is the use of contrastively stressed utterances, as well as qualitative analysis of repetition consistency and variability.

METHODS

Subjects

Four males, diagnosed as having apraxia of speech with no aphasia, and four neurologically normal males were studied. All subjects were over 50 years old and the same approximate age. McNeil et al. (1990) report the precise selection criteria used in the apraxia of speech project being conducted at the University of Wisconsin-Madison.

The speech sample included utterances from a contrastive stress task, in which stressed words are elicited by asking various questions. For example, contrastive stress was elicited for the utterance "Build a big building," by asking, "Should you *buy* a big building?", "Should you build a *small* building?", and "Should you build a big *garage?*" The same protocol was followed for the utterance "Buy Bobby a poppy." Five repetitions of each contrastive stress condition were obtained from each speaker. Results from only the sentences in which "Build," "building," "Buy," and "Bobby" were stressed are reported here.

Analysis consisted of visual evaluation of spectrographic characteristics of the utterances and auditory perceptual evaluation that yielded a broad transcription with selected diacritics for each utterance. The utterances were displayed on a Kay 5500 Workstation, and extensive notes were made of specific features of the utterance. We initially approached this analysis task with certain preconceived categories. Many of these categories were the product of the informal examination of spectrograms in the Liss and Weismer project (1989). These categories are:

Formant trajectory patterns
Segmental phenomena
Repetitions
Movement perseveration
Prosodic characteristics

Formant Trajectories

Formant trajectories were examined because they provide a straightforward qualitative index of the magnitude and speed of change in vocal tract geometry. Moreover, previous work (Kent & Rosenbek, 1983) has shown that these indices are sensitive to speech production deficits in apraxia of speech. In keeping with our aim to provide a qualitative analysis, the shapes of the selected vowel formants were described in terms of durations of the steady state and transition components of the trajectories, including direction and extent. Figures 1a–c provide examples of some unusual

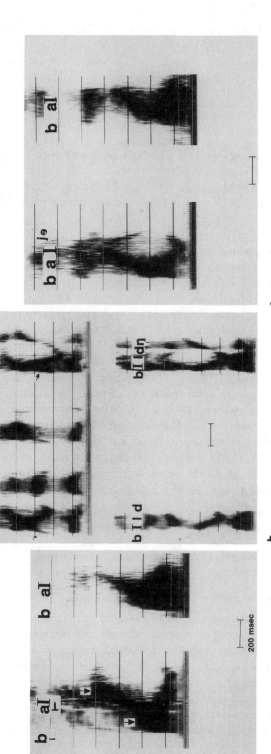

Figure 1 a–c. Spectrographic examples of formant trajectory phenomena in the speech of apraxic and normal speakers. The time bar in these figures is 200 msec. **a.** Long steady states at the beginning and end of the /aɪ/ diphthong for the apraxic speaker (left) but not the normal speaker (right). **b.** Misdirection of the initial portion of the /ɪl/ trajectories in "build" and "building" in the apraxic spectrogram (top, see arrows) compared with trajectories produced by a normal speaker (bottom). **c.** Exaggerated trajectory for an apraxic speaker (left) compared with normal production (right) of /aɪ/. Note the large range of frequencies covered by the first and second formants in the apraxic spectrogram.

phenomena observed in the spectrograms of the apraxic speakers. For example, in Figure 1a, a production of "buy" is shown for an apraxic speaker (left) and a normal speaker (right). Note that in $F2$, the apraxic speaker produces the diphthong with relatively long initial and final steady states (see arrows). In contrast, the normal speaker's diphthong is produced without any appreciable steady-state portions. Shape differences between formant trajectories of normal and apraxic speakers were likely to be located at the onsets and offsets of vocalic nuclei. Another example is seen in Figure 1b, which shows the phenomenon we have labeled "misdirected formants." Compare the $F2$ trajectories of "build" and "building" produced by the normal speaker (bottom) with those produced by the apraxic speaker (top). The normal trajectories generally follow a monotonic falling course, whereas these apraxic trajectories initially rise (see arrows), then fall. These apraxic syllables ("build") were not regarded as phonemically aberrant, but may be perceived as containing vocalic distortions. Figure 1c shows an example of an exaggerated second formant trajectory (left). The range of frequencies covered by the apraxic speaker's trajectory (Figure 1c) is much greater than that for the normal speaker.

Segmental Phenomena

Segmental observations involved: 1) the acoustic description of "off-target" articulatory events, with off-target defined as any perceptually identified substitution or distortion of vowels or consonants; and 2) identification of noise in stop-closure intervals, often referred to as spirantization. An acoustic description of segmental errors contains information about articulatory movement patterns and thus goes beyond perceptual transcription. Because it is likely that different articulatory patterns can underlie the same phonetic transcription, the acoustic analysis is more than just an alternate description of the segmental error pattern. Figures 2a – c provide examples of different segmental observations made in this analysis. Figure 2a is an example of an apraxic speaker's attempt at the word buy, transcribed as /bɪjˤlaɪ/, for which the underlying articulatory movements associated with the vocalic segmental error are revealed by formant trajectories. Although the formant trajectories at the end of the apraxic word are directed in a way consistent with the perceptual transcription and the acoustic expectations for /aɪ/ (see Figure 2a), the preceding part of the utterance shows a substantial amount of complex vocal tract behavior. A consonantal segmental error is shown in Figure 2b, where the apraxic speaker failed to make closure for the medial /b/ in "Bobby" (transcribed as /baβi/). Note in the normal example (Figure 2b, right), a clearer separation between the vocalic segments /a/ and /i/; in the apraxic production, the formant trajectory clearly extends throughout the word. In Figure 2c, a clearly spirantized stop is shown for the apraxic

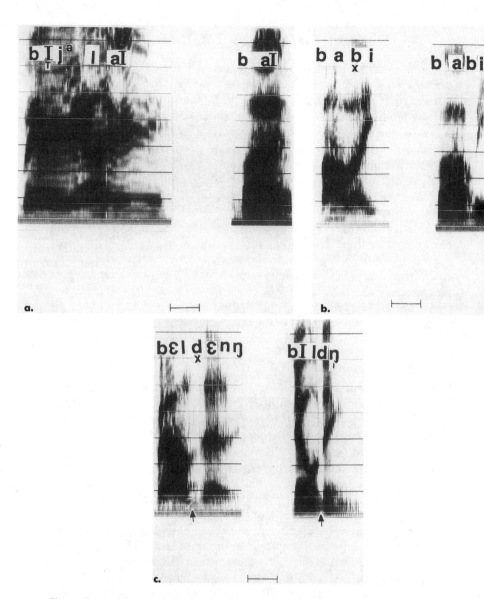

Figure 2 a–c. Spectrographic examples of segmental observations. **a.** An apraxic speaker's incorrect production of "Buy" (left). Note the complex formant trajectory movements associated with this segmental error, compared with the formant structure of /aɪ/ produced by a normal speaker (right). **b.** A consonant segmental error, in which the medial /b/ in "Bobby" by the apraxic speaker has virtually no vocal tract closure (left); a normal speaker's production is on the right. **c.** An example of a noise-filled (spirantized) /d/ closure in an apraxic speaker's "building" (see arrow, left). Compare to the relatively silent closure by a normal speaker (right). Time bar = 200 msec.

speaker, as indicated by the noise in the closure interval (arrow). There is also a small amount of noise in the closure interval of the normal spectrogram. Because experience and published observations (Liss, Weismer, & Rosenbek, 1990) suggest that spirantization may not be unusual in older speakers generally, and because some of our tapes were fairly noisy, the value of these observations is questionable[1].

Repetitions

Repetitions were examined to provide an acoustic description of the phenomenon that might be perceptually classified as "groping," or dysfluency. Articulatory groping, often cited as common among apraxic speakers, is regarded as a speaker's search for correct articulatory postures (Wertz, Lapointe, & Rosenbek, 1984). Gropes are often manifest in dysfluent initiation of utterances. For example, Figure 3a shows an apraxic speaker's attempt to produce the initial stressed word "Build" in "Build a big building." The first attempt, followed by a 2-second pause, and the second attempt, followed by a 6-second pause, appear to be accurate, although aborted, productions of the syllable, /bɪ/. That is, the center frequencies of the first and second formants of both attempts correspond with those of the initial /ɪ/ portion of the final /bɪl/ production. In Figure 3b, the same apraxic speaker produced a similar pattern in another repetition of this word. In this effort, both attempts included perceptual and spectrographic evidence of the expected sound sequence. The final /d/ in the first repetition was weaker than the final /d/ in the second repetition, however. From these examples, one might predict that some apraxic articulatory behaviors classified as groping are partial and/or aborted articulatory patterns rather than randomly varying articulatory configurations.

Movement Perseveration

Another category involved observation of movement perseveration. This term describes the carryover of particular formant trajectory shapes into the following syllable(s) that may or may not result in perceptual vocalic segment distortions. Figures 4a and 4b provide examples of the perseverance of the /aɪ/ $F2$ shape — correctly produced by both apraxic speakers for the first word "Buy" — into the second word, "Bobby." Although the $F2$ for /a/ in "Bobby" is typically flat in normal productions, the trajectories in 4a and 4b resemble those of the /aɪ/ in the preceding syllables.

Prosodic Characteristics

Prosodic characteristics, including fundamental frequency and amplitude contours and temporal patterning of vowels and consonants, were described for each utterance. Although the full set of prosodic characteristics

---

[1]Combined perceptual and acoustic analyses can identify closure intervals that are noisy because of recording conditions, compared with those that are noisy because of articulatory factors. Tape noise sounds are qualitatively different from vocal tract noise. An instrument such as the Kay 5500 Workstation allows the investigator to isolate segments and listen to noise quality. Segments with tape noise only can then be compared to segments with stop closure intervals.

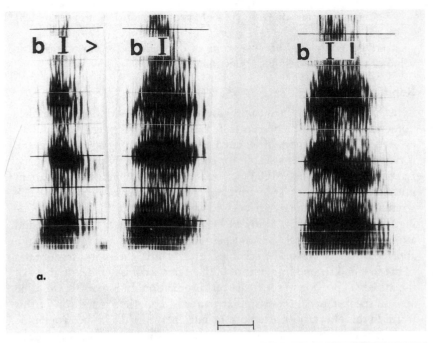

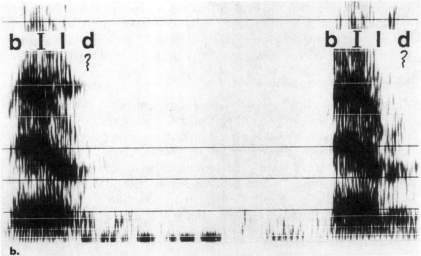

Figure 3 a–b. Spectrograms of repetition behavior in speech of an apraxic subject. **a.** Three repetitions of /bɪl/ from "Build," where formant frequencies of the initial portions of the trajectories are similar. **b.** Two repetitions of an apraxic speaker's production of "Build." Time bar = 200 msec. (/ ? / indicates weak production of a consonant.)

has not yet been analyzed, an example of temporal patterning of vowels and consonants for an apraxic and normal speaker is shown in Figure 5. In the normal spectrogram of "Build a big building" (bottom), note that the majority of the duration of the utterance is taken up by vocalic segments. The overall ratio of obstruent to vocalic durations is very small, an obser-

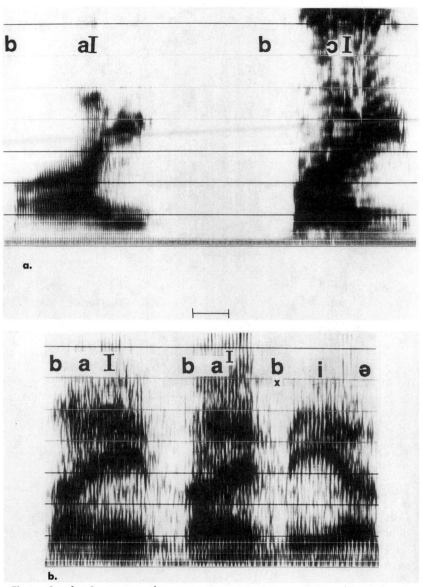

Figure 4 a–b. Spectrograms of movement perseveration in two apraxic speakers. **a.** Formant trajectories for the target syllable /ba/ in "Bobby" resemble trajectories in the previous /aɪ/ segment. **b.** A similar, but less dramatic, example for the same sequence. Time bar = 200 msec.

vation consistent with normal utterances in this study. In the apraxic utterance, however, this ratio is larger. Although the rate of speech is slower for the apraxic speaker, obstruent segments appear to be differentially lengthened relative to vocalic segments. This is particularly striking because these obstruent segments, and others in our analysis, do not contain obvious pauses.

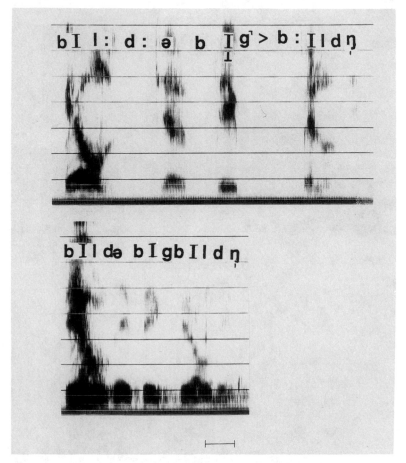

Figure 5. Temporal patterns of vowels and consonants in an apraxic speaker (top) and normal speaker (bottom). Time bar = 200 msec.

RESULTS

Data are presented in spectrographic stackplots, and examples of phenomena that occurred most frequently are shown. In analysis of these stackplots, consistency and variability of visually identified phenomena[2] were of special interest.

Normal Utterances

Figure 6 shows spectrographic stackplots for one normal speaker's production of the *"Buy"* and *"Bobby"* utterances (*"Buy* Bobby a poppy," versus

---

[2]The most productive way to analyze these data is to make simultaneous audio and visual evaluations. The audio examples obviously cannot be provided, but readers interested in obtaining the audio examples in the spectrograms can do so by sending a cassette tape to one of the authors. Also, copies of the full set of spectrograms used in this analysis are available upon request.

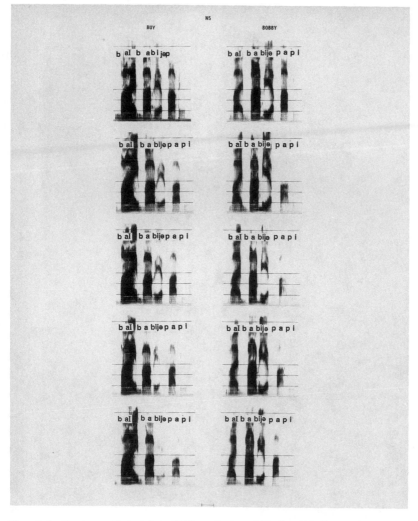

Figure 6. Spectrographic stackplots of N5's productions of "*Buy*" and "*Bobby.*" Time bar = 200 msec.

"Buy *Bobby* a poppy"). Figure 7 shows the "*Build*" and "*Building*" utterances for a different normal speaker.

In these and other displays, repetitions are aligned at the /b/ burst, or first glottal pulse associated with the initial word of the utterance. In addition, a broad transcription with selected diacritics appears at the top of each spectrogram in the stackplots. Major observations from these spectrograms are: 1) the consistency of formant characteristics across repetitions, including similarity of formant trajectories (evidenced by transition extents, durations, and rates for vocalic nuclei such as /aɪ/, /ijə/, /ɪl/) and vowel target frequency values (e.g., for the /a/ in "Bobby" and /ɪ/ in "big"); and 2) consistency of segmental and phrase-level timing charac-

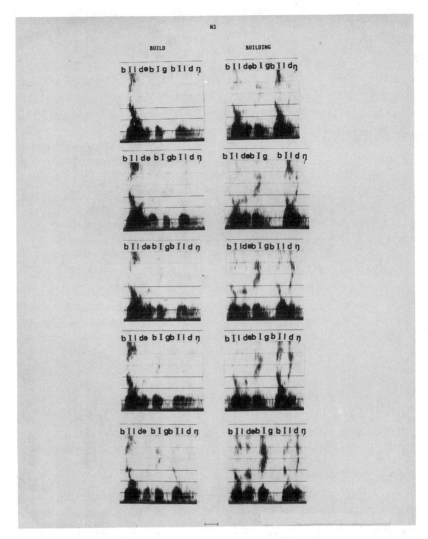

Figure 7. Spectrographic stackplots of N3's productions of *"Build"* and *"building."* Time bar = 200 msec.

teristics of the utterances, where certain stop consonants are always spirantized (e.g., medial /b/ in /babi/), and relatively long vocalic segments alternate with relatively short obstruent segments. Note also that when *"Buy"* is stressed, the formant trajectories for /aɪ/ are consistently longer and larger than when *"Bobby"* is stressed. In *"Build"* versus *"Building,"* the stressed /ɪl/ nucleus shows slightly greater transition extents than the nonstressed /ɪl/, but differences are not as obvious as in the /aɪ/ nucleus.

Apraxic Utterances

Figure 8 presents A1's productions of the *"Buy"* utterances. The formant trajectories for the stressed /aɪ/ are highly variable across repetitions,

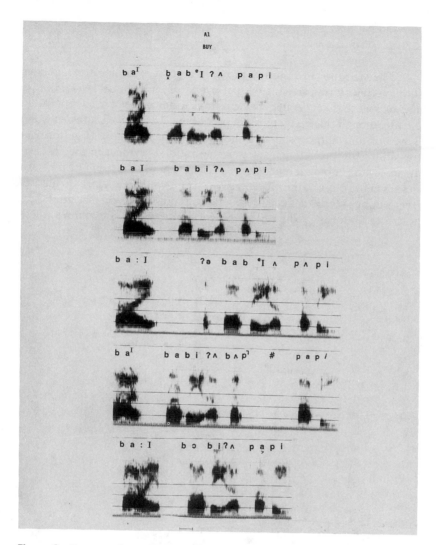

Figure 8. Spectrographic stackplots of A1's productions of *"Buy."* Time bar = 200 msec. (/#/ is a pause that does not fit an IPA juncture category.)

sometimes reflecting limited change in vocal tract configuration (repetitions 1 and 4) and sometimes relatively large change in vocal tract configuration (repetitions 3 and 5). There is also considerable variation across repetitions in duration of this vocalic nucleus. In contrast, formant trajectories for /ijə/ are relatively similar across repetitions, though the overall shape of the $F2$ trajectory is unlike that of the normal speakers. Although the first three formant frequencies for /a/ in /babi/ appear to reflect a backed tongue position (note the unusual proximity of $F1$ and $F2$, especially in repetitions 1, 3, and 5), the articulation is repeated across several repetitions.

The stackplot in Figure 9 provides a good example of exaggerated formant trajectories, articulatory perseveration, and phrase-level timing in apraxic speech. Exaggerated formant trajectories are seen in all repetitions of /aɪ/, though this segment is not part of the contrastively stressed word. Three of four apraxic speakers showed evidence of these large formant transitions for /aɪ/. Articulatory perseveration is evident in the /a/ segments (from /babi/) of repetitions 1, 4, and 5, in which F1 and F2 trajectories resemble those of the preceding /aɪ/ segments. With respect to phrase-level timing, recall that the temporal structure of the normal utterances described above is predominated by vocalic segments. In contrast, these

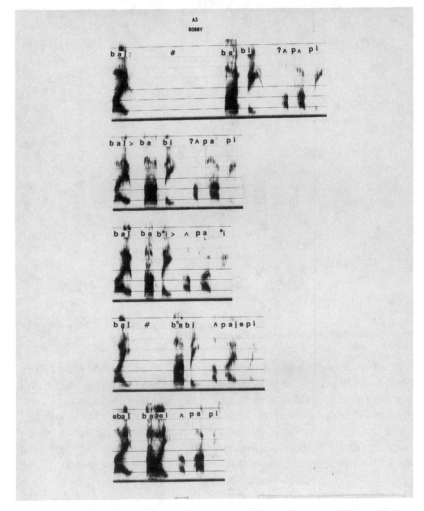

Figure 9. Spectrographic stackplots of A3's productions of "*Bobby.*" Time bar = 200 msec. (/#/ is a pause that does not fit an IPA juncture category.)

apraxic utterances (repetitions 2, 3, and 5) contained relatively larger consonantal intervals. It should be noted that the larger consonantal interval of these repetitions differ from the intervals seen in repetitions 1 and 4 (between /baɪ/ and /babi/, which probably reflect pauses.

Figure 10 contains a stackplot of the same condition for a different apraxic speaker and provides additional examples of the phenomena described in Figure 9. Note that consistently exaggerated formant trajectories for /aɪ/, articulatory perseveration for the /a/ segment, and large consonant intervals in the phrase-level timing patterns are seen again.

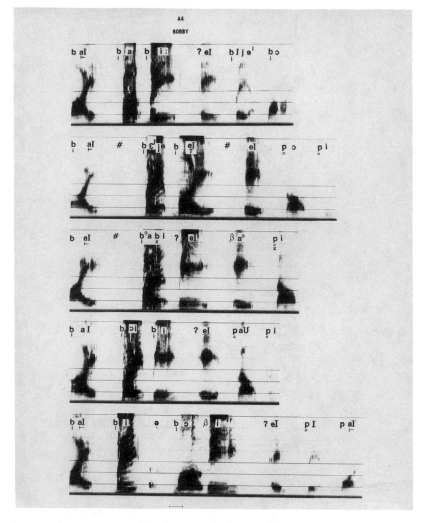

Figure 10. Spectrographic stackplots of A4's productions of "*Bobby.*" Time bar = 200 msec. (/#/ is a pause that does not fit an IPA juncture category.)

Figures 11 and 12 present repetitions of *"Build* a big building," and "Build a big *building,"* respectively, and provide examples of certain segmental phenomena evidenced by the other apraxic speakers in this investigation. Note from the transcriptions that many segments in these repetitions were "off-target," or did not contain expected sequences of sounds. By our qualitative descriptions, these were labeled as segmental errors. It is interesting to consider that the stress conditions, per se, did not result in more accurate productions of the target word. For example, comparing the accuracy of productions of "Build" in the two stress conditions reveals

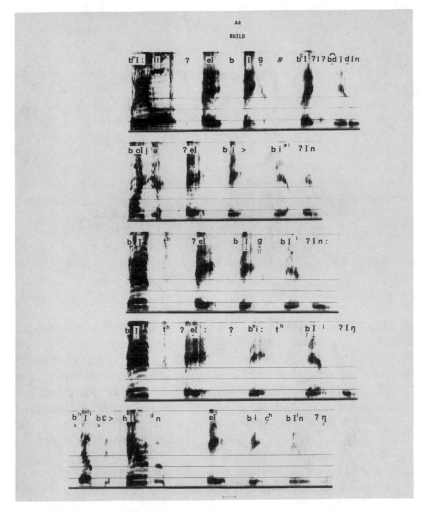

Figure 11. Spectrographic stackplots of A4's productions of *"Build."* Time bar = 200 msec. (/#/ is a pause that does not fit an IPA juncture category; / ? / indicates weak production of a consonant and doubling of the symbol corresponds to very weak production.)

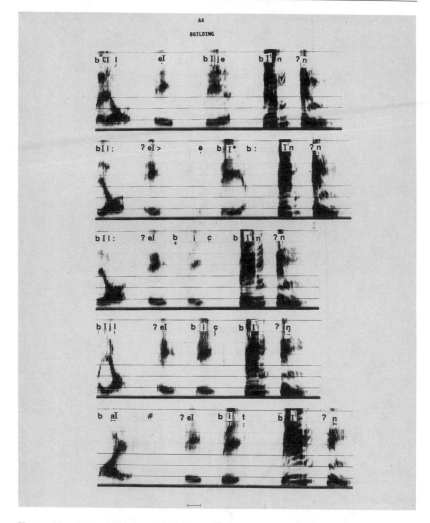

Figure 12. Spectrographic stackplots of A4's productions of *"Building."* Time bar = 200 msec. (/#/ is a pause that does not fit an IPA juncture category; / ? / indicates weak production of a consonant and doubling of the symbol corresponds to very weak production.)

that segmental errors occurred in each condition. However, slightly more segmental errors occurred in "Build" under the *Build* stress condition compared with the *building* stress condition. At the least, this example suggests that contrastively stressing a word does not result in immediate increases in articulatory accuracy.

Figures 13 and 14 contain the stackplots of A2's productions of "Build a big *building*," and "*Build* a big building," respectively. Acoustic characteristics of "Build" are fairly consistent across repetitions in Figure 13, and onsets of utterances are not characterized by repetitions and/or

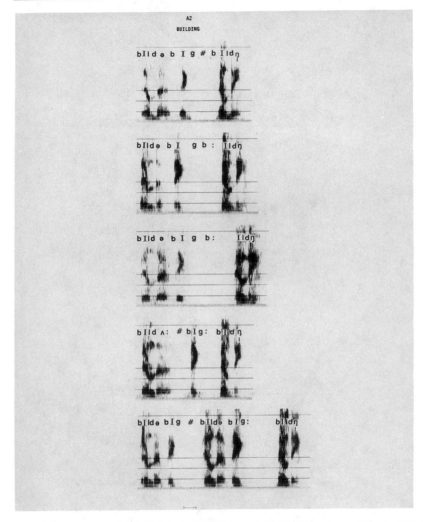

Figure 13. Spectrographic stackplots of A2's productions of *"Building."* Time bar = 200 msec. (/#/ is a pause that does not fit an IPA juncture category.)

segmental errors. In contrast, four utterances produced in the *Build* stress condition (Figure 14) contain dysfluencies at the utterance onset (repetitions 1, 2, 3, and 5). The presence of these initial dysfluencies may be additional evidence that contrastively stressing a word does not result in immediate increases in production accuracy. It is also interesting that these utterance-initial dysfluencies, which might be labeled gropes, do not appear to represent uncertain articulatory search behavior. Instead, they resemble aborted attempts or fragments of the target, as evidenced by shapes of the formant trajectories and formant frequency values.

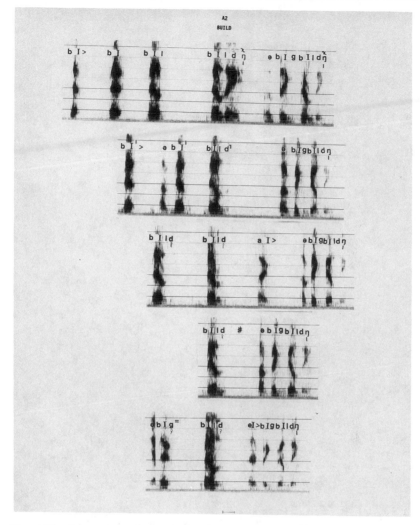

Figure 14. Spectrographic stackplots of A2's productions of "*Build.*" Time bar = 200 msec. (/#/ is a pause that does not fit an IPA juncture category; / ? / indicates weak production of a consonant.)

Figure 15 contains the repetitions of A3's "Build a big *building.*" These productions contain examples of misdirected formant trajectories in "Build" and "building." Unlike normal speakers' *F2* trajectories, described as monotonic and falling, these *F2* trajectories rise and then fall in initial portions of the words (see *F2* of "Build," repetitions 1–5; *F2* of "building," repetitions 1, 2, 4, and 5). In addition, this set of repetitions again shows the tendency for obstruent intervals to occupy a disproportionate amount of time in the temporal structure of the utterance. In

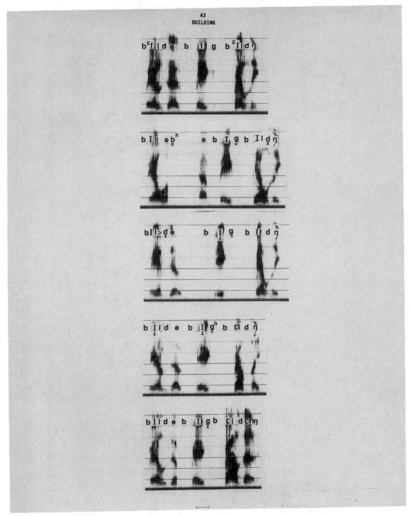

Figure 15. Spectrographic stackplots of A3's productions of *"Building."* Time bar = 200 msec.

particular, note the unusually long /gb/ obstruent intervals (/bɪg bɪld/) as compared with normal productions.

CONCLUSIONS

This chapter has presented a method for qualitatively examining and describing acoustic representations of disordered speech. This method was developed because the requirements of typical quantitative analyses of speech limit the theoretical power of the results. The aim of our analysis was to identify acoustic/perceptual phenomena that characterize speech production in apraxic speakers in an attempt to discover those important aspects described earlier. This method reverses the typical approach that assumes that the phenomena being quantified are the important ones. Other than the assumption that the acoustic waveform is important in the study of apraxia of speech, we have attempted to let the data dictate the phenomena that deserve attention. Although the speech samples for this investigation were obtained with a contrastive stress task, evaluation of the effects of contrastive stress on speech production was not a primary goal.

Major findings of this investigation include: 1) exaggerated articulatory gestures and misdirected formant trajectories for some vocalic events, 2) articulatory perseveration, 3) the "fragment" nature of groping behaviors, and 4) consistency across repetitions of many phenomena. These phenomena are highlighted because they were easily identified and occurred frequently across speakers. There were, however, other interesting observations that are not described here.

Articulomotor Integrity

Inasmuch as formant trajectories reflect the magnitude and speed of changes in vocal tract geometry, the large formant extents and misdirected formants seen for the apraxic speakers can be interpreted as evidence of unusual articulomotor behavior. The qualitative nature of the acoustic observations, together with perceptual impressions of the utterances, permits speculation regarding underlying mechanisms.

Although we did not undertake extensive perceptual characterization of these utterances for this study, a consistent impression of the sentence-level utterances was that they had an ataxic quality. In particular, the term "scanning speech" seems descriptive of many utterances. This is not a new observation (Kent & Rosenbek, 1983), but these acoustic data provide evidence for the productive correlates of the perceptual impression of scanning speech. For example, the misdirected $F2$s in "Build" (Figure 15) probably reflect a failure to overlap articulatory gestures associated with word-initial /b/ and the following vocalic segment. Although there are not much data on this matter, available observations suggest that during closure for a bilabial stop normal speakers position the tongue in anticipation of the upcoming vocalic segment (Alfonso & Baer, 1982; Perkell, 1969; Perkell & Cohen, 1987). Acoustically, this articulatory adjustment (coarticulation or coproduction, Fowler, 1985) should result in the starting frequency of the $F2$ trajectory being close to the "target" frequency of the vocalic segment. In normal speakers' spectrograms of "Build a big building," it is clear that the $F2$ onset frequency in the /bɪl/ segments is approximately the same as $F2$ values throughout the /ɪ/ portion. In the absence of this articulatory adjustment, a more prominent "locus" influence of bilabial articulation might be expected, with $F2$ rising to the "target" from a low frequency (~ 700 Hz). Many apraxic spectrograms of "Build a big building" show exactly this effect. This *decomposition* of the overlapping temporal structure of articulation is consistent with the fractionation of motor behavior in cerebellar disease (Holmes, 1939). This type of coarticulatory breakdown is not exclusive to neuromotor disorders, because the same phenomenon has been reported in the speech of hearing impaired persons (Rothman, 1976). These observations do point to the need for additional studies of interarticulator coordination in apraxic speech, similar to the case study reported by Itoh, Sasanuma, and Ushijima (1979).

The view of apraxic speech production as ataxic in nature is also supported by the occurrence of certain exaggerated segment durations, long formant steady states, and exaggerated formant trajectories. The disproportionately long /gb/ interval in "Build a big building," and the long steady states seen particularly in /aɪ/ and the /ɪl/ sequence are additional evidence of decomposition of the articulatory stream. These observations are noteworthy for the analogy to ataxia because ataxic deficits are most prominent when action is complex. The /aɪ/ and /ɪl/ vocalic nuclei and sequencing of adjoining nonhomorganic stop consonants can be viewed as requiring fairly complex articulatory behavior. As with our speculation about coarticulation effects, the articulatory complexity issue is not associated exclusively with ataxic-like deficits because parkinsonian speech movements have also been shown to be differentially affected by phonetic complexity (Forrest, Weismer, & Turner, 1989).

Exaggeration of formant trajectory extents is consistent with the ataxic characteristic of inappropriate scaling of movements, which can take the form of excessive displacement and/or velocity. If exaggeration of formant trajectories were not found also in a natural speech sample, effects seen in this study might be attributed to the artificial nature of the speech tasks. More specifically, the experimental setting may encourage certain compensatory speech production strategies, such as rate reduction, that could produce some phenomena observed in our analysis. It would be useful to determine modifications of formant trajectory and phrase-level timing that occur when normal speakers voluntarily slow their speaking rates. If the slower speaking rate produced exaggerated transitions, long steady states, and an increase in the relative amount of obstruent duration in the timing pattern, the apraxic speech phenomena identified in our analysis may be in part a function of slow speaking rates among apraxic speakers. There is evidence that slow rates do result in exaggerated transition extents in normal speakers (Fennell & Weismer, 1984; Weismer, Kimelman, & Gorman, 1985).

Repetitions examined in this investigation were characterized as fragments of the target word. Similarity of the onset spectra of repetitions to the onset spectra of target words does not indicate random variation of articulatory configurations. We did find examples, such as production of "Buy" in Figure 2a, that were not repetitions but did seem to be characterized by articulatory searching behavior. The repetitions described may be regarded as another manifestation of decomposition of movement, where production of a word is interrupted by a lack of syllable cohesion. In other words the "fragment" nature of these repetitions suggests that the interruption, or dysfluency, results from a failure to produce all segments of the syllable. (In the case of Figure 3a, there is no evidence of the first two repetitions of the word-final /ld/.) From this perspective it can be predicted that repetitions that are spectrally similar to the target will always be fragments, that is, they will not include all syllable segments (at least when the syllable is closed). This could be best tested in a spontaneous speech sample. It is not clear how this kind of articulatory attempt differs from an on-line revision of articulation such as seen in Figure 2a where the apraxic subject produced a varying vowel nucleus that eventually converged on the diphthong target. Because there is no data base regarding these kinds of errors, a likely first step is a qualitative analysis that documents the occurrence and characteristics of repetitions and on-line revisions.

Articulatory Perseveration

We have shown several examples where incorrect formant trajectories for a vowel nucleus appear to be partial or full versions of correct trajectories for the preceding vowel nucleus. In addition to this intra-utterance perseveration, there appear to be cases of inter-utterance perseveration, in which the correct formant trajectories from one of the experimental utterances are produced as an error in another of the experimental utterances (e.g., the /aɪ/ trajectories from "Buy" intruding in the vocalic nuclei for "Build").

Although the origin(s) of these perseverations are not obvious, the qualitative analysis performed here provides a basis for speculation. This phenomenon has been the focus of controversies concerning the phonetic versus phonemic origin of apraxic errors (Buckingham, 1983). From a traditional perspective, intra-utterance perseveration could be attributed (e.g., /baɪ baɪbi/) to persistence of an articulomotor pattern. Inter-utterance perseveration ("*Buy* a big building") could be interpreted as a linguistic selection error, perhaps more typical of an aphasic error than an apraxic speaking error. We would argue, however, that few theoretical advances have resulted from categorizations of errors as "motor" versus "linguistic." More can be gained from assuming that motor and linguistic components are not separable in the production of speech (see Kelso, Saltzmann, & Tuller, 1986). Identification of factors that produce the observed perseverations is more important than determination of the relative contributions of motor and linguistic mechanisms. These factors may be identified by varying the nature of sentence material and analyzing perseverations as a function of these variables.

Consistency

A theory of apraxia of speech, or of neuromotor speech disorders in general, will have to account for both variable and consistent aspects of articulation. An outstanding feature in this study was the consistent occurrence of certain nonnormal acoustic phonetic phenomena across repetitions. This finding may seem at odds with the classic view of apraxia of speech (e.g., Darley, Aronson, & Brown, 1975), where error inconsistency on repeated productions is the rule. Rather than focus on the apparent contradiction, it is more productive to regard segmental error patterns as only one component of the segmental phenomena in speech, and as only one speech production phenomenon among others such as prosody, source function, and characteristics of articulatory gestures. Categorization of apraxic speech as consistent or inconsistent should not be made by a single type of observation such as segmental error patterns. This is especially important because the differentiation of apraxia and dysarthria is held to depend in part on the variability of segmental error patterns in these respective disorders.

The idea that neuromotor speech disorders may be characterized by important consistencies is not new. In a seldom cited, but important, study, Neilson and O'Dwyer (1983) showed that patterns of electromyographic activity from the orofacial musculature of athetoid adults did not vary more across repetitions than did corresponding patterns from normal speakers. Though their EMG magnitudes were aberrant, the athetoid speakers produced muscular activity with the same degree of reproducibility as normal speakers. These results and the observations of this study suggest that it is as important for theoretical development to address consistencies in neuromotor speech disorders — especially of nonnormal phenomena — as it is to account for inconsistencies.

It is obvious from the data of this and other investigations, however, that some aspects of apraxic speech are characterized by inconsistencies. Consistency of speech in normal speakers is usually interpreted to reflect standard and cojoined linguistic and articulatory goals. Any existing variation is regarded as a combination of "motor noise" and motor flexibility (e.g., motor equivalence). Variation in disordered speakers, however, is often attributed to decreased control of the mechanism. In other words, the goals are often considered to be the same (by most), but the "loose" or deficient control of the mechanism is thought to result in the excess variability that is often observed. "Control" generally refers to neuromuscular mechanisms defined in a low-level, sensorimotor sense, without regard to other factors affecting speech production. We propose, however, from our data that the term "control" should include factors that are related to compensation strategies, linguistic set (i.e., determined by the experimental setting), and rate-adjusted phenomena. This line of thinking then extends into the traditional notion of neurogenic speech disorders, wherein the boundaries between dysarthria, apraxia of speech, and aphasia are partly defined with respect to the locus of the control deficit. When behavior is also considered, as in this study, these boundaries have little heuristic value. Thus, we conclude that there is little benefit theoretically or clinically in referring to our speakers as "pure" apraxics, as originally labeled based on the test battery. It has been shown in another study (McNeil et al., 1990) that some of these patients have static force control deficits such as those seen in dysarthric speakers. At least two apraxic subjects (A2, A4) exhibited perseverative and dysfluent behaviors that are more often associated with aphasia.

The kinds of careful physiologic hypotheses that can emerge from the qualitative analysis described above are likely to be sharper and more economical than hypotheses that are driven by statistical analyses. Moreover, this analysis permits theoretical consideration of the phenomenology of speech production *aberrancies*, which the parametric approach often suppresses because of analytic constraints. We view our approach as a first step in identification of phenomena that need to be explained by a theory of neurogenic speech disorders.

REFERENCES

Alfonso, P.J., & Baer, T. (1982). Dynamics of vowel articulation. *Language and Speech, 25,* 151–173.

Buckingham, H. (1983). Apraxia of language versus apraxia of speech. In R. A. Magill (Ed.), *Memory and control of action* (pp. 275–292). Amsterdam: North Holland.

Darley, F.L., Aronson, A.E., & Brown, J.R. (1975). *Motor speech disorders.* Philadelphia: W.B. Saunders.

Fennell, A., & Weismer, G. (1984, November). *When (if ever) does speaking rate become an inessential variable in speech production?* Paper presented at the 108th meeting of the Acoustical Society of America, Minneapolis, MN.

Forrest, K., Weismer, G., & Turner, G. (1989). Kinematic, acoustic, and perceptual analyses of connected speech produced by Parkinsonian and normal geriatric adults. *Journal of the Acoustical Society of America, 85,* 2608–2622.

Fowler, C.A. (1985). Current perspectives on language and speech production: A critical review. In R.G. Daniloff (Ed.), *Speech science* (pp. 193–278). San Diego: College-Hill Press.

Holmes, G. (1939). The cerebellum of man. *Brain, 62,* 1–30.

Itoh, M., Sasanuma, S., & Ushijima, T. (1979). Velar movements during speech in a patient with apraxia of speech. *Brain and Language, 7,* 227–239.

Kelso, J.A.S., Saltzman, E.L., & Tuller, B. (1986). The dynamic perspective on speech production: Data and theory. *Journal of Phonetics, 14,* 29–59.

Kent, R.D., & Rosenbek, J.C. (1983). Acoustic patterns of apraxia of speech. *Journal of Speech and Hearing Research, 26,* 231–249.

Liss, J.M., & Weismer, G. (1989, May). *Acoustic characteristics of contrastive stress production in normal geriatric and apraxic speakers.* Paper presented at the 117th meeting of the Acoustical Society of America, Syracuse, NY.

Liss, J.M., Weismer, G., & Rosenbek, J.C. (1990). Selected acoustic characteristics of speech production in very old males. *Journal of Gerontology: Psychological Sciences, 45,* 35–45.

McNeil, M., Weismer, G., Adams, S.G., & Mulligan, M. (1990). Oral structure nonspeech motor control in normal, dysarthric, aphasic and apraxic speakers: Isometric force and position control. *Journal of Speech and Hearing Research, 33,* 255–268.

Neilson, P.D., & O'Dwyer, N.J. (1983). Reproducibility and variability of speech muscle activity in athetoid dysarthria of cerebral palsy. *Journal of Speech and Hearing Research, 27,* 502–517.

Perkell, J.A.S. (1969). *Physiology of speech production.* Cambridge, MA: MIT Press.

Perkell, J.A.S., & Cohen, M.H. (1987). Token-to-token variation of tongue-body vowel targets: The effect of coarticulation. *Journal of the Acoustical Society of America, 82,* S17.

Rothman, H. (1976). An acoustic investigation of consonant-vowel transitions in the speech of deaf adults. *Journal of Phonetics, 4,* 95–102.

Sussman, H.M., Marquardt, T.P., MacNeilage, P.F., & Hutchinson, J.A. (1988). Anticipatory coarticulation in aphasia: Some methodological considerations. *Brain and Language, 35,* 369–379.

Weismer, G. (1984). Articulatory characteristics of parkinsonian dysarthria: Segmental and phrase-level timing, spirantization, and glottal-supraglottal coordination. In M.R. McNeil, J.C. Rosenbek, & A.E. Aronson (Eds.), *The dysarthrias: Physiology, acoustics, perception, management* (pp. 101–130). San Diego: College-Hill Press.

Weismer, G., & Ingrisano, D. (1979). Phrase-level timing patterns in English: Effects of emphatic stress location and speaking rate. *Journal of Speech and Hearing Research, 22,* 516–533.

Weismer, G., Kent, R.D., Hodge, M., & Martin, R.E. (1988). The acoustic signature for intelligibility of test words. *Journal of the Acoustical Society of America, 84,* 1281–1291.

Weismer, G., Kimelman, M.D.Z., & Gorman, S. (1985, November). *More on the speech production deficit associated with Parkinson's disease.* Paper presented at the 110th meeting of the Acoustical Society of America, Nashville, TN.

Wertz, R.T., Lapointe, L.L., & Rosenbek, J.C. (1984). *Apraxia of speech in adults: The disorder and its management.* Orlando, FL: Grune & Stratton.

*Dysarthria and Apraxia of Speech:
Perspectives on Management*
edited by Christopher A. Moore, Ph.D., Kathryn M. Yorkston, Ph.D.,
and David R. Beukelman, Ph.D.
copyright © 1991   Paul H. Brookes Publishing Co., Inc.
Baltimore · London · Toronto · Sydney

Chapter 18

An Acoustic Study of Apraxia of Speech in Patients with Different Lesion Loci

Paula A. Square-Storer and Suzanne Apeldoorn

ACOUSTIC STUDIES OF patients with apraxia of speech (AOS) are not infrequent, but with the exception of the study by Kent and Rosenbek (1983), most have described only one or two acoustic characteristics. For example, studies have focused on segment duration of consonants (DiSimoni & Darley, 1977), vowel and word durations (Collins, Rosenbek, & Wertz, 1983), and voice onset times (Freeman, Sands, & Harris, 1978; Itoh et al., 1982) as isolated acoustic parameters in patients with AOS. The study by Kent and Rosenbek (1983) was the first report of holistic acoustic patterns in the speech of patients with AOS, and the results of their study led to the hypothesis that aberrant spatial and temporal motor speech control underlies this disorder.

While the significance of the study by Kent and Rosenbek (1983) cannot be overlooked, several concerns exist in regard to subjects and limited patient descriptions. First, subject selection may have been biased toward patients who would demonstrate acoustic temporal deviancies, because all individuals demonstrated the perceptual symptom of slow, dysprosodic speech. Thus, it is not surprising that acoustic temporal deviancies were prominent. Second, the 7 AOS speakers also demonstrated mild aphasia. The effects of word-finding difficulties, literal paraphasia, and verbal repetition dysfunction due to memory disruptions might have impinged upon spatial and/or temporal acoustic speech characteristics. Finally, no neuroanatomical data were presented regarding sites and ex-

271

tents of lesions. Such information would have been extremely valuable since several studies concluded that symptoms of apraxia of speech may arise from a variety of lesion sites, both cortical and subcortical, in the language-dominant hemisphere (e.g., Square-Storer, 1987; Square-Storer, Darley, & Sommers, 1988; Square-Storer & Roy, 1989). More specifically, different clusters of AOS symptoms may arise from particular lesion sites (Square, Darley, & Sommers, 1982). Based on reports of "conditions of extremities" among their patients, it is likely that speakers studied by Kent and Rosenbek (1983) had varying sites of lesion and thus, heterogeneous clusterings of AOS symptoms. Individual patient data, however, were not reported.

The purpose of this study was to extend knowledge of the acoustic patterns of apraxia of speech. We studied AOS in its pure form, unaccompanied by clinically demonstrable aphasia and dysarthria. In addition, each patient studied had a different lesion site and so a second objective was to determine if these patients' perceptual and acoustic speech characteristics were also different.

METHOD

Patients

The patients were 1 male and 2 female adults with numerous symptoms of apraxia of speech, but no aphasia was discerned from their performances on standardized aphasia batteries. The speech of 1 normally speaking adult male was also studied for comparison.

The apraxic patients ranged in age from 49 to 72 years. Time post-onset ranged from 4 to 6 months. For patient JT, a CT scan identified a subcortical lesion in the left basal ganglia, especially at the head of the caudate nucleus, and the anterior limb of the internal capsule (Figure 1). In Figure 2 the cortex was not damaged. In Figure 3, a left parietal lesion, largely subcortical and extending to the cortex, was identified for MG. In Figure 4, the subcortical extension of the lesion did not involve the basal ganglia or internal capsule. Figure 5 shows the location of left cortical parietal involvement. For patient RS, two old parietal lesions in the right hemisphere were identified and are seen in Figure 6. No chronic neurologic sequelae resulted from them. A newer and larger lesion in the left parietal lobe, also in Figure 6, occurred 3 months later in the cortex and resulted in a speech disorder. From the CT scan in Figure 7 it can be seen that there was no subcortical lesion extension.

Pertinent descriptive information for each apraxic patient is summarized in Table 1. Both patients with subcortical lesions had chronic right hemiplegia, more severe in the patient with basal ganglia damage than in

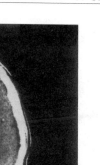

Figure 1. CT scan of JT with a subcortical lesion of the left basal ganglia, especially the head of the caudate nucleus, and anterior limb of the internal capsule.

the patient with subcortical and cortical parietal damage. The patient with cortical parietal damage had a mild sensory loss to the index and middle fingers of his right hand.

As summarized in Table 2, no patient demonstrated aphasia from the results of standardized aphasia batteries. Language function was assessed using the Porch Index of Communicative Abilities (PICA) (Porch, 1973) and a full form of the Token Test (Bollier & Vignolo, 1966) for RS and JT. For MG, the Western Aphasia Battery (WAB) (Kertesz, 1982) and a short form of the Token Test (Spellacy & Spreen, 1969) were used. With this

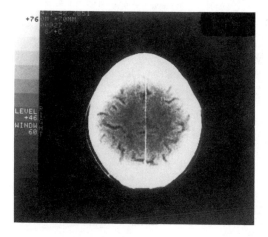

Figure 2. CT scan of JT with no cortical damage.

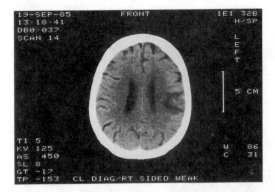

Figure 3. CT scan of MG with a left parietal lesion, largely subcortical and extending to the cortex.

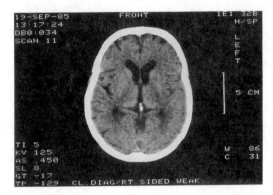

Figure 4. CT scan of MG indicating that subcortical involvement did not extend into basal ganglia or the internal capsule.

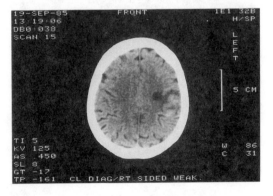

Figure 5. CT scan of MG with cortical parietal involvement.

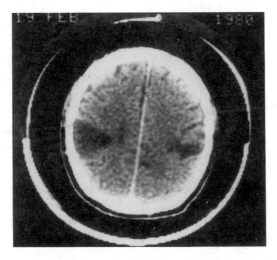

Figure 6. CT scan of RS following second stroke with two old parietal lesions in the right hemisphere, and the newer, larger left mid-parietal lesion.

information we were relatively certain that our perceptual and instrumental measures and observations were based on motor speech disturbances and not influenced by linguistic disturbances such as literal paraphasias, word-finding initiation difficulties, and acquired reading disturbances.

All 3 speakers demonstrated characteristics of apraxia of speech (Darley, Aronson, & Brown, 1975; Wertz, 1981; Wertz, LaPointe, &

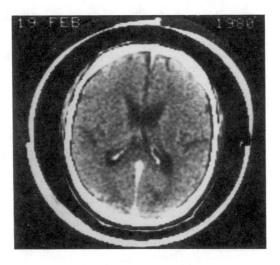

Figure 7. CT scan of RS following second stroke with no subcortical damage to the basal ganglia or internal capsule.

Table 1. Descriptive information for each apraxic speaker

Patient	Sex	Age	Months post-stroke	Lesion site	Right extremity(ies)
JT	F	49	6	Left basal ganglia	Moderate hemiplegia leg and arm
MG	F	72	4	Left parietal subcortical /cortical	Mild hemiplegia leg and arm
RS	M	57	6	Bilateral parietal	Sensory loss index and middle fingers

Rosenbek, 1984) which are summarized in Table 3. Perceptual identification of these characteristics was accomplished by two experienced clinicians based on taped performances of the Mayo Clinic Screening Battery for Apraxia of Speech (Wertz et al., 1984) and connected speech samples elicited from describing two pictures and conversational discourse from the Job task (Johnson, Darley, & Spriestersbach, 1963). Unlike Kent and Rosenbek (1983) and Robin, Bean, and Folkins (1989), patient inclusion was not based on the presence of the following four speech symptoms.

1. Effortful trial and error groping and self-correction
2. Slow rate and dysprosody unrelieved by extended periods of normal rhythm, stress, and intonation
3. Error inconsistency and self-initiated repeated productions
4. Obvious difficulty initiating utterances

In those studies, the presence of unrelieved dysprosody figured prominently. Patient RS, who had a parietal lesion, did not present with this symptom.

Results of motor speech examinations (Darley et al., 1975) revealed no clinically significant abnormalities in muscle strength or tone, or any classifiable dysarthrias (Darley et al., 1975) in our 3 patients. Six of eight experienced clinicians independently rated two speakers as having "questionable" dysarthric symptoms because of mild but pervasive resonance

Table 2. Results of aphasia testing

Patient	Token test (errors/items)	PICA[c] overall	PICA verbal	WAB aphasia quotient[d]
RS	3/62[a]	14.72	14.28	
JT	0/62[a]	14.41	14.23	
MG	1/16[b]			96.5

[a] Bollier and Vignolo (1966).
[b] Spellacy and Spreen (short form).
[c] Porch Index of Communicative Abilities (Porch, 1973).
[d] Western Aphasia Battery (Kertesz, 1982).

Table 3. Perceptual characteristics of apraxia of speech

	Speaker		
Characteristic	RS (Parietal-cortical)	JT (Basal ganglia)	MG (Parietal-subcortical /cortical)
Substitutions perceived	X	X	X
Additions	X	X	X
Repetitions	X	X	X
Off-target approximations	X	X	X
Inconsistent errors	X	X	X
Errors on phonetically complex stimuli	X	X	X
Errors on polysyllabic stimuli	X	X	X
Islands of error-free productions	X	X	X
Awareness of errors	X	X	X
Slow rate	Occasionally	Pervasive	Occasionally normal
Abnormal rhythm, stress, or intonation		X	X

abnormalities in the speech of the patients with basal ganglia and parietal subcortical lesions and mild dysphonia in the patient with a basal ganglia lesion.

The speech of 1 male, age 47, with no neurologic damage or communication deficits, was studied to observe acoustic trends, and these results are presented only for illustration. The purpose of this study was not to distinguish normal from apraxic perceptual and acoustic patterns, but focused on observing acoustic patterns between and within apraxic speakers.

Stimuli

Stimulus items for the acoustic study are shown in Table 4. They included four monosyllabic words that were each elicited three times, two bisyllabic words, each elicited three times, and five polysyllabic words, each elicited twice. These 13 words (28 productions) were randomly selected from a larger set (Square, Darley, & Sommers, 1982). Words were elicited by reading, repeating, and naming mono- and bisyllabic nouns, and reading and repeating polysyllabic words that could not be represented by objects. Speech samples were video- and audiotaped. A trained phonetician, unfamiliar with this particular study, transcribed the tokens using a modification of the system of Shriberg and Kent (1984).

Table 4. Stimuli used for acoustic analysis

Repeat	Read	Name
dice	dice	dice
dime	dime	dime
lid	lid	lid
leash	leash	leash
file	file	file
lighter	lighter	lighter
opinion	opinion	
represent	represent	
relation	relation	
population	population	
prisoner	prisoner	

Acoustic Analysis

Stimulus items were digitized from an Akai tape recorder using Mac-Speech software on a MacIntosh computer. Input levels were adjusted for each sample to ensure an optimal signal-to-noise ratio. Stimulus items were saved on diskettes, and acoustic measurements were made from these.

Wide band (300Hz) spectrograms, with frequency ranges of 0–5kHz and 0–10 kHz, and narrow band (45Hz) spectrograms, with a frequency range of 2.5 kHz, were used. Time waveforms and expanded time waveforms corresponding to the spectrogram were used to compute duration measurements, and spectral analysis was used to calculate vowel formant frequencies.

The speech parameters measured included duration of segments, syllables, words, pauses, and additions; average amplitude of syllable nuclei; relative intensity envelope; and relative syllable nuclei duration of polysyllabic words. The speech parameters were operationally defined a priori, and definitions are provided in Appendix A. Additional descriptive observations were also noted for nonmeasurable parameters (e.g., forced expirations).

Reliability

Fourteen percent of randomly selected stimulus words were re-measured on applicable parameters, and totaled 199 re-measurements. Eighty-seven percent of the re-measurements were within 10% of the originals. Deviations greater than 10% were obtained for aspiration duration, durations of vowel transition, and vowel steady state durations, calculated separately, and performance on those parameters were not studied further. Re-measurements of total duration of vowels, including transition and steady state were, however, within 10% of original measurements 90% of the time, and thus the dependent measure of total vowel duration was used.

RESULTS

Results for 2 patients were wholly consistent with those reported by Kent and Rosenbek (1983) for 7 aphasic-apraxic speakers. However, for 1 patient, measures of duration for words, syllables, and segments in longer utterances were not in accordance with earlier results (Kent & Rosenbek, 1983). Those results, as well as results for relative syllable amplitude in polysyllabic words, are highlighted.

Absolute Durations of Polysyllables and Syllabic Nuclei

Kent and Rosenbek (1983), as well as Collins et al. (1983), reported that although there was great inter-subject variability, there was consistent lengthening of utterances by their apraxic speakers. While this was true for 2 of the AOS speakers in this study, it was not for the third.

As seen in Figure 8, JT and MG, the 2 apraxic speakers with subcortical lesions, demonstrated polysyllabic word durations sometimes twice as long as those produced by the apraxic speaker with a parietal cortex lesion (RS). Furthermore, durations of polysyllabic words produced by RS were similar to those of the normal speaker, JS.

Durations of syllabic nuclei were compared across patients. Kent and Rosenbek (1983) noted that longer than normal syllabic nuclei durations were frequently produced by their apraxic speakers.

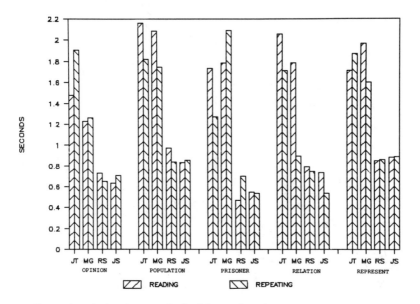

Figure 8. Absolute durations of polysyllabic words. Each word was read and repeated.

JT, with a basal ganglia lesion, demonstrated syllable durations that greatly exceeded those of the normal speaker, JS, for all polysyllabic words (Figure 9). Patient MG, with a parietal subcortical lesion, demonstrated great variability — syllable durations approximated those of the normal speaker in two polysyllables, and greatly exceeded them in the three other tokens. Patient RS, with the bilateral parietal lesion, demonstrated syllable nuclei that approximated those of the normal speaker.

Prosodic Patterns in Polysyllabic Words

Both unstressed and stressed syllables in polysyllabic words were compared regarding relative durations and intensities. Relative syllable nuclei durations are shown in Figure 10 for each patient. For "opinion" and "prisoner" all speakers showed similar patterns of relative syllabic length, with a trend toward lengthening the final syllable. (RS omitted the second syllable nucleus, /ə/, in the word "prisoner," a dialect pattern often observed in the speech of those with midwestern dialect [Allen, 1978].) However, both speakers with subcortical involvement, JT and MG, demonstrated excessive prolongation of unstressed syllables. This is seen in MG's production of the syllable /ju/ in population, which accounts for 50% of the word length. The second syllable /rɪ/ in represent for both JT and MG is similarly prolonged.

For relative syllable intensity, the mean absolute value of the voltage of each syllabic nucleus was measured, and the mean absolute voltage of

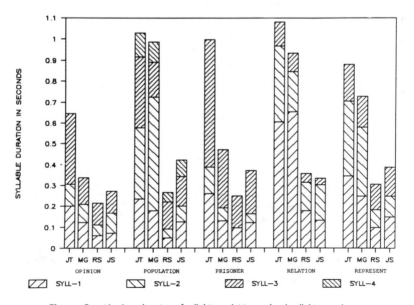

Figure 9. Absolute duration of syllabic nuclei in read polysyllabic words.

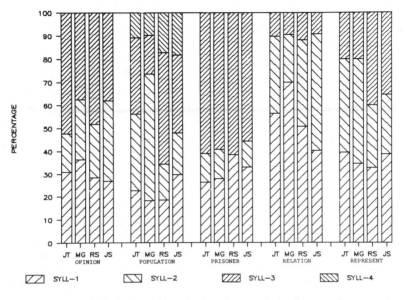

Figure 10. Relative syllable nuclei durations in read polysyllabic words.

the strongest syllable was assigned 100% and compared with other syllables in the word. Results for polysyllabic words are shown in Figure 11. RS, with the bilateral parietal lesion, demonstrated a pattern similar to JS,

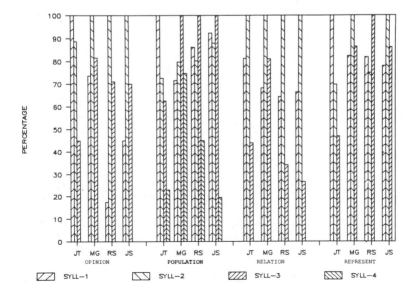

Figure 11. Relative syllable intensity in read polysyllabic words.

the normal speaker, and produced the second syllable in opinion and relation, and the third syllable in population, most intensely. MG had the same intensities as JS and RS, but this speaker with the parietal subcortical/cortical lesion showed less variation of intensity over stressed and unstressed syllables. RS and JS often produced tertiary syllables with 20% of amplitude of primary stressed ones, while MG's tertiary syllables were approximately 60% amplitude of primary stressed syllables. JT, with a basal ganglia lesion, in contrast demonstrated abnormal relative amplitude patterns in three polysyllabic words, and unlike the other speakers, gave greatest amplitude to the first syllable.

Durations of Monosyllabic Words

Results of durational measures of monosyllabic words, produced three times by each speaker, are shown in Figure 12. For MG, with the subcortical and cortical lesion, 58% absolute word durations exceeded the normal speaker's, compared with 90% for polysyllables. MG also demonstrated the greatest variability, and this is especially apparent for the words "dime" and "lid." The speaker with the basal ganglia lesion, JT, consistently demonstrated longer durations of monosyllabic words than any of the speakers, except for two of MG's abnormally long productions. JT's polysyllables were also longer than RS's, the speaker with the bilateral parietal lesion, and JS, the normal speaker, in all instances. JT, although performances varied over three trials, did not vary as much as MG. The

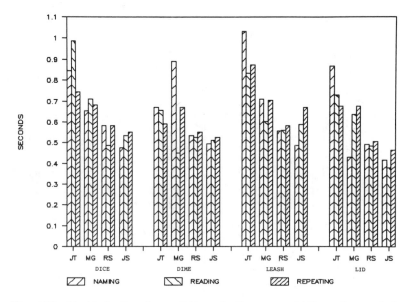

Figure 12. Absolute durations of monosyllabic words with response variability over three productions.

Table 5. Re-attempts of acoustic stimuli (in %)

Speakers	Polysyllable	Mono- and bisyllable
JT	50	11
Left basal ganglia		
MG	40	39
Left parietal		
subcortical/cortical		
RS	10	5
Bilateral cortical		
JS	0	0
Normal		

total word durations of RS approximated the normal speaker's, especially if pre-voicing was not considered. From data in Figure 12, it is apparent that RS varied less in production of these words than MG and JT.

False Starts, Reattempts, and Intra-phoneme Groping

Reattempts or false starts occurred for all 3 of our apraxic speakers (see Table 5). On polysyllabic words, JT, with a basal ganglia lesion, demonstrated re-attempts on 50% of productions; MG, with a parietal subcortical/cortical lesion, 40%; and RS, with the bilateral parietal lesion, 10%. Scrutiny of the raw data did not reveal a connection with production modes (i.e., re-attempts were not more frequent in either reading, naming, or repeating). On mono- and bisyllabic words, JT's re-attempts dropped to 11%, while MG's remained about the same at 39%, and RS's decreased to 5%.

Using electropalatography with spectrography, Washino, Casai, Uchida, and Takeda (1981) were able to demonstrate intra-phoneme groping in one apraxic speaker. In this study, independent allophonic transcriptions corroborated intra-phoneme groping in our spectrograms, particularly during fricative production. Intra-phoneme groping occurred on fricatives by JT and MG, while for RS, cessation of articulation preceding embedded fricative production occurred several times. In Figure 13, articulatory cessation is observed preceding /z/ in prisoner. A successful second attempt with a prolonged /z/ was followed by a successful third attempt in which /z/ was considerably shorter in duration. Acoustic variation, presumably due to lingual groping during vowel production, is observed for JT in Figure 14. First, /leɪd/ was produced, then /lɪəd/: Intra-phoneme groping on the terminal fricative in leash by JT is shown in Figure 15.

CONCLUSIONS

Results of this study lead to the following conclusions:

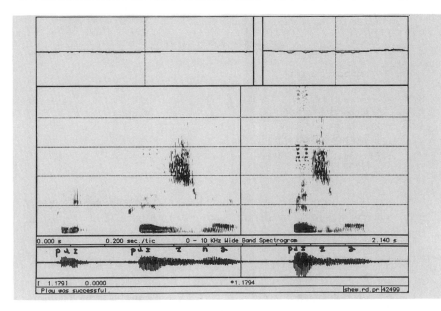

Figure 13. Spectrograms of RS's re-attempts of prisoner.

1. Apraxia of speech symptoms, discerned perceptually or acoustically, may arise from very different cortical and subcortical lesion sites.

2. The criterion of dysprosody unrelieved by extended periods of normal rhythm, stress, and intonation (Kent & Rosenbek, 1983; Robin et al., 1989) for study of apraxia of speech may not be valid because 1 of our speakers with apraxia of speech symptoms (i.e., initiation difficulty, re-attempts, and intra-phoneme groping), also demonstrated normal durations, rhythm, and stress.

3. Dysprosodic characteristics, especially slow speech and abnormal stress patterns, were characteristic of 2 speakers with subcortical in-

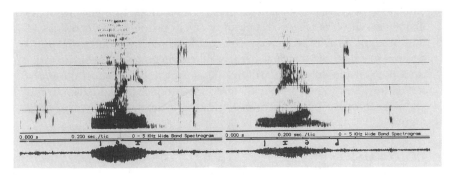

Figure 14. Spectrograms of JT's re-attempt to approximate the vowel in lid.

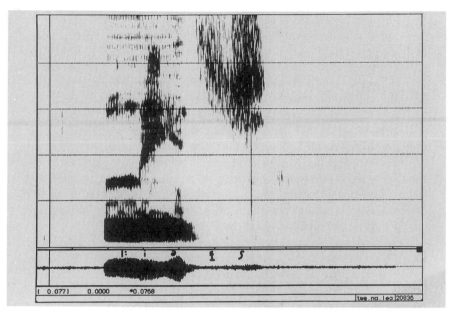

Figure 15. Spectrogram of JT's intra-phoneme groping for final fricative in leash. There is perceptual and acoustical evidence that the tongue retracted from an anterior to a more posterior position in the vocal tract during production.

volvement but not of the speaker with cortical mid-parietal involvement.

Based on the results of this preliminary investigation, we tentatively offer three hypotheses, each in need of investigation:

Hypothesis 1. The perceptual and acoustic symptom of unrelieved dysprosody characterizes the speech of patients with subcortical left hemisphere lesions and may not necessarily be a sign of apraxia of speech.

Hypothesis 2. Speakers with perceptual and acoustic apraxic symptoms, but without unrelieved dysprosody, may have less severe apraxia of speech than apraxic speakers with unrelieved dysprosody.

Hypothesis 3. The symptom complex of unrelieved dysprosody, including slow rate, excess and equal stress, or other aberrations, is consistent with unilateral upper motor neuron or pyramidal track damage (Hartman & Abbs 1989), and as such is a symptom of dysarthria. Thus, for patients with symptoms of apraxia of speech that include unrelieved dysprosody, the most appropriate diagnosis is apraxia of speech symptoms complicated by unilateral upper motor neuron dysarthria.

This last hypothesis is particularly compelling since both speakers in this study with unrelieved dysprosody also had hemiplegia. Furthermore, both demonstrated mild resonance deviancies and one, JT, mild dysphonia. Hypothesis 2, that dysprosody does not occur in mild apraxia of speech, is also worth considering since the speaker who was not dysprosodic did demonstrate less severe symptoms of apraxia of speech.

To address these hypotheses, neuroanatomic (particularly magnetic resonance imaging) and neurometabolic studies using positron emission tomography are needed, along with acoustic and perceptual investigations of speech production. Neuroanatomic and neurophysiologic bases of apraxia of speech symptomatology may be enhanced by such studies. Patients of particular interest are those with varying lesion sites in the left hemisphere who present symptoms of apraxia of speech without language disruptions or classifiable dysarthrias (Darley et al., 1975).

Furthermore, to test Hypothesis 3, neurometabolic, perceptual, and acoustic studies are needed to compare apraxic speakers with dysarthric speakers, especially those with unilateral upper motor neuron dysarthria. Finally, in future investigations of apraxia of speech, subsets of inclusionary symptoms should not be used for patient selection. Instead, speakers with any symptoms of apraxia of speech that led to a clinical diagnosis of apraxia of speech should be considered and all symptoms should be thoroughly enumerated and evaluated.

REFERENCES

Allen, H.B. (1978). *The linguistic atlas of the upper Midwest; Vol: 1–3*. Minneapolis: University of Minnesota Press.

Bollier, F., & Vignolo, L.A. (1966). Latent sensory aphasia in hemisphere-damaged patients: An experimental study with the Token Test. *Brain, 89*, 815–830.

Collins, M., Rosenbek, J., & Wertz, R. (1983). Spectrographic analysis of vowel and word duration in apraxia of speech. *Journal of Speech and Hearing Research, 26*, 224–230.

Darley, F.D., Aronson, A.E., & Brown, J. (1975). *Motor speech disorders*. Philadelphia: W.B. Saunders.

DiSimoni, F.G., & Darley, F.D. (1977). Effects on phoneme duration control of three utterance-length conditions in an apractic patient. *Journal of Speech and Hearing Disorders, 42*, 257–264.

Freeman, F.J., Sands, E.S., & Harris, K.S. (1978). Temporal coordination of phonation and articulation in a case of verbal apraxia. *Brain and Language, 6*, 106–111.

Hartman, D., & Abbs, J. (1989, November). *Perceptual and physiological characteristics of unilateral upper motor neuron (UUMN) dysarthria*. Paper presented at the annual convention of the American Speech-Language and Hearing Association, St. Louis, MO.

Itoh, M., Sasanuma, S., Tatsumi, I.F., Murakami, S., Fukusako, Y., & Suzuki, T.

(1982). Voice onset time characteristics in apraxia of speech. *Brain and Language*, *17*, 193–210.

Johnson, W., Darley, F.L., & Spriestersbach, D.(1963). *Diagnostic methods in speech pathology* (pp. 204–205). New York: Harper & Row.

Kent, R.D., & Rosenbek, J.C. (1983). Acoustic patterns of apraxia of speech. *Journal of Speech and Hearing Research*, *26*, 231–249.

Kertesz, A. (1982). *The Western Aphasia Battery (WAB)*. Orlando, FL: Grune & Stratton.

Porch, B. (1973). *Porch Index of Communicative Ability*. Palo Alto, CA: Consulting Psychologists Press.

Robin, D.A., Bean, C., & Folkins, J.W. (1989). Lip movement in apraxia of speech, *Journal of Speech and Hearing Research*, *32*, 512–523.

Shriberg, L.D., & Kent, R.D. (1984). *Clinical phonetics*. New York: John Wiley & Sons.

Spellacy, F., & Spreen, D. (1969). A short form of the Token Test. *Cortex*, *5*, 390–397.

Square, P., Darley, F.L., & Sommers, R.K. (1982). An analysis of the productive errors made by pure apraxic speakers with differing loci of lesions. In R. Brookshire (Ed.), *Clinical aphasiology conference proceedings* (pp. 245–250). Minneapolis: BRK Publishers.

Square-Storer, P.A. (1987). Acquired apraxia of speech. In H. Winitz (Ed.), *Human communication and its disorders: A review* (pp. 88–159). Norwood, NJ: Able.

Square-Storer, P., Darley, F.L., & Sommers, R.K. (1988). Speech processing abilities in patients with aphasia and apraxia of speech. *Brain and Language*, *33*, 65–85.

Square-Storer, P., & Roy, E. (1989). The apraxias: Commonalities and distinctions. In P. Square-Storer (Ed.), *Acquired apraxia of speech in adults: Theoretical and clinical issues* (pp. 20–63). London: Taylor and Francis.

Washino, K., Casai, Y., Uchida, Y., & Takeda, K. (1981). Tongue movements during speech in a patient with apraxia of speech. *Current issues in neurolinguistics: A Japanese contribution* (Supplement to *Language Sciences*). Tokyo: International Christian University.

Wertz, R.T. (1981). Neuropathologies of speech and language: An introduction to patient management. In D.G. Johns (Ed.), *Clinical management of neurogenic communicative disorders* (pp. 1–96). Boston: Little, Brown.

Wertz, R., LaPointe, L., & Rosenbek, J. (1984). *Apraxia of speech in adults: The disorder and its management*. New York: Grune & Stratton.

Appendix A

Operational Definitions

Vowel duration was measured from the first to last large amplitude, complex-shape glottal pulse. The first and last second formant striations on the spectrogram were used as a guide to the beginning and end of the vowel and then the oscillographic trace was used to precisely locate each.

Nasal duration was measured from the final second formant spectrogram striation of the preceding vowel to the beginning of the next segment (vowel or closure duration of following stop).

Fricative duration was measured from the final large amplitude, complex-shape glottal pulse preceding the aperiodic energy to the first complex-shape glottal pulse following the aperiodic waveform. If a pause occurred between the complex-shape glottal pulse and the aperiodic waveform, the duration between the first and last aperiodic energy striations on the spectrogram was measured.

Stop duration was measured from the final large amplitude, complex-shape glottal pulse preceding aperiodic energy to the first complex-shape glottal pulse following the aperiodic waveform.

Closure duration was measured from the final spectrogram striation in the region of the second formant (that indicates the boundary between an open and a closed vocal tract) and the release burst.

Syllable nuclei durations (vowel, vowel plus /r/ preceding or following, vowel plus /l/) were measured. Syllable duration was then measured from the first to last large amplitude, complex-shape glottal pulse.

Pause duration was defined as a lack of formant or aperiodic energy on the spectrogram within a word, not including stop closure durations.

Word duration was defined as the duration between the first to last aperiodic/periodic energy spectrogram striations that perceptually corresponded to the word. The waveform was also used in making measurements of duration.

Average amplitude of syllabic nuclei was calculated by placing cursors around each syllable nucleus (i.e., vowel, vowel plus /r/ preceding or following, vowel plus /l/), and the average amplitude (V) beyond this duration was determined. Due to the inability to segment vowels from /r/ and /l/ (less than 10% error), they were included in the vowel nucleus.

288

Chapter 19

A Discussion of
Classification in
Motor Speech Disorders
Dysarthria and Apraxia of Speech

John C. Rosenbek and Malcolm R. McNeil

NAMES AND DEFINITIONS, if carefully chosen and constructed, define a discipline's boundaries and offer clues to its conceptual underpinnings. The definition of a pathologic condition is a first approach to a general theory governing that condition. In neurogenic speech-language pathology, as in most disciplines, definitions determine appropriate experimental questions and methods for answering them. Thus, a definition can serve as a paradigm in the Kuhnian (1970) sense. If carelessly, idiosyncratically, or prematurely chosen, names and definitions obscure boundaries, disturb or repudiate concepts, and frustrate experimentation. Such an indictment of "dysarthria" and "apraxia of speech" is not really intended, but the purpose of this chapter is to urge a re-examination of these terms.

The Mayo group (Darley, Aronson, & Brown, 1975) made a prodigious attempt to develop definitions and descriptions of dysarthria and apraxia of speech. The re-examination being suggested here relies heavily on the work of these three clinical scientists, not because their work was flawed, but because it was developed within the identifiable conceptual framework of behavioral neurology.

Darley et al. (1975) define dysarthria as: "a collective name for a group of related speech disorders that are due to disturbances in muscular control of the speech mechanism resulting from impairment of any of the basic motor processes involved in the execution of speech" (p. 2).

Apraxia of speech was, in their view, an articulatory disorder resulting from impairment of "certain brain circuits devoted specifically to the
programming of articulatory movements" (p. 2). For the Mayo group,
dysarthria resulted from impaired muscle control or execution, and apraxia of speech was a disorder of programming. These authors felt that the
two conditions could be differentiated at several levels: speech processes,
neuromuscular functions, and signs.

SPEECH PROCESSES

For Darley et al. (1975), the speech processes are respiration, phonation,
resonation, articulation, and prosody. Dysarthria can exist to some extent
in all processes, although flaccid dysarthria can be present only in one.
Apraxia of speech is present only in articulation, but it can be accompanied by compensatory prosodic disturbances. Among the challenges to
diagnosis at this level is Marshall, Gandour, and Windsor's (1988) report
of a chronic apraxia confined to the larynx.

Prosody deserves special attention. Prosodic disturbances, presumably as primary signs, are assumed to be universal in dysarthria, but in
apraxia of speech, they have been minimized and are usually described as
compensatory. Concepts about differences between execution (dysarthria)
and programming (apraxia) may explain the relative importance assigned
to prosodic disturbances in each condition. Many practitioners have ignored the idea that prosody in some dysarthric types could be compensatory, and that prosodic disturbances could be significant and primary in
apraxia of speech. The acoustic analyses of Kent and Rosenbek (1983) are
typical of data documenting significant prosodic disturbance in apraxia of
speech. Their acoustic profile of apraxic speech includes: slow speaking
rate with prolongations of transitions, steady states, and inter-syllabic
pauses; reduced intensity variations across syllables; and slow inaccurate
movements of the articulators. As another example, McNeil, Liss, Tseng,
and Kent (1990) replicated an earlier study (Kent & McNeil, 1987) and
reported that acoustic data on utterance and segment durations, and vowel
formant trajectories at normal, fast, and slow speaking rates, suggest that
apraxic speech is slower than normal speech. The apraxic speakers in the
latter study also had significantly greater difficulty than the normal speakers in adjusting, especially increasing, their speaking rate. It might be
expected that if the slowness in apraxic speech is merely compensatory,
these speakers would have been better at achieving faster rates.

Data now suggest similar patterns of prosodic disturbance in apraxia
of speech and some types of dysarthria. Kent and Rosenbek (1982), for
example, comment on similarities of ataxic and apraxic speakers, including
articulatory prolongations, syllable segregation, and lengthening of un-

stressed syllables. Similarities in aspects of dysprosody were also discovered through narrow phonetic transcriptions of ataxic and apraxic single word imitations by Odell, McNeil, Rosenbek, and Hunter (1990b). Both types of speakers produced syllabic stress errors that included perceived deviation in expected relative syllable weights in two- or three-syllable words, and similar difficulties with speech initiation and open juncture and long stop closure. Even if replication confirms and extends the findings (and not all studies confirm that apraxic speech is slow), the data do not support the conclusion that some dysarthric and some apraxic speakers have the same prosodic profiles, or even that similar patterns are present for the same reasons. The data do support the need for continuing re-evaluation of traditional concepts about process disturbances in dysarthria and apraxia of speech.

NEUROMUSCULAR FUNCTIONS

It is reasonably easy to document the concept that the dysarthric individual must demonstrate clinical evidence of impairment to one or more neuromuscular functions (statistically related to perceptual speech signs): strength, speed, range, accuracy, tone, and steadiness of muscle contraction. Apraxic speakers do not. A related idea (with somewhat more obscure origins) is that to qualify as dysarthric, a speaker must have deficits in nonspeech movements. The apraxic speaker does not have deficits in nonspeech movements, except for the occasional concomitant oral, nonverbal apraxia.

Development and application of instrumental measures of acoustic and physiologic functions have increased detection of neuromuscular deficits. The relation of these deficits to the original list (Darley et al., 1975) is somewhat unclear, a consideration in evaluating these data. Even with this caution, however, the data are intriguing. Abnormal force and position control have been documented for both apraxic and ataxic speakers (McNeil, Weismer, Adams, & Mulligan, 1990). Kinematic measures have documented increased speech movement durations by both apraxic and ataxic dysarthric speakers (McNeil, Caligiuri, & Rosenbek, 1989). McNeil et al. (1989) and Robin, Bean, and Folkins (1989), however, documented that some apraxic speakers can produce movement velocities that are within the range of normal speakers. Itoh, Sasanuma, Hirose, Yoshioka, and Ushijima (1980) report similar velocities of lower lip elevations for an apraxic speaker and a dysarthric speaker with amyotrophic lateral sclerosis, but they are quick to admit that patterns of difficulty are different. Discoordination of articulators is a frequent finding (Freeman, Sands, & Harris, 1978; Itoh et al., 1980) but not universal (Robin et al., 1989) in apraxia of speech and is a cardinal feature of ataxic dysarthria.

Problems with these data are not limited to those of inconsistency and small sample sizes. Measures need refinement. Adams, McNeil, and Weismer (1989) proposed solutions to the inadequacies of velocity measurements of neurogenic speakers, and preliminary data suggest abnormal, but distinct, profiles for apraxic, ataxic, and conduction aphasic subjects. These studies deserve replication. Forrest, Adams, and McNeil (1990) suggest that abnormalities such as antagonistic muscle co-contraction reported in apraxia of speech may be characteristic of normal performance as well. Interpretations need refinement. Studies by McNeil (McNeil, 1989; 1990) include data on conduction aphasic speakers who are remarkably similar to apraxic speakers on several measures. One interpretation of these data is that conduction aphasic speakers, like apraxic ones, have a motor component to their deficit. Another interpretation is that some sophisticated measures provide what Forrest et al. call a "general index of neuropathology."

Even with these caveats, it is possible that at least some apraxic and dysarthric speakers share features of neuromuscular dysfunction. We need not conclude that apraxia is dysarthria, or the reverse. Nor do we benefit from grouping both disorders under the rubric of movement disorder or even speech production disorder, which shifts attention from the perceptual signs that are the critical features of all speech disorders. We should consider that some of the "salient features of neuromuscular function" (Darley et al., 1975) disturbed in dysarthria may also be disturbed in apraxia, and we should explore the relation of each to speech signs.

PERCEIVED SPEECH ERRORS

A distinction between dysarthria and apraxia of speech offered by Darley et al. (1975) and Johns and Darley (1970) based on speech errors is often used as evidence when other arguments for distinction have failed. Dysarthric speech is characterized (though not defined) primarily by errors of distortion, while apraxic speech errors are reported to be primarily substitutions. Distortions are the so-called simplification errors that Darley et al. (1975) attribute to slowness, weakness, and other neuromuscular deficits of dysarthria. Substitutions were assumed to be symptomatic of the apraxic programming deficit. Approached with those assumptions and the method of broad phonetic transcription, data confirming these assumptions emerged.

Additional data, however, are forcing re-assessment. Square, Darley, and Sommers (1982), using a form of broad phonetic transcription, describe distortion as the "predominant phonetic error" in purely apraxic speakers. Odell, McNeil, Rosenbek, and Hunter (1990a), using narrow phonetic transcription of initiative speech, report that distortions were the most frequent errors made by all 4 purely apraxic speakers. Distortion in an apraxic utterance does not necessarily mean that the speaker has two problems — apraxia of speech and dysarthria. Speakers with such errors, however, do compel us to consider that a pattern of distortion and substitution supports the diagnostic hypothesis of apraxia of speech. The challenge is to quantify the mixture of substitutions and distortions and the nature (perhaps) of both that distinguish dysarthria and apraxia of speech.

CONCLUSION

According to Mayr, Linsley, and Usinger (1953), biologic taxonomy begins with the task of separating "the almost unlimited and confusing diversity of individuals in nature into easily recognizable groups, to work out the significant characters of these groups, and to find constant differences between similar ones" (p. 17). We believe that aphasiologists have made significant strides in separating speakers into groups, though not always distinctive ones. The problem, however, is working out the significant characters of the groups and finding constant differences between similar ones. In our view, a partial explanation is that the profession has used labels — dysarthria and apraxia, which carry with them inadequately tested assumptions borrowed from neurology. These assumptions, in turn, have biased the search for significant characters and constant differences.

One solution may be to set aside assumptions about dysarthria and apraxia until more data are available from several levels of analysis and from a larger number of normal and disordered speakers. Such data may reveal one or more strong neuromotor syndromes in dysarthria and apraxia of speech. A strong syndrome is one in which neuromuscular abnormalities are identified in predictable distribution across functional components and are related to a pattern of perceptual speech abnormalities with sufficient frequency to suggest a causal relationship. If the pattern is unique, the syndrome is stronger yet. Some strong syndromes may emerge. Flaccid dysarthria is most likely. Apraxia of speech is likely too, but less so. At issue will be what to do with what is left. We can consider redefining dysarthria and even apraxia of speech, which would require a massive change in attitude and procedure. We can keep the definitions, exclude subtypes of dysarthria that do not meet the test of coherence of neuromuscular deficit and perceptual symptoms, and perhaps add subtypes to apraxia. These possibilities would benefit from better physiologic data on motor control, and from models that predict the pattern and nature of disturbance from the deficits in neuromotor control, as well as the effects of interactions of cognitive, linguistic, and motor systems.

REFERENCES

Adams, J.G., McNeil, M.R., & Weismer, G. (1989, November). *Speech movement velocity profiles in neurogenic speech disorders.* Paper presented at the meeting of the American Speech and Hearing Association, St. Louis, MO.

Darley, F.L., Aronson, A.E., & Brown, J.R. (1975). *Motor speech disorders.* Philadelphia: W.B. Saunders.

Forrest, K., Adams, S., & McNeil, M.R. (1990, January). *Perioral EMG activity in aphasic, apraxic, and dysarthric speakers.* Paper presented at the meeting of the Clinical Dysarthria Conference, San Antonio, TX.

Freeman, F.J., Sands, E.S., & Harris, K.S. (1978). Temporal coordination of phonation and articulation in a case of verbal apraxia: A voice onset time study. *Brain and Language, 6,* 106–111.

Itoh, M., Sasanuma, S., Hirose, H., Yoshioka, H., & Ushijima, T. (1980). Abnormal articulatory dynamics in a patient with apraxia of speech: X-ray microbeam observation. *Brain and Language, 11,* 66–75.

Johns, D.F., & Darley, F.L. (1970). Phonemic variability in apraxia of speech. *Journal of Speech and Hearing Research, 13,* 556–583.

Kent, R.D., & McNeil, M.R. (1987). Relative timing of sentence repetition in apraxia of speech and conduction aphasia. In J. Ryalls (Ed.), *Phonetic approaches to speech production in aphasia and related disorders* (pp. 181–220). San Diego: College Hill Press.

Kent, R.D., & Rosenbek, J.C. (1982). Prosodic disturbance and neurologic lesion. *Brain and Language, 15,* 259–291.

Kent, R.D., & Rosenbek, J.C. (1983). Acoustic patterns of apraxia of speech. *Journal of Speech and Hearing Research, 26,* 231–249.

Kuhn, T. (1970). *The structure of scientific revolutions* (2nd ed.). Chicago: University of Chicago Press.

Marshall, R.C., Gandour, J., & Windsor, J. (1988). Selective impairment of phonation: A case study. *Brain and Language, 35,* 313–339.

Mayr, E., Linsley, E.G., & Usinger, R.L. (1953). *Methods and principles of systematic zoology.* New York: McGraw-Hill.

McNeil, M.R., Caligiuri, M., & Rosenbek, J.C. (1989). A comparison of labiomandibular kinematic durations, displacements, velocities and dysmetrias in apraxic and normal adults. In T.E. Prescott (Ed.), *Clinical aphasiology* (Vol.18., pp. 173–179). Boston: College-Hill Press.

McNeil, M.R., Liss, J., Tseng, C-H., & Kent, R.D. (1990). Effects of speech rate on the absolute and relative timing of apraxic and conduction aphasic sentence production. *Brain and Language, 38,* 135–158.

McNeil, M.R., Weismer, G., Adams, S., & Mulligan, M. (1990). Oral structure nonspeech motor control in normal, dysarthric, aphasic and apraxic speakers: Isometric force and static fine position control. *Journal of Speech and Hearing Research, 33,* 255–268.

Odell, K.H., McNeil, M.R., Rosenbek, J.C., & Hunter, L. (1990a). Perceptual characteristics of consonant productions by apraxic speakers. *Journal of Speech and Hearing Disorders, 55,* 345–359.

Odell, K.H., McNeil, M.R., Rosenbek, J.C., & Hunter, L. (1990b). A perceptual comparison of prosodic features in apraxia of speech and conduction aphasia. In T.E. Prescott (Ed.), *Clinical aphasiology.* Austin, TX: PRO-ED.

Robin, D.A., Bean, C., & Folkins, J.W. (1989). Lip movement in apraxia of speech. *Journal of Speech and Hearing Research, 32,* 512–523.

Square, P.A., Darley, F.L., & Sommers, R.K. (1982). An analysis of the productive errors made by pure apractic speakers with differing loci of lesions. In R.H. Brookshire (Ed.), *Clinical aphasiology* (Vol.19., pp. 245–250). Minneapolis: BRK Publishers.

Dysarthria and Apraxia of Speech:
Perspectives on Management
edited by Christopher A. Moore, Ph.D., Kathryn M. Yorkston, Ph.D.,
and David R. Beukelman, Ph.D.
copyright © 1991   Paul H. Brookes Publishing Co., Inc.
Baltimore · London · Toronto · Sydney

Index

Voicing errors, in apraxia of speech,
148
Von Recklinghausen's disease, *see*
Neurofibromatosis
Vowel approximation, and perceptual
analysis of intelligibility, 58, 63

Weakness, muscle, sources of, 9–10
Western Aphasia Battery (WAB), 273
Whispered diadochokinetic rate, in
spasmodic dysphonia, 210, 211
Wood's syndrome, 227
see also Orolingual-mandibular dystonia (OLMD)
Word(s)
monosyllabic, durations of,
282–283

polysyllabic, *see* Polysyllabic
utterances
Word characteristics, and perceptual
analysis of intelligibility, 58
Word durations, 282–283, 288
orolingual-mandibular dystonia and,
botulinum treatment for, 234,
236–239
Word-final voicing, apraxia of speech
and, 148
Word-level analysis, Reye's syndrome
and, 100–101, 104–105
Word positions, neurofibromatosis
and, 141–142
Word production, adequacy of, and
perceptual analysis of intelligibility, 58–59